Casarett & Doull's
Essentials of Toxicology

NOTICE

Medicine is an ever-changing science. As new research and clinical experience broaden our knowledge, changes in treatment and drug therapy are required. The authors and the publisher of this work have checked with sources believed to be reliable in their efforts to provide information that is complete and generally in accord with the standards accepted at the time of publication. However, in view of the possibility of human error or changes in medical sciences, neither the authors nor the publisher nor any other party who has been involved in the preparation or publication of this work warrants that the information contained herein is in every respect accurate or complete, and they disclaim all responsibility for any errors or omissions or for the results obtained from use of the information contained in this work. Readers are encouraged to confirm the information contained herein with other sources. For example and in particular, readers are advised to check the product information sheet included in the package of each drug they plan to administer to be certain that the information contained in this work is accurate and that changes have not been made in the recommended dose or in the contraindications for administration. This recommendation is of particular importance in connection with new or infrequently used drugs.

Casarett & Doull's
Essentials of Toxicology

Third Edition

Editors

Curtis D. Klaassen, PhD

University Distinguished Professor
Division of Gastroenterology
Department of Internal Medicine
University of Kansas Medical Center
Kansas City, Kansas

John B. Watkins III, PhD

Associate Dean and Director
Professor of Pharmacology and Toxicology
Medical Sciences Program
Indiana University School of Medicine
Bloomington, Indiana

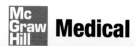 **Medical**

New York   Chicago   San Francisco   Lisbon   London   Madrid   Mexico City
Milan   New Delhi   San Juan   Seoul   Singapore   Sydney   Toronto

Casarett & Doull's Essentials of Toxicology, 3ed.

3 4 5 6 7 8 9 10 LWI 21 20 19 18 17

ISBN 978-0-07-184708-7
MHID 0-07-184708-1

This book was set in Minion Pro by MPS Limited
The editors were Michael Weitz and Christie Naglieri.
The production supervisor was Richard Ruzycka.
Project management was provided by Charu Khanna, MPS Limited.
The index was prepared by Edwin Durbin
LSC Communications was the printer and binder.

This book is printed on acid-free paper.

Library of Congress Cataloging-in-Publication Data

Casarett & Doull's essentials of toxicology / Curtis D. Klaassen and John B. Watkins, editors. — 3E.
     p. ; cm.
   Casarett and Doull's essentials of toxicology
   Essentials of toxicology
   Includes index.
   ISBN 978-0-07-184708-7 (alk. paper) — ISBN 0-07-184708-1 (alk. paper)
   I. Klaassen, Curtis D., editor.   II. Watkins, John B. (John Barr), III, editor.   III. Title: Casarett and Doull's essentials of toxicology.   IV. Title: Essentials of toxicology.
   [DNLM: 1. Poisons—toxicity.   2. Toxicology—methods.   QV 600]
   RA1211
   615.9—dc23
                                                  2015000090

International Edition ISBN 978-1-25-925535-9; MHID 1-25-925535-2.

Contents

Contributors

S. Satheesh Anand, PhD, DABT
Senior Research Toxicologist
Haskell Global Centers for Health and Environmental
Sciences
Newark, Delaware
Chapter 24

Michael Aschner, PhD
Professor
Department of Pediatrics
Vanderbilt University Medical Center
Nashville, Tennessee
Chapter 16

Thomas M. Badger, PhD
Distinguished Faculty Scholar
Professor
Departments of Pediatrics and Physiology/Biophysics
University of Arkansas for Medical Sciences
Director
Arkansas Children's Nutrition Center
Little Rock, Arkansas
Chapter 27

John C. Bloom, VMD, PhD
President
Bloom Consulting Services, LLC
Special Government Employee
FDA
Adjunct Professor of Pathology
Schools of Veterinary Medicine
University of Pennsylvania and Purdue University
Indianapolis, Indiana
Chapter 11

Windy A. Boyd, PhD
Biologist
Biomolecular Screening Branch
National Toxicology Program Division
National Institute of Environmental Health Sciences, NIH
Research Triangle Park, North Carolina
Chapter 23

William K. Boyes, PhD
Neurotoxicology Branch
Toxicity Assessment Division
National Health and Environmental Effects Research
Laboratory
Office of Research and Development
US Environmental Protection Agency
Research Triangle Park, North Carolina
Chapter 17

John T. Brandt, MD
Eli Lilly & Co. (retired)
Indianapolis, Indiana
Chapter 11

James V. Bruckner, PhD
Professor of Pharmacology & Toxicology
Department of Pharmaceutical & Biomedical
Sciences
College of Pharmacy
University of Georgia
Athens, Georgia
Chapter 24

David B. Buckley, PhD
Chief Scientific Officer
XenoTech, LLC
Lenexa, Kansas
Chapter 6

George A. Burdock, PhD, DABT, FACN
President
Burdock Group Consultants
Orlando, Florida
Chapter 31

Louis R. Cantilena Jr., MD, PhD
Professor, Medicine and Pharmacology
Department of Medicine
Uniformed Services University
Bethesda, Maryland
Chapter 33

Daniel L. Costa, PhD
Office of Research and Development
National Program Director for Air, Climate, and Energy
Research Program
US Environmental Protection Agency
Research Triangle Park, North Carolina
Chapter 29

Lucio G. Costa, PhD
Professor
Department of Environmental and Occupational
Health Sciences
School of Public Health
University of Washington
Seattle, Washington
Chapter 22

Maciej Czerwinski, PhD
Principal Scientist
XenoTech, LLC
Lenexa, Kansas
Chapter 6

Richard T. Di Giulio, PhD
Professor
Nicholas School of the Environmental
Duke University
Durham, North Carolina
Chapter 30

David L. Eaton, PhD
Professor
Department of Environmental and Occupational
Health Sciences
Associate Vice Provost for Research
University of Washington
Seattle, Washington
Chapter 2

Elaine M. Faustman, PhD
Professor
Institute for Risk Analysis and Risk Communication
Department of Environmental and Occupational
Health Sciences
School of Public Health
University of Washington
Seattle, Washington
Chapter 4

Jodi A. Flaws, PhD
Professor
Department of Comparative Biosciences
University of Illinois
Urbana, Illinois
Chapter 21

Paul M.D. Foster, PhD
Chief
Toxicology Branch
Division of the National Toxicology Program
National Institute of Environmental Health Sciences
Research Triangle Park, North Carolina
Chapter 20

Donald A. Fox, PhD
Professor of Vision Sciences
Biology and Biochemistry, Pharmacology, and Health and
Human Performance
University of Houston
Houston, Texas
Chapter 17

Jonathan H. Freedman, PhD
Laboratory of Toxicology and Pharmacology
National Institute of Environmental Health Sciences
Research Triangle Park, North Carolina
Chapter 23

Michael A. Gallo, PhD
Environmental and Occupational Health Sciences
Institute
Rutgers-The State University of New Jersey
UMDNJ-Robert Wood Johnson Medical School
Piscataway, New Jersey
Chapter 1

Steven G. Gilbert, PhD
Director
Institute of Neurotoxicology & Neurological Disorders
Seattle, Washington
Chapter 2

Bruce A. Goldberger, PhD
Professor and Director of Toxicology
Departments of Pathology and Psychiatry
University of Florida College of Medicine
Gainesville, Florida
Chapter 32

Terry Gordon, PhD
Professor
Department of Environmental Medicine
NYU School of Medicine
Tuxedo, New York
Chapter 29

L. Earl Gray Jr., PhD
Reproductive Toxicology Branch
United States Environmental Protection Agency
Adjunct Professor
North Carolina State University
Raleigh, North Carolina
Chapter 20

Zoltán Gregus, MD, PhD, DSc, DABT
Professor
Department of Pharmacology and Therapeutics
Toxicology Section
University of Pecs
Medical School
Pecs, Hungary
Chapter 3

David G. Hoel, PhD
Principal Scientist
Exponent, Inc
Alexandria, Virginia
Distinguished University Professor
Department of Medicine
Medical University of South Carolina
Charleston, South Carolina
Chapter 25

George R. Hoffmann, PhD
Professor
Department of Biology
College of the Holy Cross
Worcester, Massachusetts
Chapter 9

Michael P. Holsapple, PhD, ATS
Senior Research Leader
Systems Toxicology
Health and Life Sciences Global Business
Battelle Memorial Institute
Columbus, Ohio
Chapter 12

Patricia B. Hoyer, PhD
Professor
Department of Physiology
College of Medicine
The University of Arizona
Tucson, Arizona
Chapter 21

Robert H. Hurt, PhD
Professor
School of Engineering
Director
Institute for Molecular and Nanoscale Innovation
Brown University
Providence, Rhode Island
Chapter 28

Hartmut Jaeschke, PhD, ATS
Professor and Chair
Department of Pharmacology, Toxicology & Therapeutics
University of Kansas Medical Center
Kansas City, Kansas
Chapter 13

Norbert E. Kaminski, PhD
Professor
Department of Pharmacotherapy and Toxicology
Director
Center for Integrative Toxicology
Michigan State University
East Lansing, Michigan
Chapter 12

Agnes B. Kane, MD, PhD
Professor
Department of Pathology and Laboratory Medicine
Brown University
Providence, Rhode Island
Chapter 28

Y. James Kang, DVM, PhD, FATS
Professor and Distinguished University Scholar
Department of Pharmacology and Toxicology
University of Louisville School of Medicine
Louisville, Kentucky
Chapter 18

Barbara L.F. Kaplan, PhD
Assistant Professor
Center for Integrative Toxicology
Department of Pharmacology and Toxicology and Neuroscience
Program
Michigan State University
East Lansing, Michigan
Chapter 12

Faraz Kazmi, BS
Senior Scientist
XenoTech, LLC
Lenexa, Kansas
Chapter 6

Rebecca D. Kapler, PhD
School of Freshwater Sciences
University of Wisconsin-Milwaukee
Milwaukee, Wisconsin
Chapter 28

James E. Klaunig, PhD, ATS, IATP
Professor
Environmental Health
Indiana University
Bloomington, Indiana
Chapter 8

Frank N. Kotsonis, PhD
Retired Corporate Vice President
Worldwide Regulatory Sciences
Monsanto Corporation
Skokie, Illinois
Chapter 31

Lois D. Lehman-McKeeman, PhD
Distinguished Research Fellow
Discovery Toxicology
Bristol-Myers Squibb Company
Princeton, New Jersey
Chapter 5

George D. Leikauf, PhD
Professor
Department of Environmental and Occupational Health
Graduate School of Public Health
University of Pittsburgh
Pittsburgh, Pennsylvania
Chapter 15

Theodora M. Mauro, MD
Professor and Vice-Chair
Dermatology Department
University of California, San Francisco
Service Chief
Dermatology
San Francisco Veterans Medical Center
San Francisco, California
Chapter 19

Virginia C. Moser, PhD, DABT, FATS
Toxicologist
Toxicity Assessment Division
National Health and Environmental Effects Research
Laboratory
US Environmental Protection Agency
Research Triangle Park, North Carolina
Chapter 16

Michael C. Newman, MS, PhD
A. Marshall Acuff Jr. Professor
Virginia Institute of Marine Science
College of William & Mary
Gloucester Point, Virginia
Chapter 30

Gunter Oberdörster, DVM, PhD
Professor
Department of Environmental Medicine
University of Rochester
School of Medicine & Dentistry
Rochester, New York
Chapter 28

Brian W. Ogilvie, BA
Principal Scientist
XenoTech, LLC
Lenexa, Kansas
Chapter 6

Gilbert S. Omenn, MD, PhD
Professor of Internal Medicine, Human Genetics
and Public Health
Director
Center for Computational Medicine and Bioinformatics
University of Michigan Department of Computational
Medicine and Bioinformatics
Ann Arbor, Michigan
Chapter 4

Oliver Parkinson, PhD
XPD Consulting, LLC
Shawnee, Kansas
Chapter 6

Andrew Parkinson, PhD
CEO
XPD Consulting, LLC
Shawnee, Kansas
Chapter 6

Martin A. Philbert, PhD
Professor of Toxicology and Dean
School of Public Health
University of Michigan
Ann Arbor, Michigan
Chapter 16

R. Julian Preston, MA, PhD
Associate Director for Health
National Health and Environmental Effects Research
Laboratory
US Environmental Protection Agency
Research Triangle Park, North Carolina
Chapter 9

Robert H. Rice, PhD
Professor
Department of Environmental Toxicology
University of California
Davis, California
Chapter 19

Rudy J. Richardson, ScD, DABT
Toxicology Program
University of Michigan School of Public Health
Neurology Department
University of Michigan School of Medicine
Ann Arbor, Michigan
Chapter 16

John M. Rogers, PhD
Toxicity Assessment Division
National Health and Environmental Effects Research
Laboratory
Office of Research and Development
United States Environmental Protection Agency
Research Triangle Park, North Carolina
Chapter 10

Martin J. Ronis, BA, MA, PhD
Professor
Department of Pharmacology & Toxicology
College of Medicine
University of Arkansas for Medical Sciences
Associate Director for Basic Research
Arkansas Children's Nutrition Center
Arkansas Children's Hospital Research Institute
Little Rock, Arkansas
Chapter 27

Andrew E. Schade, MD, PhD
Senior Director
Clinical Diagnostics Laboratory
Diagnostics Research and Development
Eli Lilly and Co.
Indianapolis, Indiana
Chapter 11

Rick G. Schnellmann, PhD
Professor and Chair
Department of Pharmaceutical and Biomedical Sciences
Medical University of South Carolina
Charleston, South Carolina
Chapter 14

Kartik Shankar, PhD, DABT
Arkansas Children's Nutrition Center
Department of Pediatrics
University of Arkansas for Medical Sciences
Little Rock, Arkansas
Chapter 27

Danny D. Shen, PhD
Professor
Departments of Pharmaceuticals and Pharmacy
School of Pharmacy
University of Washington
Seattle, Washington
Chapter 7

Courtney E.W. Sulentic, PhD
Associate Professor
Department of Pharmacology & Toxicology
Boonshoft School of Medicine
Wright State University
Dayton, Ohio
Chapter 12

Peter S. Thorne, MS, PhD
Professor and Head
Department of Occupational and Environmental Health
College of Public Health
The University of Iowa
Iowa City, Iowa
Chapter 34

Erik J. Tokar, PhD
Biologist
Inorganic Toxicology Group
Division of the National Toxicology Program
National Toxicology Program
National Institute of Environmental Health Sciences
Research Triangle Park, North Carolina
Chapter 23

Michael P. Waalkes, PhD
Chief
National Toxicology Group
Division of the National Toxicology Program
National Toxicology Program
National Institute of Environmental Health Sciences
Research Triangle Park, North Carolina
Chapter 23

D. Alan Warren, MPh, PhD
Program Director
Environmental Health Science
University of South Carolina Beaufort
Beaufort, South Carolina
Chapter 24

John B. Watkins, III, PhD
Associate Dean and Director
Professor of Pharmacology and Toxicology
Medical Sciences Program
Indiana University School of Medicine
Bloomington, Indiana
Chapter 26

Diana G. Wilkins, MS, PhD
Director
Center for Human Toxicology
Research Associate Professor
Department of Pharmacology and Toxicology
University of Utah
Salt Lake City, Utah
Chapter 32

Preface

This updated full-color edition of *Essentials of Toxicology* distills the major principles and concepts of toxicology that were described in detail in the eighth edition of *Casarett & Doull's Toxicology: The Basic Science of Poisons*. We are grateful to the authors who contributed to the eighth edition of *Casarett & Doull's Toxicology: The Basic Science of Poisons*; their chapters in the parent text provided the foundation for the chapters in this edition of *Essentials of Toxicology*.

Essentials of Toxicology concisely describes the expansive science of toxicology, and includes important concepts from anatomy, physiology, and biochemistry to facilitate the understanding of the principles and mechanisms of toxicant action on specific organ systems. We trust that this book will assist students in undergraduate and graduate courses in toxicology, as well as students from other disciplines, to develop a strong foundation in the concepts and principles of toxicology.

The book is organized into seven units: (1) General Principles of Toxicology; (2) Disposition of Toxicants; (3) Nonorgan-directed Toxicity; (4) Target Organ Toxicity; (5) Toxic Agents; (6) Environmental Toxicology; and (7) Applications of Toxicology. A summary of key points is included at the beginning of each chapter, and a set of review questions is provided at the end of each chapter. We invite readers to send us suggestions of ways to improve this text and we appreciate the thoughtful recommendations that we received on the last edition.

We would like to acknowledge all individuals who were involved in this project. We particularly give a heartfelt and sincere thanks to our families for their love, patience, and support during the preparation of this book. We especially appreciate Richard J. Batka and Alyssa Shapiro who provided invaluable assistance on this project. The capable advice, guidance, and assistance of the McGraw-Hill staff is gratefully acknowledged. Finally, we thank our students for their enthusiasm for learning and what they have taught us during their time with us.

Curtis D. Klaassen
John B. Watkins III

UNIT 1 GENERAL PRINCIPLES OF TOXICOLOGY

History and Scope of Toxicology

Michael A. Gallo

HISTORY OF TOXICOLOGY	20TH CENTURY TOXICOLOGY: THE AWAKENING OF UNDERSTANDING
Antiquity	
Middle Ages	AFTER WORLD WAR II
Renaissance	
Age of Enlightenment	21ST CENTURY TOXICOLOGY

KEY POINTS

- Toxicology is the study of the adverse effects of xenobiotics on living systems.
- Toxicology assimilates knowledge and techniques from biochemistry, biology, chemistry, genetics, mathematics, medicine, pharmacology, physiology, and physics.
- Toxicology applies safety evaluation and risk assessment to the discipline.

HISTORY OF TOXICOLOGY

Modern toxicology goes beyond the study of the adverse effects of exogenous agents by assimilating knowledge and techniques from most branches of biochemistry, biology, chemistry, genetics, mathematics, medicine, pharmacology, physiology, and physics and applies safety evaluation and risk assessment to the discipline. In all branches of toxicology, scientists explore the mechanisms by which chemicals produce adverse effects in biological systems. Activities in these broad subjects complement toxicologic research.

Antiquity

Knowledge of animal venoms and plant extracts for hunting, warfare, and assassination presumably predate recorded history. One of the oldest known writings, the Ebers Papyrus (circa 1500 B.C.), contains information pertaining to many recognized poisons, including hemlock, aconite, opium, and metals such as lead, copper, and antimony. The *Book of Job* (circa 1400 B.C.) speaks of poison arrows (Job 6:4) and Hippocrates (circa 400 B.C.) added a number of poisons and clinical toxicology principles pertaining to bioavailability in therapy and overdosage. Theophrastus (370–286 B.C.), a student of Aristotle, included numerous references to poisonous plants in *De Historia Plantarum*. Dioscorides, a Greek physician in the court of the Roman emperor Nero, made the first attempt at classifying poisons as plant, animal, and mineral in his book *De Materia Medica*, which contains reference to some 600 plants.

One legend tells of Roman King Mithridates VI of Pontus, who was so fearful of poisons that he regularly ingested a mixture of 36 ingredients as protection against assassination. On the occasion of his imminent capture by enemies, his attempts to kill himself with poison failed because of his successful antidote concoction. This tale leads to use of the word mithridatic as an antidote or protective mixture. Because poisonings in politics became so extensive, Sulla issued the *Lex Cornelia* (circa 82 B.C.), which appears to be the first law against poisoning and later became a regulatory statute directed at careless dispensers of drugs.

Middle Ages

The writings of Maimonides (Moses ben Maimon, A.D. 1135–1204) included a treatise on the treatment of poisonings from insects, snakes, and mad dogs (*Treatise on Poisons and Their Antidotes*, 1198). Maimonides described the subject of bioavailability, noting that milk, butter, and cream could delay intestinal absorption. In the early Renaissance and under the guise of delivering provender to the sick and the poor, Catherine de Medici tested toxic concoctions, carefully noting the rapidity of the toxic response (onset of action), the effectiveness of the compound (potency), the degree of response of the parts of the body (specificity and site of action), and the complaints of the victim (clinical signs and symptoms).

Renaissance

All substances are poisons; there is none that is not a poison. The right dose differentiates a poison from a remedy.

Paracelsus

Philippus Aureolus Theophrastus Bombastus von Hohenheim-Paracelsus (1493–1541) was pivotal, standing between the philosophy and magic of classic antiquity and the philosophy and science willed to us by figures of the seventeenth and eighteenth centuries. Paracelsus, a physician-alchemist, formulated many revolutionary views that remain integral to the structure of toxicology, pharmacology, and therapeutics today. He focused on the primary toxic agent as a chemical entity, and held that (1) experimentation is essential in the examination of responses to chemicals, (2) one should make a distinction between the therapeutic and toxic properties of chemicals, (3) these properties are sometimes but not always indistinguishable except by dose, and (4) one can ascertain a degree of specificity of chemicals and their therapeutic or toxic effects. These principles led Paracelsus to articulate the dose–response relation as a bulwark of toxicology.

Come bitter pilot, now at once run on
The dashing rocks thy seasick weary bark!
Here's to my love! O true apothecary!
Thy drugs are quick. Thus with a kiss I die.

Romeo and Juliet, act 5, scene 3

Although Ellenbog (circa 1480) warned of the toxicity of mercury and lead from goldsmithing and Agricola published a short treatise on mining diseases in 1556, the major work on the subject, *On the Miners' Sickness and Other Diseases of Miners* (1567), was published by Paracelsus. This treatise addressed the etiology of miners' disease, along with treatment and prevention strategies. Occupational toxicology was further advanced by the work of Bernardino Ramazzini when he published in 1700 his *Discourse on the Diseases of Workers*, which discussed occupations ranging from miners to midwives and including printers, weavers, and potters. Percival Pott's (1775) recognition of the role of soot in scrotal cancer among chimney sweeps was the first report of polyaromatic hydrocarbon carcinogenicity. These findings led to improved medical practices, particularly in prevention.

Age of Enlightenment

Experimental toxicology accompanied the growth of organic chemistry and developed rapidly during the nineteenth century. Magendie (1783–1885), Orfila (1787–1853), and Bernard (1813–1878) laid the groundwork for pharmacology, experimental therapeutics, and occupational toxicology.

Orfila, a Spanish physician in the French court, used autopsy material and chemical analysis systematically as legal proof of poisoning. His introduction of this detailed type of analysis survives as the underpinning of forensic toxicology. Orfila published a major work devoted expressly to the toxicity of natural agents in 1815. Magendie, a physician and experimental physiologist, studied the mechanisms of action of emetine and strychnine. His research determined the absorption and distribution of these compounds in the body. One of Magendie's more famous students, Claude Bernard, contributed the classic treatise, *An Introduction to the Study of Experimental Medicine*.

German scientists Oswald Schmiedeberg (1838–1921) and Louis Lewin (1850–1929) made many contributions to the science of toxicology. Schmeideberg trained approximately 120 students who later populated the most important laboratories of pharmacology and toxicology throughout the world. Lewin published much of the early work on the toxicity of narcotics, methanol, glycerol, acrolein, and chloroform.

20TH CENTURY TOXICOLOGY: THE AWAKENING OF UNDERSTANDING

Toxicology has drawn its strength and diversity from its proclivity to borrowing from almost all the basic sciences to test its hypotheses. This fact, coupled with the health and occupational regulations that have driven toxicology research since 1900, has made this discipline exceptional in the history of science.

With the advent of anesthetics and disinfectants in the late 1850s, toxicology as it is currently understood began. The prevalent use of "patent" medicines led to several incidents of poisonings from these medicaments, which, when coupled with the response to Upton Sinclair's exposé of the meatpacking industry in *The Jungle,* culminated in the passage of the Wiley Bill in 1906, the first of many U.S. pure food and drug laws.

During the 1890s and early 1900s, the discovery of radioactivity and the vitamins, or "vital amines," led to the use of the first large-scale bioassays (multiple animal studies) to determine whether these "new" chemicals were beneficial or harmful to laboratory animals.

One of the first journals expressly dedicated to experimental toxicology, *Archiv für Toxikologie,* began publication in Europe in 1930. That same year the National Institutes of Health (NIH) was established in the United States. As a response to the tragic consequences of acute kidney failure after taking sulfanilamide in glycol solutions, the Copeland bill was passed in 1938. This was the second major bill involving the formation of the U.S. Food and Drug Administration (FDA). The first major U.S. pesticide act was signed into law in 1947. The significance of the initial Federal Insecticide, Fungicide, and Rodenticide Act was that for the first time in U.S. history a substance that was neither a drug nor a food had to be shown to be safe and efficacious for approval.

AFTER WORLD WAR II

You too can be a toxicologist in two easy lessons, each of ten years.
Arnold Lehman (circa 1955)

The mid-1950s witnessed the strengthening of the U.S. FDA's commitment to toxicology. The U.S. Congress passed and the president of the United States signed the additives amendments to the Food, Drug, and Cosmetic Act. The Delaney clause (1958) of these amendments stated broadly that any chemical found to be carcinogenic in laboratory animals or humans could not be added to the U.S. food supply. Delaney became a battle cry for many groups and resulted in the inclusion at a new level of biostatisticians and mathematical modelers in the field of toxicology. Shortly after the Delaney amendment, the first American journal dedicated to toxicology, *Toxicology and Applied Pharmacology,* was launched. The founding of the Society of Toxicology followed shortly afterward.

The 1960s started with the tragic thalidomide incident, in which several thousand children were born with serious birth defects, and the publication of Rachel Carson's *Silent Spring* (1962). Attempts to understand the effects of chemicals on the embryo and fetus and on the environment as a whole gained momentum. New legislation was passed, and new journals were founded. Cellular and molecular toxicology developed as a subdiscipline, and risk assessment became a major product of toxicologic investigations.

Currently, many dozens of professional, governmental, and other scientific organizations with thousands of members and over 120 journals are dedicated to toxicology and related disciplines. In addition, the International Congress of Toxicology is composed of toxicology societies from Europe, South America, Asia, Africa, and Australia, which brings together the broadest representation of toxicologists.

21ST CENTURY TOXICOLOGY

The sequencing of the human genome and that of several other organisms has markedly affected all biological sciences, including toxicology. Genetically modifying organisms is now commonplace and those possessing orthologs of human genes (e.g., zebrafish [*Danio rerio*], roundworms [*Caenorhabditis elegans*], and fruit flys [*Drosophila melanogaster*]) are widely used in toxicology. Deeper understanding of epigenetics has provided novel approaches to studying the fetal origin of adult diseases including cancers, diabetes, and neurodegenerative diseases and disorders.

Toxicology has an interesting and varied history. Perhaps as a science that has grown and prospered by borrowing from many disciplines, it has suffered from the absence of a single goal, but its diversification has allowed for the interspersion of ideas and concepts from higher education, industry, and government. This has resulted in an exciting, innovative, and diversified field that is serving science and the community at large. Few disciplines can point to both basic sciences and direct applications at the same time. Toxicology—the study of the adverse effects of xenobiotics—may be unique in this regard.

BIBLIOGRAPHY

Bryan CP: *The Papyrus Ebers.* London: Geoffrey Bales, 1930.

Carson R: *Silent Spring.* Boston, MA: Houghton Mifflin, 1962.

Gunther RT: *The Greek Herbal of Dioscorides.* New York: Oxford University Press, 1934.

Guthrie DA: *A History of Medicine.* Philadelphia, PA: Lippincott, 1946.

Hays HW: *Society of Toxicology History, 1961–1986.* Washington, DC: Society of Toxicology, 1986.

Munter S (ed.): *Treatise on Poisons and Their Antidotes. Vol. II of the Medical Writings of Moses Maimonides.* Philadelphia, PA: Lippincott, 1966.

Pagel W: *Paracelsus: An Introduction to Philosophical Medicine in the Era of the Renaissance.* New York: Karger, 1958.

Thompson CJS: *Poisons and Poisoners: With Historical Accounts of Some Famous Mysteries in Ancient and Modern Times.* London: Shaylor, 1931.

http://www.toxipedia.org/display/toxipedia/History+of+Toxicology

QUESTIONS

1. Which one of the following statements regarding toxicology is true?
   a. Modern toxicology is concerned with the study of the adverse effects of chemicals on ancient forms of life.
   b. Modern toxicology studies embrace principles from such disciplines as biochemistry, botany, chemistry, physiology, and physics.
   c. Modern toxicology has its roots in the knowledge of plant and animal poisons, which predates recorded history and has been used to promote peace.
   d. Modern toxicology studies the mechanisms by which inorganic chemicals produce advantageous as well as deleterious effects.
   e. Modern toxicology is concerned with the study of chemicals in mammalian species.

2. Knowledge of the toxicology of poisonous agents was published earliest in the:
   a. Ebers papyrus.
   b. *De Historia Plantarum.*
   c. *De Materia Medica.*
   d. *Lex Cornelia.*
   e. *Treatise on Poisons and Their Antidotes.*

3. Paracelsus, a physician-alchemist, formulated many revolutionary views that remain integral to the structure of toxicology, pharmacology, and therapeutics today. He focused on the primary toxic agent as a chemical entity and articulated the dose–response relation. Which one of the following statements is not attributable to Paracelsus?
   a. Natural poisons are quick in their onset of actions.
   b. Experimentation is essential in the examination of responses to chemicals.
   c. One should make a distinction between the therapeutic and toxic properties of chemicals.
   d. These properties are sometimes but not always indistinguishable except by dose.
   e. One can ascertain a degree of specificity of chemicals and their therapeutic or toxic effects.

4. The art of toxicology requires years of experience to acquire, even though the knowledge base of facts may be learned more quickly. Which modern toxicologist is credited with saying that "you can be a toxicologist in two easy lesions, each of 10 years?"
   a. Claude Bernard.
   b. Rachel Carson.
   c. Upton Sinclair.
   d. Arnold Lehman.
   e. Oswald Schmiedeberg.

5. Which of the following statements is correct?
   a. Claude Bernard was a prolific scientist who trained over 120 students and published numerous contributions to the scientific literature.
   b. Louis Lewin trained under Oswald Schmiedeberg and published much of the early work on the toxicity of narcotics, methanol, and chloroform.
   c. *An Introduction to the Study of Experimental Medicine* was written by the Spanish physician Orfila.
   d. Magendie used autopsy material and chemical analysis systematically as legal proof of poisoning.
   e. Percival Potts was instrumental in demonstrating the chemical complexity of snake venoms.

specifically studying the impacts of chemicals on nonhuman organisms such as fish, birds, terrestrial animals, and plants. *Ecotoxicology,* a specialized area within environmental toxicology, focuses specifically on the impacts of toxic substances on population dynamics in an ecosystem (see Chapter 29).

Developmental toxicology is the study of adverse effects on the developing organism that may result from exposure to chemical or physical agents before conception (either parent), during prenatal development, or postnatally until the time of puberty. *Teratology* is the study of defects induced during development between conception and birth (see Chapter 10).

Reproductive toxicology is the study of the occurrence of adverse effects on the male or female reproductive system that may result from exposure to chemical or physical agents (see Chapter 20).

Toxicology and Society

Knowledge about the toxicologic effect of a compound affects consumer products, drugs, manufacturing processes, waste cleanup, regulatory action, civil disputes, and broad policy decisions. The expanding influence of toxicology on societal issues is accompanied by the responsibility to be increasingly sensitive to the ethical, legal, and social implications of toxicologic research and testing.

There are several ethical dilemmas in toxicology. First, experience and new discoveries in the biological sciences have emphasized the need for well-articulated visions of human, animal, and environmental health. Second, experience with the health consequences of exposure to such things as lead, asbestos, and tobacco has precipitated many regulatory and legal actions and public policy decisions. Third, we have an increasingly well-defined framework for discussing our social and ethical responsibilities. Fourth, all research involving humans or animals must be conducted in a responsible and ethical manner. Fifth, the uncertainty and biological variability inherent in the biological sciences requires decision making with limited or uncertain information.

General Characteristics of the Toxic Response

Virtually every known chemical has the potential to produce injury or death if it is present in a sufficient amount. Table 2–1 shows the wide spectrum of dosages needed to produce death in 50% of treated animals (lethal dose 50, LD_{50}). Chemicals producing death in microgram doses are often considered extremely poisonous. Note that measures of acute lethality such as LD_{50} may not accurately reflect the full spectrum of toxicity, or hazard, associated with exposure to a chemical. For example, some chemicals with low acute toxicity may have carcinogenic or teratogenic effects at doses that produce no evidence of acute toxicity. For a given chemical, each of the various effects that may occur in a given organism will have their own dose–response relationship.

TABLE 2–1 Approximate acute LD$_{50}$ of some representative chemical agents.

Agent	LD$_{50}$, mg/kg*
Ethyl alcohol	10 000
Sodium chloride	4 000
Ferrous sulfate	1 500
Morphine sulfate	900
Phenobarbital sodium	150
Picrotoxin	5
Strychnine sulfate	2
Nicotine	1
Tubocurarine	0.5
Hemicholinium-3	0.2
Tetrodotoxin	0.10
Dioxin (TCDD)	0.001
Botulinum toxin	0.00001

*LD_{50} is the dosage (mg/kg body weight) causing death in 50% of exposed animals.

CLASSIFICATION OF TOXIC AGENTS

Toxic agents are classified depending on the interests and needs of the classifier. These agents may be discussed in terms of their target organs, use, source, and effects. The term *toxin* generally refers to toxic substances that are produced by biological systems such as plants, animals, fungi, or bacteria. The term *toxicant* is used in speaking of toxic substances that are produced by or are a by-product of human activities. Toxic agents may be classified in terms of their physical state, chemical stability or reactivity, general chemical structure, or poisoning potential. No single classification is applicable to the entire spectrum of toxic agents and, therefore, a combination of classifications is needed to provide the best characterization of a toxic substance.

SPECTRUM OF UNDESIRED EFFECTS

The spectrum of undesired effects of chemicals is broad. In therapeutics, e.g., each drug produces a number of effects, but usually only one effect is associated with the primary objective of the therapy; all the other effects are referred to as *undesirable* or *side effects*. However, some of these side effects may be desired for another therapeutic indication. Some side effects of drugs are always deleterious to the well-being of humans. These are referred to as the *adverse, deleterious,* or *toxic* effects of the drug.

Allergic Reactions

Chemical allergy is an immunologically mediated adverse reaction to a chemical resulting from previous sensitization to that chemical or to a structurally similar one. The terms *hypersensitivity, allergic reaction,* and *sensitization reaction* are used to describe this situation (see Chapter 12). Once sensitization has occurred, allergic reactions may result from exposure to relatively very low doses of chemicals. Importantly, for a given allergic individual, allergic reactions are dose-related. Sensitization reactions are sometimes very severe and may be fatal.

Most chemicals and their metabolic products are not sufficiently large to be recognized by the immune system as a foreign substance and thus must first combine with an endogenous protein to form an antigen (or immunogen). Such a molecule is called a *hapten*. The hapten–protein complex (antigen) is then capable of eliciting the formation of antibodies. Subsequent exposure to the chemical results in an antigen–antibody interaction, which provokes the typical manifestations of an allergy that range in severity from minor skin disturbance to fatal anaphylactic shock.

Idiosyncratic Reactions

Chemical idiosyncrasy refers to a genetically determined abnormal reactivity to a chemical. The response observed is usually qualitatively similar to that observed in all individuals but may take the form of extreme sensitivity to low doses or extreme insensitivity to high doses of the chemical. For example, some individuals are abnormally sensitive to nitrites and other substances capable of oxidizing the iron in hemoglobin. This produces methemoglobin, which is incapable of binding and transporting oxygen to tissues. Consequently, they may suffer from tissue hypoxia after exposure to doses of methemoglobin-producing chemicals, whereas normal individuals would be unaffected. It is now recognized that many idiosyncratic drug reactions are due to the interplay between an individual's ability to form a reactive intermediate, detoxify that intermediate, and/or mount an immune response to adducted proteins. Specific genetic polymorphisms in drug-metabolizing enzymes, transporters, or receptors are responsible for many of these observed differences.

Immediate versus Delayed Toxicity

Immediate toxic effects occur or develop rapidly after a single administration of a substance, whereas delayed toxic effects occur after the lapse of some time. Most substances produce immediate toxic effects. However, carcinogenic effects of chemicals usually have long latency periods, often 20 to 30 years after the initial exposure, before tumors are observed in humans.

Reversible versus Irreversible Toxic Effects

Some toxic effects of chemicals are reversible, and others are irreversible. If a chemical produces pathological injury to a tissue, the ability of that tissue to regenerate largely determines whether the effect is reversible or irreversible. Liver tissue has high regeneration ability and most injuries are, therefore, reversible. However, CNS injury is largely irreversible because its cells are differentiated and cannot be replaced. Carcinogenic and teratogenic effects of chemicals, once they occur, are usually considered irreversible toxic effects.

Local versus Systemic Toxicity

Another distinction between types of effects is made on the basis of the general site of action. Local effects occur at the site of first contact between the biological system and the toxicant. In contrast, systemic effects require absorption and distribution of a toxicant from its entry point to a distant site, at which deleterious effects are produced. Most substances, except for highly reactive materials, produce systemic effects. Some materials can produce both effects.

Most chemicals that produce systemic toxicity usually elicit their major toxicity in only one or two organs, which are referred to as the *target organs* of toxicity of a particular chemical. Paradoxically, the target organ of toxicity is often not the site of the highest concentration of the chemical.

Target organs in order of frequency of involvement in systemic toxicity are the CNS; the circulatory system; the blood and hematopoietic system; visceral organs such as the liver, kidney, and lung; and the skin. Muscle and bone are seldom target tissues for systemic effects.

Interaction of Chemicals

Chemical interactions can occur via various mechanisms, such as alterations in absorption, protein binding, and the biotransformation and excretion of one or both of the interacting toxicants. In addition to these modes of interaction, the response of the organism to combinations of toxicants may be increased or decreased because of toxicologic responses at the site of action.

An *additive* effect, most commonly observed when two chemicals are given together, occurs when the combined effect of two chemicals is equal to the sum of the effects of each agent given alone (e.g.: $2 + 3 = 5$). A *synergistic* effect occurs when the combined effects of two chemicals are much greater than the sum of the effects of each agent given alone (e.g.: $2 + 2 = 20$). *Potentiation* occurs when one substance does not have a toxic effect on a certain organ or system but when added to another chemical makes that chemical much more toxic (e.g.: $0 + 2 = 10$). Isopropanol, e.g., is not hepatotoxic, but when it is administered in addition to carbon tetrachloride, the hepatotoxicity of carbon tetrachloride is much greater than that when it is given alone.

Antagonism occurs when two chemicals administered together interfere with each other's actions or one interferes with the action of the other (e.g.: $4 + 6 = 8$; $4 + (-4) = 0$; $4 + 0 = 1$). There are four major types of antagonism: functional, chemical, dispositional, and receptor. *Functional antagonism* occurs when two chemicals counterbalance each other by producing opposite effects on the same physiologic function.

Mechanisms of Toxicity

Zoltán Gregus

- Toxicity involves toxicant delivery to its target or targets and interactions with endogenous target molecules that may trigger perturbations in cell function and/or structure or that may initiate repair mechanisms at the molecular, cellular, and/or tissue levels.
- Biotransformation to harmful products is called *toxication* or *metabolic activation*.
- Biotransformations that eliminate the ultimate toxicant or prevent its formation are called *detoxications*.
- Apoptosis, or programmed cell death, is a tightly controlled, organized process whereby individual cells break into small fragments that are phagocytosed by adjacent cells or macrophages without producing an inflammatory response.

- Sustained elevation of intracellular Ca^{2+} is harmful because it can result in (1) depletion of energy reserves by inhibiting the ATPase used in oxidative phosphorylation, (2) dysfunction of microfilaments, (3) activation of hydrolytic enzymes, and (4) generation of reactive oxygen and nitrogen species (ROS and RNS).
- Cell injury progresses toward cell necrosis (death) if molecular repair mechanisms are inefficient or the molecular damage is not readily reversible.
- Chemical carcinogenesis involves insufficient function of various repair mechanisms, including (1) failure of DNA repair, (2) failure of apoptosis (programmed cell death), and (3) failure to terminate cell proliferation.

An understanding of the mechanisms of toxicity provides a rational basis for interpreting descriptive toxicity data. The cellular mechanisms that contribute to the manifestation of toxicities are overviewed by relating a series of events that begins with exposure, involves a multitude of interactions between the invading toxicant and the organism, and culminates in a toxic effect.

As a result of the huge number of potential toxicants and the multitude of biological structures and processes that can be impaired, there are a tremendous number of possible pathways that may lead to toxicity (Figure 3–1). Commonly, a toxicant is delivered to its target, reacts with it, and the resultant cellular dysfunction manifests itself in toxicity. Sometimes a xenobiotic does not react with a specific target molecule but rather adversely influences the biological environment, causing molecular, organellar, cellular, or organ dysfunction leading to deleterious effects.

The most complex path to toxicity involves more steps (Figure 3–1). First, the toxicant is delivered to its target or targets (step 1), interacting with endogenous target molecules (step 2a) or altering the environment (step 2b), triggering perturbations in cell function and/or structure (step 3), which initiate repair mechanisms at the molecular, cellular, and/or tissue levels (step 4). When the perturbations induced by the toxicant exceed repair capacity or when repair becomes malfunctional, toxicity occurs. Tissue necrosis, cancer, and fibrosis are examples of chemically induced toxicities that follow this four-step course.

STEP 1—DELIVERY: FROM THE SITE OF EXPOSURE TO THE TARGET

Theoretically, the intensity of a toxic effect depends on the concentration and persistence of the ultimate toxicant at its site of action. The ultimate toxicant is the chemical species that reacts with the endogenous target molecule or critically alters the biological environment, initiating structural and/or functional alterations that result in toxicity. The ultimate toxicant can be the original chemical to which the organism is exposed (parent compound), a metabolite, or a reactive oxygen or nitrogen species (ROS or RNS) generated during the biotransformation of the toxicant, or an endogenous molecule.

The concentration of the ultimate toxicant at the target molecule depends on the relative effectiveness of the processes that increase or decrease its concentration at the target site (Figure 3–2). Increased concentration is facilitated by absorption, distribution to the site of action, reabsorption, and toxication, while presystemic elimination, distribution away from the site of action, excretion, and detoxication will decrease the toxicant concentration at its target.

Absorption versus Presystemic Elimination

Absorption—Transfer of a chemical from the site of exposure, usually an external or internal body surface, into the systemic circulation is called *absorption*. Transporters contribute to gastrointestinal (GI) absorption of some chemicals; however, the vast majority of toxicants traverse epithelial barriers via diffusion. Factors that influence absorption include concentration, surface area of exposure, characteristics of the epithelial layer through which the toxicant is being absorbed, and, usually most important, lipid solubility because lipid-soluble molecules are absorbed most easily into cells.

Presystemic Elimination—During transfer from the site of exposure to the systemic circulation, toxicants may be eliminated. This is common for chemicals absorbed from the gastrointestinal (GI) tract because they must first pass through the GI mucosal cells, into the liver (enterohepatic circulation), and then

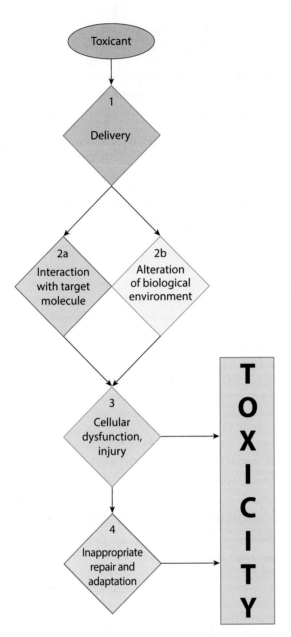

FIGURE 3–1 Potential stages in the development of toxicity after chemical exposure.

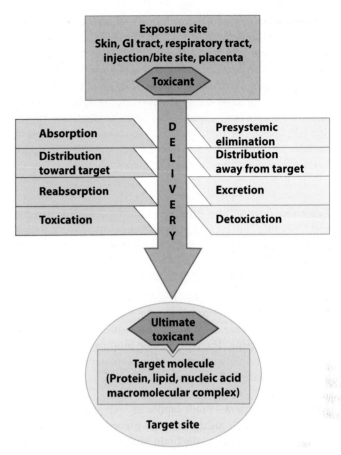

FIGURE 3–2 **The process of toxicant delivery is the first step in the development of toxicity.** Delivery—that is, movement of the toxicant from the site of exposure to the site of its action in an active form—is promoted by the processes listed on the left and opposed by the events indicated on the right.

lung (pulmonary circulation) before being distributed to the rest of the body (systemic circulation). The GI mucosa and the liver may eliminate a significant fraction of a toxicant during its passage through these tissues. Presystemic or first-pass elimination generally reduces the toxic effects of chemicals that reach their target sites by way of the systemic circulation, but may contribute to injury of the digestive mucosa, the liver, and the lungs because these processes necessitate toxicant delivery to those sites.

Distribution to and away from the Target

Toxicants exit the blood during the distribution phase, enter the extracellular space, and reach their site or sites of action, usually a macromolecule on either the surface or the interior of a particular type of cell. Chemicals also may be distributed to the site or sites of toxication, usually an intracellular enzyme, where the ultimate toxicant is formed through biotransformation.

Mechanisms Facilitating Distribution to a Target

Porosity of the Capillary Endothelium—There are three types of capillaries (continuous, fenestrated, and sinusoidal), each with varying degrees of porosity. Endothelial cells in the hepatic sinusoids and in the renal peritubular capillaries have large fenestrae (50 to 150 nm in diameter) that permit passage of even protein-bound xenobiotics. This relatively free filtration promotes the accumulation of chemicals in the liver and kidneys.

Specialized Transport across the Plasma Membrane—Specialized ion channels and membrane transporters can contribute to the intracellular delivery of toxicants, making those cells targets. Na^+,K^+-ATPase, voltage-gated Ca^{2+} channels, carrier-mediated uptake, endocytosis, and membrane recycling are some examples of methods that facilitate the entry of toxicants into specific cells. Further, endocytosis of some toxicant–protein complexes also occurs in some cells.

Accumulation in Cell Organelles—Amphipathic xenobiotics with a protonatable amine group and lipophilic character accumulate in lysosomes as well as mitochondria. Lysosomal accumulation occurs by pH trapping, that is, diffusion of the amine in unprotonated form into the acidic interior of the organelle, where the amine is protonated, preventing its efflux, so that it impairs phospholipid degradation. Mitochondrial accumulation takes place electrophoretically. The amine is protonated in the intermembrane space and then sucked into the matrix space by the strong negative potential ($-220\,mV$), where it may impair β-oxidation of fatty acids and oxidative phosphorylation.

Reversible Intracellular Binding—Chemicals such as organic and inorganic cations and polycyclic aromatic hydrocarbons accumulate in melanin-containing cells by binding to melanin.

Mechanisms Opposing Distribution to a Target

Binding to Plasma Proteins—Hydrophobic xenobiotics generally bind proteins or lipoproteins in the plasma. In order to leave the blood and enter cells, these xenobiotics must dissociate from these proteins. Therefore, strong binding to plasma proteins delays xenobiotics movement across membranes and prolongs their effects and elimination.

Specialized Barriers—Brain capillaries lack fenestrae and are joined by extremely tight junctions, preventing the access of hydrophilic chemicals to the brain except by active transport. The spermatogenic cells are supported by Sertoli cells that are tightly joined to form the blood–testis barrier. Transfer of hydrophilic toxicants across the placenta is also restricted. However, none of these barriers are effective against lipophilic substances.

Distribution to Storage Sites—Some chemicals accumulate in tissues (i.e., storage sites) where they do not exert significant effects. Such storage decreases toxicant availability for their target sites.

Association with Intracellular Binding Proteins—Binding to nontarget intracellular sites, such as metallothionein, temporarily reduces the concentration of toxicants at the target site.

Export from Cells—Intracellular toxicants may be transported back into the extracellular space. Some ATP-dependent membrane transporters, also known as the multidrug-resistance (mdr) proteins, extrude chemicals from cells.

Excretion versus Reabsorption

Excretion—Excretion is the removal of xenobiotics from blood and their return to the external environment. Excretion is a physical mechanism, whereas biotransformation is a chemical mechanism for eliminating the toxicant.

The route and speed of excretion depend largely on the physicochemical properties of the toxicant. The major excretory organs—the kidney and the liver—efficiently remove highly hydrophilic chemicals such as organic acids and bases.

There are no efficient elimination mechanisms for nonvolatile, highly lipophilic chemicals. If they are resistant to biotransformation, such chemicals are eliminated very slowly and tend to accumulate in the body on repeated exposure. Three rather inefficient processes are available for the elimination of such chemicals: (1) excretion from the mammary gland in breast milk, (2) excretion in bile, and (3) excretion into the intestinal lumen from blood. Volatile, nonreactive toxicants such as gases and volatile liquids diffuse from pulmonary capillaries into the alveoli and are exhaled.

Reabsorption—Toxicants in the blood are filtered at the glomerulus into the renal tubules. These filtered toxicants may reenter the blood by diffusing through peritubular capillaries. This reentry is facilitated by tubular fluid reabsorption which increases intratubular fluid concentration and residence time of non-reabsorbed chemical by slowing urine flow.

Reabsorption by diffusion is dependent on the lipid solubility of the chemical and inversely related to the extent of ionization, because the nonionized molecule is more lipid soluble. Therefore, pH of the tubular fluid affects reabsorption such that acidification favors excretion of weak organic bases and alkalinization favors the elimination of weak organic acids.

Toxicants delivered to the GI tract by biliary, gastric, and intestinal excretion and secretion by salivary glands and exocrine pancreas may be reabsorbed by diffusion across the intestinal mucosa. Reabsorption of compounds excreted into bile is possible only if they are sufficiently lipophilic or are converted to more lipid-soluble forms in the intestinal lumen.

Toxication versus Detoxication

Toxication—A number of xenobiotics are directly toxic, whereas other xenobiotics exert a toxic effect through their metabolites. Biotransformation to harmful products is called *toxication* or *metabolic activation*. With some xenobiotics, toxication confers physicochemical properties that adversely alter the microenvironment of biological processes or structures. Occasionally, chemicals acquire structural features and reactivity by biotransformation that allows for a more efficient interaction with specific receptors or enzymes. Most often, however, toxication renders xenobiotics and occasionally other molecules in the body, such as nitric oxide, indiscriminately reactive toward endogenous molecules with susceptible functional groups. This increased reactivity may be due to conversion into (1) electrophiles, (2) free radicals, (3) nucleophiles, or (4) redox-active reactants.

Electrophiles are molecules that contain an electron-deficient atom with a partial or full positive charge that allows it to react by sharing electron pairs with the electron-rich atoms in nucleophiles. A free radical is a molecule or molecular fragment that contains one or more unpaired electrons. One of the more biologically relevant free radicals is superoxide anion ($O_2^{\bullet-}$), which is formed both endogenously and exogenously. The immune system produces $O_2^{\bullet-}$ and transforms it into hypochorous acid (aka bleach, HOCl) through a series of reactions in order to combat pathogens. The most reactive metabolites are electron-deficient molecules and molecular fragments such as electrophiles and neutral or cationic free radicals. Some nucleophiles are inherently reactive (e.g., HCN and CO); however, many are activated by conversion into electrophiles.

Detoxication—Biotransformations that eliminate the ultimate toxicant or prevent its formation are called *detoxications*. In some cases, detoxication may compete with toxication.

Detoxication of Toxicants with No Functional Groups—In general, chemicals without functional groups, such as benzene and toluene, are detoxicated in two phases. Initially, a functional group such as hydroxyl or carboxyl is introduced into the molecule, most often by cytochrome P450 enzymes. Next, an endogenous acid, such as glucuronic acid, sulfuric acid, or an amino acid, is added to the functional group by a transferase. With some exceptions, the final products are inactive, highly hydrophilic organic acids that are readily excreted.

Detoxication of Nucleophiles—Nucleophiles generally are detoxicated by conjugation of a functional group to the nucleophilic atom. Sulfonation, glucuronidation, methylation, and acetylation are common reactions. Conjugation prevents peroxidase-catalyzed conversion of the nucleophiles to free radicals and biotransformation of phenols, aminophenols, catechols, and hydroquinones to electrophilic quinines and quinoneimines. Alternative mechanisms of nucleophile detoxication exist, including oxidation by flavin-containing monooxygenases and oxidation to carboxylic acids, as is the case with ethanol.

Detoxication of Electrophiles—Generally, detoxication of electrophilic toxicants involves conjugation with the nucleophile, glutathione. This reaction may occur spontaneously or can be facilitated by glutathione S-transferases. Covalent binding of electrophiles to proteins can be regarded as detoxification, provided that the protein has no critical function and does not become a neoantigen or otherwise harmful.

Detoxication of Free Radicals—Detoxication and elimination of $O_2^{\bullet-}$ is important because it can be converted into much more reactive compounds (Figure 3–3) such as the hydroxyl radical (HO•), nitrogen dioxide (•NO$_2$), and the carbonate anion radical (CO$_3^{\bullet-}$). Superoxide dismutases (SODs), located in the cytosol (Cu, Zn-SOD) and the mitochondria (Mn-SOD), convert $O_2^{\bullet-}$ to hydrogen peroxide (HOOH) (Figure 3–4). Subsequently, HOOH is reduced to water by cytosolic glutathione peroxidase or peroxisomal catalase (Figure 3–4). No enzyme eliminates HO• owing to its extremely short half-life (10^{-9} s). The only effective protection against HO• is to prevent its formation by converting its precursor, HOOH, to water (Figure 3–4).

Peroxynitrite (ONOO$^-$), like HOOH, is an intermediate of $O_2^{\bullet-}$ toxication and is not a free radical oxidant itself. It is significantly more stable than HO•, and rapidly reacts with CO$_2$ to form the reactive free radicals, •NO$_2$ and CO$_3^{\bullet-}$ (Figure 3–3). Glutathione peroxidase can reduce ONOO$^-$ to nitrite (ONO$^-$), thereby preventing free radical production. In addition,

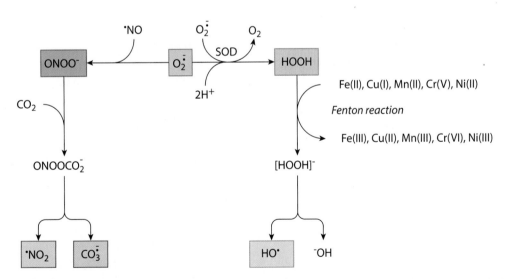

FIGURE 3–3 **Two pathways for toxication of superoxide anion radical ($O_2^{\bullet-}$) via nonradical products (ONOO— and HOOH) to radical products (•NO$_2$, CO$_3^{\bullet-}$, and HO•).** In one pathway, conversion of ($O_2^{\bullet-}$) to HOOH is spontaneous or is catalyzed by SOD. Homolytic cleavage of HOOH to hydroxyl radical and hydroxyl ion is called the Fenton reaction and is catalyzed by the transition metal ions shown. Hydroxyl radical formation is the ultimate toxication for xenobiotics that form $O_2^{\bullet-}$ or for HOOH, the transition metal ions listed, and some chemicals that form complexes with these transition metal ions. In the other pathway, $O_2^{\bullet-}$ reacts avidly with nitric oxide (•NO), the product of •NO synthase (NOS), forming peroxynitrite (ONOO$^-$). Spontaneous reaction of ONOO$^-$ with carbon dioxide (CO$_2$) yields nitrosoperoxy carbonate (ONOOCO$_2^-$) that is homolytically cleaved to nitrogen dioxide (•NO$_2$) and carbonate anion radical (CO$_3^{\bullet-}$). All three radical products indicated in this figure are oxidants, whereas •NO$_2$ is also a nitrating agent.

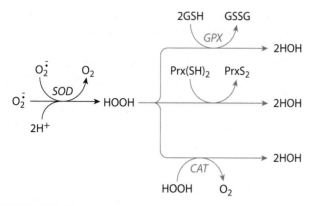

FIGURE 3-4 Detoxication of superoxide anion radical ($O_2^{\bullet-}$) by superoxide dismutase (SOD), glutathione peroxidase (GPX), and catalase (CAT).

$ONOO^-$ reacts with oxyhemoglobin, heme-containing peroxidases, and albumin, all of which could be important binding sites for $ONOO^-$. Furthermore, elimination of the two $ONOO^-$ precursors—that is, $^{\bullet}NO$ by reaction with oxyhemoglobin and $O_2^{\bullet-}$ by SODs—is a significant mechanism in preventing $ONOO^-$ buildup.

Peroxidase-generated free radicals are eliminated by electron transfer from glutathione. This results in the oxidation of glutathione, which is reversed by NADPH-dependent glutathione reductase (Figure 3–5). Thus, glutathione plays an important role in the detoxication of both electrophiles and free radicals.

Detoxication of Protein Toxins—Extra- and intracellular proteases are involved in the inactivation of toxic polypeptides. Several toxins found in venoms, such as α- and β-bungarotoxin, erabutoxin b, and phospholipase, contain intramolecular disulfide bonds that are required for their activity. These proteins become inactivated by the enzyme thioredoxin, which reduces the essential disulfide bond.

When Detoxication Fails—Detoxication may be insufficient for several reasons: (1) the toxicant overwhelms the detoxication processes, (2) a reactive toxicant inactivates a detoxicating enzyme, (3) the detoxication is reversed after transfer to other tissues, or (4) harmful by-products are produced by the detoxication process.

STEP 2—REACTION OF THE ULTIMATE TOXICANT WITH THE TARGET MOLECULE

Toxicity is typically mediated by a reaction of the ultimate toxicant with a target molecule (step 2a in Figure 3–1). Subsequently, a series of secondary biochemical events occur, leading to dysfunction or injury that is manifest at various levels of biological organization, such as at the target molecule itself, cell organelles, cells, tissues and organs, and even the whole organism.

Attributes of Target Molecules

Practically all endogenous compounds are potential targets for toxicants. The most prevalent and toxicologically relevant targets are nucleic acids (especially DNA), proteins, and membranes. The first target for reactive metabolites is often the enzyme responsible for their production or the adjacent intracellular structures. Not all targets for chemicals contribute harmful effects. Covalent binding to proteins without adverse consequences may even represent a form of detoxication by sparing toxicologically relevant targets. Thus, to conclusively identify a target molecule as being responsible for toxicity, it should be demonstrated that the ultimate toxicant (1) reacts with the target and adversely affects its function, (2) reaches an effective concentration at the target site, and (3) alters the target in a way that is mechanistically related to the observed toxicity.

Types of Reactions

The ultimate toxicant may bind to the target molecules noncovalently or covalently and may alter it by hydrogen abstraction, electron transfer, or enzymatically.

Noncovalent Binding—Hydrophobic interactions, hydrogen bonding, and ionic bonding are forms of noncovalent binding through which a toxicant can interact with targets such as membrane receptors, intracellular receptors, ion channels, and certain enzymes. Noncovalent binding usually is reversible because of the comparatively low bonding energy.

Covalent Binding—Being practically irreversible, covalent binding permanently alters endogenous molecules. Covalent adduct formation is common with electrophilic toxicants such

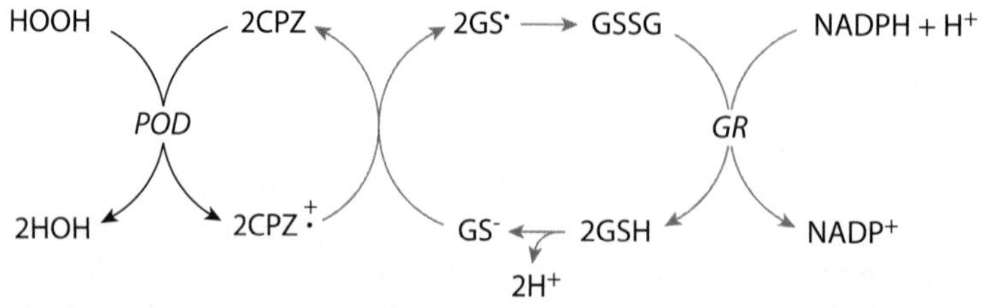

FIGURE 3-5 Detoxication of peroxidase (POD)-generated free radicals such as chlorpromazine free radical ($CPZ^{\bullet+}$) by glutathione (GSH). The by-products are glutathione thiyl radical ($GS^{\bullet}$) and glutathione disulfide (GSSG), from which GSH is regenerated by glutathione reductase (GR).

as nonionic and cationic electrophiles and radical cations. These toxicants react with nucleophilic atoms that are abundant in biological macromolecules, such as proteins and nucleic acids. Neutral free radicals such as $HO^\bullet$, $^\bullet NO_2$, and $Cl_3C^\bullet$ also can bind covalently to biomolecules. Nucleophilic toxicants are, in principle, reactive toward electrophilic endogenous compounds. However, such reactions are infrequent due to the rarity of electrophilic biomolecules. Carbon monoxide, cyanide, hydrogen sulfide, and azide are examples of nucleophiles that form coordinate covalent bonds with iron in various heme proteins.

Hydrogen Abstraction—Neutral free radicals can readily abstract H atoms from endogenous compounds, subsequently converting those compounds into radicals. Radicals can also remove hydrogen from methylene groups (CH_2) of free amino acids or from amino acid residues in proteins and convert them to carbonyls (C=O), forming cross-links with DNA or other proteins.

Electron Transfer—Chemicals can exchange electrons to oxidize or reduce other molecules, leading to formation of harmful by-products. For example, chemicals can oxidize Fe(II) in hemoglobin to Fe(III), producing methemoglobinemia.

Enzymatic Reactions—A few toxins act enzymatically on specific target proteins. For example, diphtheria toxin blocks the function of elongation factor 2 in protein synthesis and cholera toxin activates a G protein through such a mechanism.

In summary, most ultimate toxicants act on endogenous molecules on the basis of their chemical reactivity. Those with more than one type of reactivity may react by different mechanisms with various target molecules.

Effects of Toxicants on Target Molecules

Dysfunction of Target Molecules—Some toxicants activate protein target molecules, mimicking endogenous ligands. More commonly, chemicals inhibit the function of target molecules by blocking neurotransmitter receptors or ion channels, inhibiting enzymes, and interfering with cytoskeleton dynamics.

Protein function is impaired when conformation or structure is altered by interaction with the toxicant. Many proteins possess critical moieties that are essential for catalytic activity or assembly to macromolecular complexes. Covalent and/or oxidative modification of these moieties by xenobiotics can cause aberrant signal transduction and/or impaired maintenance of the cell's energy and metabolic homeostasis. Toxicants may also interfere with the template function of DNA. The covalent binding of chemicals to DNA causes nucleotide mispairing during replication.

Destruction of Target Molecules—In addition to adduct formation, toxicants alter the primary structure of endogenous molecules by means of cross-linking and fragmentation. Cross-linking imposes both structural and functional constraints on the linked molecules.

Other target molecules are susceptible to spontaneous degradation after chemical attack. Free radicals such as $Cl_3COO^\bullet$ and $HO^\bullet$ can initiate peroxidative degradation of lipids by hydrogen abstraction from fatty acids. This not only destroys lipids in cellular membranes but also generates endogenous toxicants, free radicals, and electrophiles, which can go on to harm adjacent molecules (e.g., membrane proteins) or more distant molecules (e.g., DNA). Several forms of DNA fragmentation can be caused by toxicants, including imidazole ring-opening on purines, imidazole ring-contraction on pyrimidines, single-strand breaks (SSBs), phosphodiester bond cleavage, and double-strand breaks (DSBs).

Neoantigen Formation—Covalent binding of xenobiotics or their metabolites to proteins may evoke an immune response (Chapter 12). Some chemicals (e.g., dinitrochlorobenzene, penicillin, and nickel) bind to proteins spontaneously. Others may obtain reactivity by autooxidation to quinones (e.g., urushiols, the allergens in poison ivy) or by enzymatic biotransformation.

Toxicity Not Initiated by Reaction with Target Molecules

Some xenobiotics alter the biological microenvironment (see step 2b in Figure 3–1), leading to a toxic response. Included here are (1) chemicals that alter H^+ ion concentrations in the aqueous biophase, (2) solvents and detergents that physicochemically alter the lipid phase of cell membranes and destroy transmembrane solute gradients, and (3) xenobiotics that cause harm merely by occupying a site or space.

STEP 3—CELLULAR DYSFUNCTION AND RESULTANT TOXICITIES

Reaction of toxicants with a target molecule may result in impaired cellular function as the third step in the development of toxicity (Figures 3–1). Each cell in a multicellular organism carries out defined programs, some of which determine whether cells undergo division, differentiation, or apoptosis. Other programs control the ongoing (momentary) activity of differentiated cells, determining whether they secrete more or less of a substance, whether they contract or relax, and whether they transport and metabolize nutrients at higher or lower rates. For regulation of these cellular programs, cells possess signaling networks that can be activated and inactivated by external signaling molecules.

As outlined in Figure 3–6, the nature of the primary cellular dysfunction caused by toxicants, but not necessarily the ultimate outcome, depends on the role of the target molecule affected. The reaction of a toxicant with targets serving external functions can influence the operation of other cells and integrated organ systems. However, if the target molecule is involved predominantly in the cell's internal maintenance, the resultant dysfunction can ultimately compromise survival of the cell.

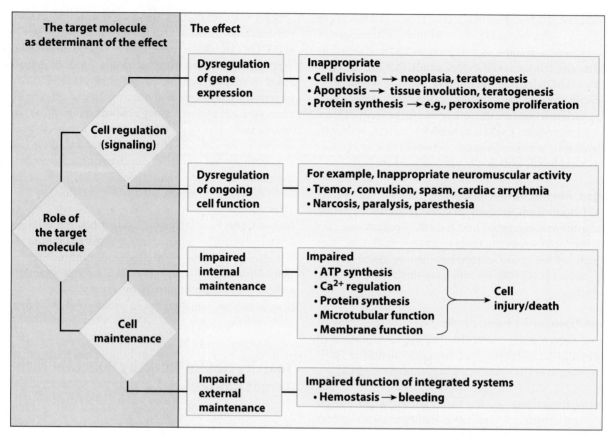

FIGURE 3–6 The third step in the development of toxicity: alteration of the regulatory or maintenance function of the cell.

Toxicant-induced Cellular Dysregulation

Cells are regulated by signaling molecules that activate specific cellular receptors linked to signal-transducing networks that transmit the signals to the regulatory regions of genes and/or functional proteins. Receptor activation may ultimately lead to altered gene expression and/or a chemical modification of specific proteins, typically by phosphorylation. Programs controlling the destiny of cells primarily affect gene expression, whereas those regulating the ongoing activities primarily influence the activity of functional proteins. However, one signal often evokes both responses because of branching and interconnection of signaling networks.

Dysregulation of Gene Expression—Gene expression is the process by which information from a gene is used to synthesize a functional gene product. The central dogma of molecular biology is that information from DNA is transcribed into messenger RNA (mRNA), which is then translated into a protein product. Genes that are transcribed into other types of RNA but not into proteins are called nonprotein-coding genes and they are one source of posttranscriptional control of protein synthesis. Among the alternative RNA types is the recently discovered small silencing RNA, called microRNA (miRNA), which can repress translation of mRNA into proteins. Dysregulation of gene expression may occur at elements that are directly responsible for transcription, at components of the intracellular signal-transduction pathway, and at the synthesis, storage, or release of the extracellular signaling molecules.

Dysregulation of Transcription—Transcription of genetic information from DNA to mRNA is controlled largely by interplay between transcription factors (TFs) and the regulatory or promoter region of genes. By binding to distinctive nucleotide sequences in the promoter or regulatory regions, TFs can facilitate or impede formation of the preinitiation complex, thereby either promoting or repressing transcription of the adjacent gene. Xenobiotics may interact with the promoter region of the gene, the TFs, or other components of the transcription initiation complex. However, altered activation of TFs appears to be the most common modality.

Several endogenous compounds, such as hormones, and vitamins, influence gene expression by binding to and activating TFs or intracellular receptors; xenobiotics may mimic these natural ligands. Either natural or xenobiotic ligands may cause toxicity when present at extreme doses or during critical periods of organism development. In addition to altering the fate of specific cells, compounds that act on ligand-activated TFs can also evoke changes in the metabolism of endogenous and foreign substances by inducing overexpression of relevant enzymes. The effects of endobiotics and xenobiotics that act on TFs may also be mediated by transcriptional up- or down-regulation of protein-coding genes (i.e., genes transcribed into mRNA) and/or nonprotein-coding genes (i.e., genes transcribed into miRNA). Xenobiotics may also dysregulate transcription by altering the regulatory gene regions and the promoter methylation pattern.

Dysregulation of Signal Transduction—Extracellular signaling molecules, such as growth factors, cytokines, hormones, and neurotransmitters, can ultimately activate TFs by utilizing cell surface receptors and intracellular signal-transducing networks. Figure 3–7 depicts such networks and identifies some important signal-activated TFs that control transcriptional activity of genes that influence cell cycle progression and thus determine the fate of cells. An example is the c-Myc protein, which, on dimerizing with Max protein and binding to its cognate nucleotide sequence, transactivates cyclin D and E genes. The cyclins, in turn, accelerate the cell-division cycle by activating cyclin-dependent protein kinases, which are involved in regulating the cell cycle. Mitogenic signaling molecules thus induce cellular proliferation.

The signal from the cell surface receptors to the TFs is relayed by successive protein–protein interactions and protein phosphorylations, that is, a signal molecule phosphorylates another protein like mitogen-activated protein kinase (MAPK), which activates that protein to phosphorylate and activate another. For example, ligands induce growth factor receptors (item 4 in Figure 3–7) on the surface of all cells to self-phosphorylate, and these phosphorylated receptors then bind to adapter proteins through which they activate Ras. The active Ras initiates the MAPK cascade, involving serial phosphorylations of protein kinases, which finally reaches the TFs. These signal transducers are typically, but not always, activated by phosphorylation, which is catalyzed by protein kinases, and are usually inactivated by dephosphorylation, which is carried out by protein phosphatases.

Chemicals most often cause aberrant signal transduction by altering protein phosphorylation, and occasionally by interfering with the GTPase activity or signal termination activity of G proteins (e.g., Ras), disrupting normal protein–protein interactions, establishing abnormal ones, or by altering the synthesis or degradation of signaling proteins. Such interventions may ultimately influence cell cycle progression.

Chemically Altered Signal Transduction with Proliferative Effect: Xenobiotics that facilitate phosphorylation of signal transducers often promote mitosis and tumor formation. For example, the phorbol esters and fumonisin B activate protein kinase C (PKC) by mimicking diacylglycerol (DAG), one of the physiologic activators of PKC (item 6 in Figure 3–7). The other physiologic PKC activator, Ca^{2+}, is mimicked by Pb^{2+}. Activated PKC promotes mitogenic signaling by starting a cascade that activates other kinases and allows certain TFs to bind to DNA. Protein kinases may also be activated by interacting with proteins that have been altered by a xenobiotic.

Aberrant phosphorylation of proteins may result from decreased dephosphorylation by phosphatases or by increased phosphorylation by kinases. Inhibition of phosphatases appears to be the underlying mechanism of the mitogenic effect of various chemicals, oxidative stress, and ultraviolet (UV) irradiation. Soluble protein phosphatase 2A (PP2A) in cells is likely responsible for reversing the growth factor–induced stimulation of MAPK, thereby controlling the extent and duration of MAPK activity. PP2A also removes an activating phosphate from a mitosis-triggering protein kinase. Several natural toxins are extremely potent inhibitors of PP2A, including the blue-green algae poison microcystin-LR and the dinoflagellate-derived okadaic acid.

Apart from phosphatases, there are also other inhibitory binding proteins that can keep signaling under control. For example, IκB binds to NF-κB, subsequently preventing its transfer into the nucleus and its function as a TF (Figure 3–7). Upon phosphorylation, IκB becomes degraded and NF-κB is set free. NF-κB is an important contributor to proliferative and prolife signaling, as well as the acute and chronic inflammatory response. IκB degradation which leads to NF-κB activation can also be induced by oxidative stress.

Chemically Altered Signal Transduction with Antiproliferative Effect: Downturning of increased proliferative signaling after cell injury may compromise replacement of injured cells (follow the path in Figure 3–7: inhibition of Raf → diminished degradation of IκB → diminished binding of NF-κB to DNA → diminished expression of c-Myc mRNA). Down-regulation of a normal mitogenic signal is a step away from survival and toward apoptosis.

Dysregulation of Extracellular Signal Production—Hormones of the anterior pituitary exert mitogenic effects on endocrine glands in the periphery by acting on cell surface receptors. Pituitary hormone production is under negative feedback control by hormones of the peripheral glands. Perturbation of this circuit adversely affects pituitary hormone secretion and, in turn, the peripheral glands. Decreased secretion of pituitary hormone produces apoptosis followed by involution of the peripheral target gland.

Dysregulation of Ongoing Cellular Activity—Toxicants can adversely affect ongoing cellular activity in specialized cells by disrupting any step in signal coupling.

Dysregulation of Electrically Excitable Cells—Many xenobiotics influence cellular activity in excitable cells, such as neurons, skeletal, cardiac, and smooth muscle cells. Release of neurotransmitters and muscle contraction are controlled by transmitters and modulators synthesized and released by adjacent neurons. Chemicals that interfere with these mechanisms are listed in Table 3–1.

Perturbation of ongoing cellular activity by chemicals may be due to an alteration in (1) the concentration of neurotransmitters, (2) receptor function, (3) intracellular signal transduction, or (4) the signal-terminating processes.

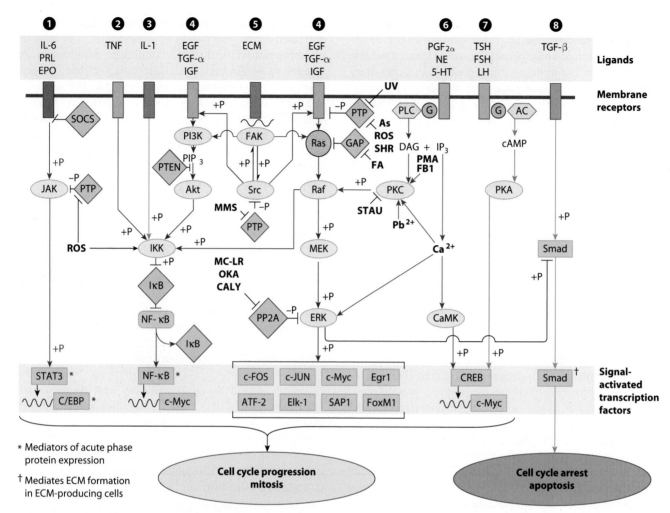

FIGURE 3–7 **Signal-transduction pathways from cell membrane receptors to signal-activated nuclear transcription factors that influence transcription of genes involved in cell-cycle regulation.** The symbols of cell membrane receptors are numbered 1 to 8 and some of their activating ligands are indicated. Circles represent G proteins, oval symbols protein kinases, rectangles transcription factors, wavy lines genes, and diamond symbols inhibitory proteins, such as protein phosphatases (PTP and PP2A) and the lipid phosphatase PTEN, the GTPase-activating protein GAP, and the inhibitory binding protein IκB. Arrowheads indicate stimulation or formation of second messengers (e.g., DAG, IP_3, PIP_3, cAMP, and Ca^{2+}), whereas blunt arrows indicate inhibition. Phosphorylation and dephosphorylation are indicated by +P and –P, respectively. Abbreviations for interfering chemicals are printed in black (As = arsenite; CALY = calyculin A; FA = fatty acids; FB1 = fumonisin B; MC-LR = microcystin-LR; OKA = okadaic acid; MMS = methylmethane sulfonate; PMA = phorbol miristate acetate; ROS = reactive oxygen species; SHR = SH-reactive chemicals, such as iodoacetamide; STAU = staurosporin).

In the center of the depicted networks is the pathway activated by growth factors, such as EGF, that acts on a tyrosine kinase receptor (#6), which uses adaptor proteins (Shc, Grb2, and SOS; not shown) to convert the inactive GDP-bound Ras to active GTP-bound form, which in turn activates the MAP-kinase phosphorylation cascade (Raf, MAPKK, and MAPK). The phosphorylated MAPK moves into the nucleus and phosphorylates transcription factors, thereby enabling them to bind to cognate sequences in the promoter regions of genes to facilitate transcription. There are numerous interconnections between the signal-transduction pathways. Some of these connections permit the use of the growth factor receptor (#6)–MAPK "highway" for other receptors (e.g., 4, 5, and 7) to send mitogenic signals. For example, receptor (#4) joins in via its G protein β/γ subunits and tyrosine kinase Src; the integrin receptor (#5), whose ligands are constituents of the extracellular matrix (ECM), possibly connects via G-protein Rho (not shown) and focal adhesion kinase (FAK); and the G-protein-coupled receptor (#7) via phospholipase C (PLC)-catalyzed formation of second messengers and activation of protein kinase C (PKC). The mitogenic stimulus relayed along the growth factor receptor (#6)–MAPK axis can be amplified by, e.g., the Raf-catalyzed phosphorylation of IκB, which unleashes NF-κB from this inhibitory protein, and by the MAPK-catalyzed inhibitory phosphorylation of Smad that blocks the cell-cycle arrest signal from the TGF-β receptor (#9). Activation of protein kinases (PKC, CaMK, and MAPK) by Ca^{2+} can also trigger mitogenic signaling. Several xenobiotics that are indicated in the figure may dysregulate the signaling network. Some may induce cell proliferation by either activating mitogenic protein kinases (e.g., PKC) or by inhibiting inactivating proteins, such as protein phosphatases (PTP and PP2A), GAP, or IκB. Others, e.g., inhibitors of PKC, oppose mitosis and facilitate apoptosis.

This scheme is oversimplified and tentative in several details. Virtually all components of the signaling network (e.g., G proteins, PKCs, and MAPKs) are present in multiple, functionally different forms whose distribution may be cell specific. The pathways depicted are not equally relevant for all cells. In addition, these pathways regulating gene expression not only determine the fate of cells, but also control certain aspects of the ongoing cellular activity.

TABLE 3–1 Agents acting on signaling systems for neurotransmitters and causing dysregulation of the momentary activity of electrically excitable cells such as neurons and muscle cells.*

Receptor/Channel/Pump		Agonist/Activator		Antagonist/Inhibitor	
Name	**Location**	**Agent**	**Effect**	**Agent**	**Effect**
1. Acetyl-choline nicotinic receptor	Skeletal muscle	Nicotine	Muscle fibrillation, and then paralysis	Tubocurarine, lophotoxin	Muscle paralysis
		Anatoxin-a		α-Bungarotoxin	
		Cytisine		α-Cobrotoxin	
		Ind: ChE inhibitors		α-Conotoxin	
				Erabutoxin b	
				Ind: botulinum toxin	
	Neurons	See above	Neuronal activation	Pb^{2+}, general anesthetics	Neuronal inhibition
2. Glutamate receptor	CNS neurons	*N*-Methyl-D-aspartate	Neuronal activation → convulsion, neuronal injury ("excitotoxicity")	Phencyclidine	Neuronal inhibition → anesthesia
		Kainate, domoate		Ketamine	Protection against "excitotoxicity"
		Quinolinate		General anesthetics	
		Quisqualate			
		Ind: hypoxia, HCN → glutamate release			
3. GABA$_A$ receptor	CNS neurons	Muscimol, Avermectins, Sedatives (barbiturates, benzodiazepines)	Neuronal inhibition → sedation, general anesthesia, coma, depression of vital centers	Bicuculline	Neuronal activation → tremor, convulsion
		General anesthetics (halothane)		Picrotoxin	
		Alcohols (ethanol)		Pentylenetetrazole	
				Cyclodiene insecticides	
				Lindane, TCAD	
				Ind: isoniazid	
4. Glycine receptor	CNS neurons, motor neurons	Avermectins (?)	Inhibition of motor neurons → paralysis	Strychnine	Disinhibition of motor neurons → tetanic convulsion
		General anesthetics		*Ind*: tetanus toxin	
5. Acetylcholine M$_2$ muscarinic receptor	Cardiac muscle	*Ind*: ChE inhibitors	Decreased heart rate and contractility	Belladonna alkaloids (e.g., atropine), atropine-like drugs (e.g., TCAD)	Increased heart rate
6. Opioid receptor	CNS neurons, visceral neurons	Morphine and congeners (e.g., heroin, meperidine)	Neuronal inhibition → analgesia, central respiratory depression, constipation, urine retention	Naloxone	Antidotal effects in opiate intoxication
		Ind: clonidine			
7. Voltage-gated Na$^+$ channel	Neurons, muscle cells, etc.	Aconitine, veratridine	Neuronal activation → convulsion	Tetrodotoxin, saxitoxin	Neuronal inhibition → paralysis, anesthesia
		Grayanotoxin		μ-Conotoxin	Anticonvulsive action
		Batrachotoxin		Local anesthetics	
		Scorpion toxins		Phenytoin	
		Ciguatoxin		Quinidine	
		DDT, pyrethroids			

(Continued)

TABLE 3–1 **Agents acting on signaling systems for neurotransmitters and causing dysregulation of the momentary activity of electrically excitable cells such as neurons and muscle cells.*** (*Continued*)

Receptor/Channel/Pump		Agonist/Activator		Antagonist/Inhibitor	
Name	**Location**	**Agent**	**Effect**	**Agent**	**Effect**
8. Voltage-gated Ca^{2+} channel	Neurons, muscle cell, etc.	Maitotoxin (?) Atrotoxin (?) Latrotoxin (?)	Neuronal/muscular activation, cell injury	ω-Conotoxin Pb^{2+}	Neuronal inhibition → paralysis
9. Voltage/Ca^{2+}-activated K$^+$ channel	Neurons, smooth and skeletal muscle, cardiac muscle	Pb^{2+}	Neuronal/muscular inhibition	Ba^{2+}, apamin (bee venom), dendrotoxin, 20-HETE, hERG inhibitors (e.g., cisapride, terfenadine)	Neuronal/muscular activation → convulsion/spasm vasoconstriction, PMV tachycardia (torsade de pointes)
10. Na$^+$,K$^+$-ATPase	Universal			Digitalis glycosides	Increased cardiac contractility, excitability
				Oleandrin Chlordecone	Increased neuronal excitability → tremor
11. Acetylcholine M$_3$ muscarinic receptor	Smooth muscle, glands	*Ind*: ChE inhibitors	Smooth muscle spasm	Belladonna alkaloids (e.g., atropine)	Smooth muscle relaxation → intestinal paralysis, decreased salivation, decreased perspiration
			Salivation, lacrimation	Atropine-like drugs (e.g., TCAD)	
Acetylcholine M$_1$ muscarinic receptor	CNS neurons	Oxotremorine *Ind*: ChE inhibitors	Neuronal activation → convulsion	See above	
12. Adrenergic α$_1$ receptor	Vascular smooth muscle	(Nor)epinephrine *Ind*: cocaine, tyramine, amphetamine, TCAD	Vasoconstriction → ischemia, hypertension	Prazosin	Antidotal effects in intoxication with α$_1$-receptor agonists
13. 5-HT$_2$ receptor	Smooth muscle	Ergot alkaloids (ergotamine, ergonovine)	Vasoconstriction → ischemia, hypertension	Ketanserine	Antidotal effects in ergot intoxication
14. Adrenergic β$_1$ receptor	Cardiac muscle	(Nor)epinephrine *Ind*: cocaine, tyramine, amphetamine, TCAD	Increased cardiac contractility and excitability	Atenolol, metoprolol	Antidotal effects in intoxication with β$_1$-receptor agonists

*Numbering of the signaling elements in this table corresponds to the numbering of their symbols in Figure 3–7. This tabulation is simplified and incomplete. Virtually all receptors and channels listed occur in multiple forms with different sensitivity to the agents. The reader should consult the pertinent literature for more detailed information. CNS, central nervous system; ChE, cholinesterase; *Ind*, indirectly acting (i.e., by altering neurotransmitter level); 20-HETE, 20-hydroxy-5,8,11,14-eicosatetraenoic acid; PMV, polymorphic ventricular; TCAD, tricyclic antidepressant.
The ? indicates there is some uncertainty regarding this action.

chronically injured tissue. As discussed above, cellular injury initiates a surge in cellular proliferation and extracellular matrix production, which normally ceases when the injured tissue is remodeled. If increased production of extracellular matrix is not halted, fibrosis develops.

TGF-β appears to be a major mediator of fibrogenesis. The increased expression of TGF-β is a common response mediating regeneration of the extracellular matrix after an acute injury. Normally, TGF-β production ceases when repair is complete. Failure to halt TGF-β overproduction, which leads to fibrosis, could be caused by continuous injury or a defect in the regulation of TGF-β.

The fibrotic action of TGF-β is due to (1) stimulation of the synthesis of individual matrix components by specific target cells and (2) inhibition of matrix degradation. Interestingly, TGF-β induces transcription of its own gene in target cells, suggesting that the TGF-β produced by these cells can amplify in an autocrine manner the production of the extracellular matrix. This positive feedback may facilitate fibrogenesis.

Fibrosis involves not only excessive accumulation of the extracellular matrix, but also changes in its composition. Basement membrane components, such as collagens and laminin, increase disproportionately during fibrogenesis.

Carcinogenesis—Chemical carcinogenesis involves inappropriate function of various repair mechanisms, including (1) failure of DNA repair, (2) failure of apoptosis, and (3) failure to terminate cell proliferation.

Failure of DNA Repair: Mutation, the Initiating Event in Carcinogenesis—Chemical and physical insults may induce neoplastic transformation of cells by genotoxic and nongenotoxic mechanisms. Chemicals that react with DNA may cause damage such as adduct formation, oxidative alteration, and strand breakage. If these lesions are not repaired or injured cells are not eliminated, a lesion in the parental DNA strand may induce a heritable alteration, or mutation, in the daughter strand during replication. The most unfortunate scenario for the organism occurs when the altered genes express mutant proteins that reprogram cells for multiplication. When such cells undergo mitosis, their descendants also have a similar propensity for proliferation. Moreover, because enhanced cell division increases the likelihood of mutations, these cells eventually acquire additional mutations that may further increase their growth advantage over their normal counterparts. The final outcome of this process is a tumor consisting of transformed, rapidly proliferating cells.

Mutation of Proto-oncogenes: Proto-oncogenes are highly conserved genes encoding proteins that stimulate progression of cells through the cell cycle or oppose apoptosis. The products of proto-oncogenes that accelerate the cell cycle include (1) growth factors; (2) growth factor receptors; (3) intracellular signal transducers such as G proteins, protein kinases, cyclins, and cyclin-dependent protein kinases; and (4) nuclear TFs.

Transient increases in the production or activity of proto-oncogene proteins are required for regulated growth, as during embryogenesis, tissue regeneration, and stimulation of cells by growth factors or hormones. In contrast, permanent activation and/or overexpression of these proteins favor neoplastic transformation. One mechanism whereby genotoxic carcinogens induce neoplastic cell transformation is by producing an activating mutation of a proto-oncogene. The altered gene (called an *oncogene*) encodes a permanently active protein that forces the cell into the division cycle.

An example of mutational activation of an oncogene protein is that of the Ras proteins. Ras proteins are localized on the inner surface of the plasma membrane and function as crucial mediators in responses initiated by growth factors (see Figure 3–7). Ras serves as a molecular switch, being active in the GTP-bound form and inactive in the GDP-bound form. Some mutations of the Ras gene dramatically lower the GTPase activity of the protein, which, in turn, locks Ras in the permanently active GTP-bound form. Continual, rather than signal-dependent, activation of Ras can lead eventually to uncontrolled proliferation and transformation.

Mutation of Tumor Suppressor Genes: Tumor-suppressor genes ncode proteins that inhibit the progression of cells in the division ycle, or promote DNA repair or apoptosis upon irreparable DNA damage. Some examples include cyclin-dependent protein kinase nhibitors, TFs that transactivate genes encoding cyclin-dependent protein kinase inhibitors, and proteins that block TFs involved in NA synthesis and cell division (Figure 3–12).

The p53 tumor-suppressor gene encodes a 53-kDa protein with multiple functions. Acting as a TF, the p53 protein transactivates genes whose products arrest the cell cycle, repair damaged DNA, or promote apoptosis. It also activates miRNA-coding genes whose products repress translation of mitogenic TFs and cell cycle accelerator proteins, and the genes that encode cell cycle accelerators or antiapoptotic proteins. DNA damage activates protein kinases to phosphorylate and stabilize the p53 protein, which causes it to accumulate and either induce cell cycle arrest or apoptosis. In addition to aberrations in critical protein-coding genes, damage in genes coding for miRNA may also contribute to carcinogenesis.

Epigenetic Mechanisms in Carcinogenesis: Inappropriate Activation or Responsiveness of the Regulatory Region of Critical Genes—Some chemicals cause cancer by reacting with DNA and inducing a mutation, whereas others that do not damage DNA yet still induce cancer after prolonged exposure are designated nongenotoxic (or epigenetic) carcinogens. Five examples include (1) xenobiotic mitogens that promote proliferative signaling, (2) endogenous mitogens such as growth factors, (3) toxicants that cause sustained cell injury, (4) xenobiotics that are display differing carcinogenicity between species, and (5) ethionine and diethanolamine, which interfere with formation of the endogenous methyl donor S-adenosyl-methionine (SAM).

Nongenotoxic chemicals eventually influence the expression of proto-oncogenes and/or tumor suppressor genes by

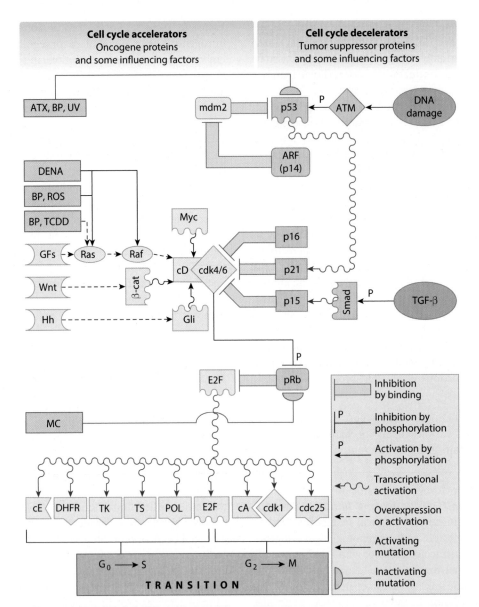

FIGURE 3–12   Key regulatory proteins controlling the cell-division cycle with some signaling pathways and xenobiotics affecting them. Proteins on the left, represented by blue symbols, accelerate the cell cycle and are oncogenic if permanently active or expressed at high level. In contrast, proteins on the right, represented by salmon symbols, decelerate or arrest the cell cycle and thus suppress oncogenesis, unless they are inactivated (e.g., by mutation).

Accumulation of cyclin D (cD) is a crucial event in initiating the cell division cycle. cD activates cyclin-dependent protein kinases 4 and 6 (cdk4/6), which in turn phosphorylate the retinoblastoma protein (pRb) causing dissociation of pRb from transcription factor E2F. Then the unleashed E2F is able to bind to and transactivate genes whose products are essential for DNA synthesis, such as dihydrofolate reductase (DHFR), thymidine kinase (TK), thymidylate synthetase (TS), and DNA polymerase (POL), or are regulatory proteins, such as cyclin E (cE), cyclin A (cA), and cyclin-dependent protein kinase 1 (cdk1), which promote further progression of the cell cycle. Expression of cD is increased, e.g., by growth factors signaling through Ras proteins and the MAPK pathway as well as by Wnt and Hedgehog (Hh) ligands that ultimately signal through B-cat and Gli transcription factors, respectively. Some carcinogens, e.g., benzpyrene (BP) and reactive oxygen species (ROS), and diethylnitrosamine (DENA) may cause mutation of the *Ras* or *Raf* gene that results in permanently active mutant Ras or Rab protein, but BP as well as TCDD may also induce simple overexpression of normal Ras protein.

Cell cycle progression is counteracted, e.g., by pRb (which inhibits the function of E2F), by cyclin-dependent protein kinase inhibitors (such as p15, p16, and p21), by p53 (which transactivates the *p21* gene), and by ARF (also called p14 that binds to mdm2, thereby neutralizing the antagonistic effect of mdm2 on p53). Signals evoked by DNA damage and TGF-β will ultimately result in accumulation of p53 and p15 proteins, respectively, and deceleration of the cell cycle. In contrast, mutations that disable the tumor suppressor proteins facilitate cell cycle progression and neoplastic conversion and are common in human tumors. Aflatoxin B_1 (ATX), BP, and UV light cause such mutations of the *p53* gene, whereas *pRb* mutations occur invariably in methylcholanthrene (MC)–induced transplacental lung tumors in mice.

increasing synthesis of normal proto-oncogene proteins and/or repressing normal tumor suppressor genes. This is in contrast to genotoxic chemicals, which induce the synthesis of permanently active mutant proto-oncogene proteins or permanently inactive mutant tumor suppressor proteins. Secondarily, nongenotoxic carcinogens may also increase mutation of critical genes, which is initiated by genotoxic agents or spontaneous DNA damage. Spontaneous DNA damage commonly occurs in normal human cells at a rate of 1 out of 10^8 to 10^{10} base pairs. Nongenotoxic carcinogens increase the frequency of spontaneous mutations through a mitogenic effect and by inhibiting apoptosis, thereby increasing the number of cells with DNA damage and mutations.

Failure of Apoptosis: Promotion of Mutation and Clonal Growth: Preneoplastic cells, or cells with mutations, have much higher apoptotic activity than do normal cells. Therefore, apoptosis counteracts clonal expansion of the initiated cells and tumor cells. Facilitation of apoptosis can induce tumor regression, whereas inhibition of apoptosis is detrimental because mutations and clonal expansion of preneoplastic cells are facilitated.

Failure to Terminate Proliferation: Promotion of Mutation, Proto-oncogene Expression, and Clonal Growth: Transformation of normal cells with controlled proliferative activity to malignant cells with uncontrolled proliferative activity is driven by three major factors: (1) accumulation of genetic damage in the form of mutant proto-oncogenes and mutant tumor suppressor genes, (2) increased transcription and/or translation of normal proto-oncogenes, and (3) silencing of normal tumor suppressor genes at the transcriptional and/or translational level. Uncontrolled proliferation results from an imbalance between mitosis and apoptosis.

1. Enhanced mitotic activity increases the probability of mutations. With activation of the cell-division cycle, a substantial shortening of the G1 phase occurs, and less time is available for the repair of injured DNA before replication.
2. Enhanced mitotic activity may compromise DNA methylation, which occurs early in the postreplication period. DNA cytosine methyltransferases (DNMTs) copy the methylation pattern of the parental DNA strand to the daughter strand. Limitations of DNMTs by shortened G2 phase or by the presence of other transacting factors might impair methylation and contribute to overexpression of proto-oncogenes.
3. Cell-to-cell communication through gap junctions and intercellular adhesion through cadherins are temporarily disrupted during proliferation, which contributes to the invasiveness of tumor cells.
4. Proliferation also promotes carcinogenesis through clonal expansion of the initial cells to form nodules (foci) and tumors.

Nongenotoxic Carcinogens: Promoters of Mitosis and Inhibitors of Apoptosis: Many chemicals do not alter DNA or induce mutations yet induce cancer after chronic administration. Designated *nongenotoxic* or *epigenetic carcinogens*, these chemicals cause cancer by promoting carcinogenesis initiated by genotoxic agents or spontaneous DNA damage.

According to an emerging theory, cancers may form by genotoxic and/or epigenetic mechanisms in pluripotent stem cell populations. Such cells are characterized by quiescence, self-renewal, and conditional immortality, and thus would potentially supply a lifelong, latent neoplastic population after carcinogenic attack. Finally, further changes in gene expression may occur in these proliferating cells, making them capable of invading other tissues (metastasis).

CONCLUSIONS

Selective or altered toxicity may be due to different or altered (1) exposure; (2) delivery, thus resulting in a different concentration of the ultimate toxicant at the target site; (3) target molecules; (4) biochemical processes triggered by the reaction of the chemical with the target molecules; (5) repair at the molecular, cellular, or tissue level; or (6) mechanisms such as circulatory and thermoregulatory reflexes by which the affected organism can adapt to some of the toxic effects. Although a simplified scheme outlines the development of toxicity (Figure 3–1), the route to toxicity can be considerably more diverse and complicated. An organism has mechanisms that (1) counteract the delivery of toxicants, such as detoxication; (2) reverse the toxic injury, such as repair mechanisms; and (3) offset some dysfunctions, such as adaptive responses. Thus, toxicity is not an inevitable consequence of toxicant exposure because it may be prevented, reversed, or compensated for by such mechanisms. Toxicity develops if the toxicant exhausts or impairs the protective mechanisms and/or overrides the adaptability of biological systems.

BIBLIOGRAPHY

Cribb AE, Peyrou M, Muruganandan S, Schneider L: The endoplasmic reticulum in xenobiotic toxicity. *Drug Metab Rev* 37:405–442, 2005.

Giordano A: *Cell Cycle Control and Dysregulation Protocols: Cyclins, Cyclin-dependent Kinases, and Other Factors.* Totowa, NJ: Humana Press, 2004.

Hancock JT: *Cell Signalling,* 3rd ed. New York: Oxford University Press, 2010.

Hansen JM, Go Y-M, Jones DP: Nuclear and mitochondrial compartmentation of oxidative stress and redox signaling. *Annu Rev Pharmacol Toxicol* 46:215–234, 2006.

Leung L, Kalgutkar AS, Obach RS: Metabolic activation in drug-induced liver injury. *Drug Metab Rev* 44:18–33, 2012.

Liu X, Van Fleet T, Schnellmann RG: The role of calpain in oncotic cell death. *Annu Rev Pharmacol Toxicol* 44:349–370, 2004.

Orrenius S, Nicotera P, Zhivotovsky B: Cell death mechanisms and their implications in toxicology. *Tox Sci* 119:3–19, 2011.

Pober JS, Min W, Bradley JR: Mechanisms of endothelial dysfunction, injury and death. *Annu Rev Pathol* 4:71–95, 2009.

Wallace KB: Mitochondrial off targets of drug therapy. *Trends Pharmacol Sci* 29:361–366, 2008.

Yokoi T, Nakajima M: Toxicological implications of modulation of gene expression by microRNAs. *Tox Sci* 123:1–14, 2011.

QUESTIONS

1. The severity of a toxin depends, in large part, on the concentration of the toxin at its site of action. Which of the following will decrease the amount of toxin reaching its site of action?
   a. absorption across the skin.
   b. excretion via the kidneys.
   c. toxication.
   d. reabsorption across the intestinal mucosa.
   e. discontinuous endothelial cells of hepatic sinusoids.

2. Toxication (or metabolic activation) is the biotransformation of a toxin to a more toxic and reactive species. Which of the following is not a reactive chemical species commonly formed by toxication?
   a. electrophiles.
   b. nucleophiles.
   c. superoxide anions.
   d. hydroxy radicals.
   e. hydrophilic organic acids.

3. Which of the following is not an important step in detoxication of chemicals?
   a. formation of redox-active reactants.
   b. reduction of hydrogen peroxide by glutathione peroxidase.
   c. formation of hydrogen peroxide by superoxide dismutase.
   d. reduction of glutathione disulfide (GSSG) by glutathione reductase (GR).
   e. conversion of hydrogen peroxide to water and molecular oxygen by catalase.

4. Regarding the interaction of the ultimate toxicant with its target molecule, which of the following is false?
   a. Toxins often oxidize or reduce their target molecules, resulting in the formation of a harmful by-product.
   b. The covalent binding of a toxin with its target molecule permanently alters the target's function.
   c. The noncovalent binding of a toxin to an ion channel irreversibly inhibits ion flux through the channel.
   d. Abstraction of hydrogen atoms from endogenous compounds by free radicals can result in the formation of DNA adducts.
   e. Several toxins can act enzymatically on their specific target proteins.

5. All of the following are common effects of toxicants on target molecules EXCEPT:
   a. blockage of neurotransmitter receptors.
   b. interference with DNA replication due to adduct formation.
   c. cross-linking of endogenous molecules.
   d. opening of ion channels.
   e. mounting of an immune response.

6. Which of the following proteins functions to prevent the progression of the cell cycle?
   a. NF-κB.
   b. MAPK.
   c. CREB.
   d. c-Myc.
   e. IκB.

7. Which of the following would have the largest negative impact on intracellular ATP levels?
   a. moderately decreased caloric intake.
   b. interference with electron delivery to the electron transport chain.
   c. inability to harvest ATP from glycolysis.
   d. increased synthesis of biomolecules.
   e. active cell division.

8. What happens when a toxin induces elevation of cytoplasmic calcium levels?
   a. Mitochondrial uptake of calcium dissipates the electrochemical gradient needed to synthesize ATP.
   b. Formation of actin filaments increases the strength and integrity of the cytoskeleton.
   c. It decreases the activity of intracellular proteases, nucleases, and phospholipases.
   d. The cell becomes dormant until the calcium is actively pumped from the cell.
   e. The generation of reactive oxygen species slows because of calcium-induced decrease in activity of the TCA cycle.

9. Cytochrome c is an important molecule in initiating apoptosis in cells. All of the following regarding cytochrome c are true EXCEPT:
   a. The release of cytochrome c into the cytoplasm is an important step in apoptosis initiation.
   b. The loss of cytochrome c from the electron transport chain blocks ATP synthesis by oxidative phosphorylation.
   c. Loss of cytochrome c from the inner mitochondrial membrane results in increased formation of reactive oxygen species.
   d. Bax proteins mediate cytochrome c release.
   e. Caspases are proteases that increase cytoplasmic levels of cytochrome c.

10. All of the following regarding DNA repair are true EXCEPT:
    a. In a lesion that does not cause a major distortion of the double helix, the incorrect base is cleaved and the correct base is inserted in its place.
    b. Base excision repair and nucleotide excision repair are both dependent on a DNA polymerase and a DNA ligase.
    c. In nucleotide excision repair, only the adduct is cleaved, and the gap is then filled by DNA polymerase.
    d. Pyrimidine dimers can be cleaved and repaired directly by DNA photolyase.
    e. Recombinational repair requires that a sister strand serve as a template to fill in missing nucleotides.

11. Apoptosis can serve as a tissue repair process in a number of cell types. In which of the following cell types would this be a plausible mechanism of tissue repair?
    a. female germ cells.
    b. gastrointestinal epithelium.
    c. neurons.
    d. retinal ganglion cells.
    e. cardiac muscle cells.

12. Which of the following is NOT associated with carcinogenesis?
    a. mutation.
    b. normal p53 function.
    c. Ras activation.
    d. inhibition of apoptosis.
    e. DNA repair failure.

Risk Assessment

Elaine M. Faustman and Gilbert S. Omenn

KEY POINTS

- *Risk assessment* is the systematic scientific characterization of potential adverse health effects resulting from human exposures to hazardous agents or situations.

- *Risk* is defined as the probability of an adverse outcome under specified conditions.
- *Risk management* refers to the process by which policy actions are chosen to control hazards.

INTRODUCTION AND HISTORICAL CONTEXT

Toxicologic research and toxicity testing conducted and interpreted by toxicologists constitute the scientific core of an important activity known as *risk assessment* for chemical exposures. In 1983, the National Research Council detailed the steps of hazard identification, dose–response assessment, exposure analysis, and characterization of risks in *Risk Assessment in the Federal Government: Managing the Process* (widely known as *The Red Book*). The scheme shown in Figure 4–1 provides a consistent framework for risk assessment across agencies with bidirectional arrows showing an ideal situation where mechanistic research feeds directly into risk assessments and critical data uncertainty drives research. Often, public policy objectives require extrapolations that go far beyond the observation of

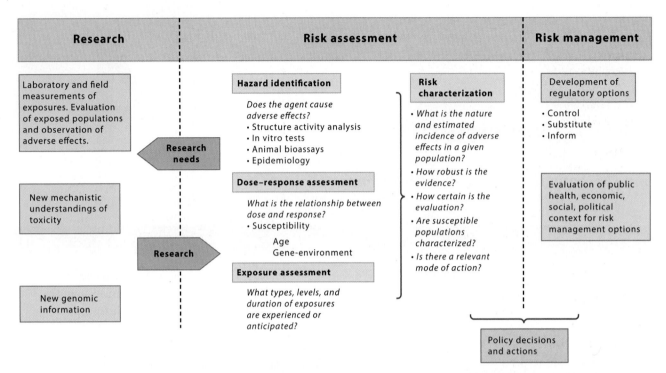

FIGURE 4–1 **Risk assessment/risk management framework.** This framework shows in blue the four key steps of risk assessment: hazard identification, dose–response assessment, exposure assessment, and risk characterization. It shows an interactive, two-way process where research needs from the risk assessment process drive new research, and new research findings modify risk assessment outcomes. (Adapted with permission from *Risk Assessment in the Federal Government: Managing the Process*, Washington, DC: National Academies Press; 1983.)

actual effects and reflect different tolerances for risks, generating controversy.

A comprehensive framework that applies two crucial concepts: (1) putting each environmental problem or issue into public health and/or ecological context and (2) proactively engaging the relevant stakeholders, affected or potentially affected community groups, from the very beginning of the six-stage process shown in Figure 4–2. Particular exposures and potential health effects must be evaluated across sources and exposure pathways and in light of multiple end points, and not the current general approach of evaluating one chemical in one environmental medium (air, water, soil, food, and products) for one health effect at a time.

DEFINITIONS

Risk assessment is the systematic scientific evaluation of potential adverse health effects resulting from human exposures to hazardous agents or situations. *Risk* is defined as the probability of an adverse outcome based on the exposure and potency of the hazardous agent(s). The term *hazard* refers to intrinsic toxic properties, whereas exposure becomes an essential consideration along with hazard for risk determination. Risk assessment requires qualitative information about the strength of the evidence and the nature of the outcomes—as well as quantitative

assessment of the exposures, host susceptibility factors, and potential magnitude of the hazard—and then a description of the uncertainties in the estimates and conclusions. The objectives of risk assessment are outlined in Table 4–1.

The phrase *characterization of risk* reflects the combination of qualitative and quantitative analyses. Unfortunately, many users tend to equate risk assessment with quantitative risk assessment, generating a number for an overly precise risk estimate, while ignoring crucial information about the uncertainties of risk assessment, mode of action (MOA), and type of effect across species or context.

Risk management refers to the process by which policy actions are chosen to control hazards identified in the risk assessment/risk characterization stage of the framework (Figure 4–2). Risk managers consider scientific evidence and risk estimates—along with statutory, engineering, economic, social, and political factors—in evaluating alternative options and choosing among those options.

Risk communication is the challenging process of making risk assessment and risk management information comprehensible to community groups, lawyers, local elected officials, judges, business people, labor, environmentalists, etc. A crucial, too-often neglected requirement for communication is listening to the fears, perceptions, priorities, and proposed remedies of these "stakeholders."

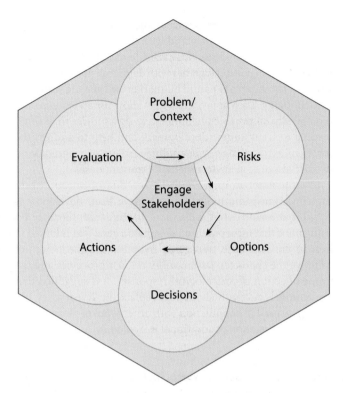

FIGURE 4–2 Risk management framework for environmental health from the U.S. Commission on Risk Assessment and Risk Management. The framework comprises six stages: (1) formulating the problem in a broad public health context, (2) analyzing risks, (3) defining options, (4) making risk-reduction decisions, (5) implementing those actions, and (6) evaluating the effectiveness of the taken actions. Interactions with stakeholders are critical and thus have been put at the center of the framework.

DECISION MAKING

Risk management decisions are reached under diverse statutes in the United States and many other countries. Some statutes specify reliance on risk alone, whereas others require a balancing of risks and benefits of the product or activity (Table 4–1). Risk assessments provide a valuable framework for priority setting within regulatory and health agencies, in the chemical development process within companies, and in resource allocation by environmental organizations. Currently, there are significant efforts toward a global harmonization of testing protocols and the assessment of risks and standards.

A major challenge for risk assessment, risk communication, and risk management is to work across disciplines to demonstrate the biological plausibility and clinical significance of the conclusions from studies of chemicals thought to have potential adverse effects. Biomarkers of exposure, effect, or individual susceptibility can link the presence of a chemical in various environmental compartments to specific sites of action in target organs and to host responses. Individual behavioral and social risk factors may be critically important to both the characterization of risk and the reduction of risk. Finally, public and media

TABLE 4–1 Objectives of risk assessment.

1. Protect human and ecological health   Toxic substances

2. Balance risks and benefits
    Drugs
    Pesticides

3. Set target levels of risk
    Food contaminants
    Water pollutants

4. Set priorities for program activities
    Regulatory agencies
    Manufacturers
    Environmental/consumer organizations

5. Estimate residual risks and extent of risk reduction after steps are taken to reduce risks

attitudes toward local polluters, other responsible parties, and relevant government agencies can greatly influence the communication process and the choices for risk management.

HAZARD IDENTIFICATION

Assessing Toxicity of Chemicals—Introduction

In order to assess toxicity of chemicals, information from four types of studies is used: structure-activity relationships (SAR), in vitro or short-term studies, in vivo animal bioassays, and information from human epidemiologic studies. In many cases, toxicity information for chemicals is limited; however, recent efforts to mitigate this gap in understanding have been successful.

Assessing Toxicity of Chemicals—Methods

Structure/Activity Relationships (SARs)—Given the cost of $2 to $4 million and the 3 to 5 years required for testing a single chemical in a lifetime rodent carcinogenicity bioassay, initial decisions on whether to continue development of a chemical, submit a premanufacturing notice, or require additional testing may be based largely on SARs and limited short-term assays. A chemical's structure, solubility, stability, pH sensitivity, electrophilicity, volatility, and chemical reactivity can be important information for hazard identification.

SARs have been used for assessment of complex mixtures of structurally related compounds. However, it is difficult to predict activity across chemical classes and especially across multiple toxic end points using a single biological response. Pharmaceutical companies are now using computerized combinatorial chemistry and three-dimensional (3D) molecular modeling approaches to design new drugs (ligands) that can sterically fit into the "receptors of interest." However, computerized SAR methods have given disappointing results because it is rare for environmental pollutants to exhibit selective ligand-receptor binding.

In Vitro and Short-term Tests—The next approach for hazard identification comprises using tests ranging from in vitro bacterial mutation assays to more elaborate short-term tests such as skin-painting studies in mice or altered rat liver-foci assays conducted in vivo, as well as other assays that evaluate developmental, reproductive, neuro-, and immunotoxicity.

Short-term assay validation and application is particularly important to risk assessment because such assays can provide information about mechanisms of effects while being faster and less expensive than lifetime bioassays. Validation requires determination of their sensitivity (ability to identify true carcinogens), specificity (ability to recognize noncarcinogens as noncarcinogens), and predictive value for the toxic end point under evaluation. Considerable effort to improve the utility of these tests is continually expended due to their value in providing chemical-specific mechanistic information.

Animal Bioassays—Animal bioassay data are key components of the hazard identification process. A basic premise of risk assessment is that chemicals that cause tumors in animals can cause tumors in humans. All human carcinogens that have been adequately tested in animals produce positive results in at least one animal model. Although this association cannot establish that all agents and mixtures that cause cancer in experimental animals also cause cancer in humans, nevertheless, in the absence of adequate data on humans, it is biologically plausible and prudent to regard agents and mixtures for which there is sufficient evidence of carcinogenicity in experimental animals as if they presented a carcinogenic risk to humans—a reflection of the "precautionary principle." In general, the most appropriate rodent bioassays are those that test exposure pathways of most relevance to predicted or known human exposure pathways. Bioassays for reproductive and developmental toxicity and other noncancer end points have a similar rationale.

Consistent features in the design of standard cancer bioassays include testing in two species and both sexes, with 50 animals per dose group and near-lifetime exposure. Important choices include the strains of rats and mice, the number of doses, and dose levels (typically 90%, 50%, and 10% to 25% of the maximally tolerated dose [MTD]), and the details of the required histopathology (number of organs to be examined, choice of interim sacrifice pathology, etc.). Positive evidence of chemical carcinogenicity can include increases in number of tumors at a particular organ site, induction of rare tumors, earlier induction (shorter latency) of commonly observed tumors, and/or increases in the total number of observed tumors.

Critical problems exist in using the hazard identification data from rodent bioassays for quantitative risk assessments. This is because of the limited dose–response data available from these rodent bioassays and nonexistent response information for environmentally relevant exposures. Results thus have traditionally been extrapolated from a dose–response curve in the 10% to 100% biologically observable tumor response range down to 10^{-6} risk estimates (upper confidence limit) or to a benchmark or reference dose-related risk.

Lifetime bioassays have been enhanced with the collection of additional mechanistic data and with the assessment of multiple noncancer end points. It is feasible and desirable to integrate such information together with data from mechanistically oriented short-term tests and biomarker and genetic studies in epidemiology. Such approaches may allow for an extension of biologically observable phenomena to doses lower than those leading to frank tumor development and help to address the issues of extrapolation over multiple orders of magnitude to predict response at environmentally relevant doses.

In an attempt to improve the prediction of cancer risk to humans, transgenic mouse models have been developed as possible alternatives to the standard 2-year cancer bioassay. By using mice that incorporate or eliminate a gene that is linked to human cancer, these transgenic models have the power to improve the characterization of key cellular processes and the mode of action of toxicological responses. It is suggested that these models currently should not replace the 2-year assay, but should be used in conjunction with other types of data to assist in the interpretation of additional toxicological and mechanistic evidence.

Use of Epidemiologic Data in Risk Assessment—The most convincing line of evidence for human risk is a well-conducted epidemiologic study in which a positive association between exposure and disease has been observed. Table 4–2 shows examples of epidemiologic study designs and provides clues on types of outcomes and exposures evaluated. There are important inherent limitations in epidemiologic studies. When the study is exploratory, hypotheses are often weak. Exposure estimates are often crude and retrospective, especially for conditions with long latency before clinical manifestations appear. Generally, there are multiple exposures, especially when a lifetime is considered. There is always a trade-off between detailed information on relatively few persons and very limited information on large numbers of persons. Contributions from lifestyle factors, such as smoking and diet, are a challenge to sort out. Humans are highly outbred, so the method must consider variation in susceptibility among those who are exposed.

Nevertheless, human epidemiology studies provide very useful information for hazard identification and sometimes quantitative information for data characterization. Three major types of epidemiology study designs are available: cross-sectional studies, cohort studies, and case–control studies (Table 4–2). Cross-sectional studies survey groups of humans to identify risk factors (exposure) and disease but are not useful for establishing cause and effect. Cohort studies evaluate individuals selected on the basis of their exposure to an agent under study. These prospective studies monitor over time individuals who initially are disease-free to determine the rates at which they develop disease. In case–control studies, subjects are selected on the basis of disease status: disease cases and matched cases of disease-free individuals. Exposure histories of the two groups are compared to determine key consistent features in their exposure histories. All case–control studies are retrospective studies.

TABLE 4–2 Attributes of three types of epidemiologic study designs.

Methodological Attributes	Type of Study		
	Cohort	Case–Control	Cross-sectional
Initial classification	Exposure–nonexposure	Disease–nondisease	Either one
Time sequence	Prospective	Retrospective	Present time
Sample composition	Nondiseased individuals	Cases and controls	Survivors
Comparison	Proportion of exposed with disease	Proportion of cases with exposure	Either one
Rates	Incidence	Fractional (percent)	Prevalence
Risk index	Relative risk–attributable risk	Relative odds	Prevalence
Advantages	Lack of bias in exposure, yields rates of incidence and risk	Inexpensive, small number of subjects, rapid results, suitable for rare diseases, no attrition	Quick results
Disadvantages	Large number of subjects required, long follow-up, attrition, change in time of criteria and methods, costly, inadequate for rare diseases	Incomplete information, biased recall, problem in selecting control and matching, yields only relative risk—cannot establish causation, population of survivors	Cannot establish causation (antecedent consequence), population of survivors, inadequate for rare diseases

Epidemiologic findings are judged by the following criteria: strength of association, consistency of observations (reproducibility in time and space), specificity (uniqueness in quality or quantity of response), appropriateness of temporal relationship (did the exposure precede responses?), dose-responsiveness, biological plausibility and coherence, verification, and analogy (biological extrapolation). In addition, epidemiologic study designs should be evaluated for their power of detection, appropriateness of outcomes, verification of exposure assessments, completeness of assessing confounding factors, and general applicability of the outcomes to other populations at risk. Power of detection is calculated using study size, variability, accepted detection limits for end points under study, and a specified significance level.

Recent advances from the human genome project, increased sophistication of molecular biomarkers, and improved mechanistic bases for epidemiologic hypotheses have allowed epidemiologists to expand our understanding of biological plausibility and clinical relevance. "Molecular epidemiology" with improved molecular biomarkers of exposure, effect, and susceptibility has allowed investigators to more effectively link molecular events in the causative disease pathway. The range of biomarkers has grown dramatically and includes identification of single nucleotide polymorphisms (SNPs), genomic profiling, transcriptome analysis, and proteomic analysis.

Integrating Qualitative Aspects of Risk Assessment

Qualitative assessment of hazard information should include consideration of the consistency and concordance of findings, including a determination of the consistency of the toxicological findings across species and target organs, an evaluation of consistency across duplicate experimental conditions, and a determination of the adequacy of the experiments to consistently detect the adverse end points of interest. Many agencies use similar evidence classification for both animal and human studies. These classifications include levels of sufficient, limited, inadequate, no evidence, or evidence suggesting lack of carcinogenicity. An overall weight-of-evidence approach to carcinogenicity uses these evidence classifications, and considers the quality and quantity of data as well as any underlying assumptions.

DOSE–RESPONSE ASSESSMENT

Integrating Quantitative Aspects of Risk Assessment

Quantitative considerations in risk assessment include dose-response assessment, exposure assessment, variation in susceptibility, and characterization of uncertainty.

The fundamental basis of the quantitative relationships between exposure to an agent and the incidence of an adverse response is the dose–response assessment. Analysis of dose-response relationships must start with the determination of the critical effects to be quantitatively evaluated. It is usual practice to choose the data sets with adverse effects occurring at the lowest levels of exposure from studies using the most relevant exposure routes. The "critical" adverse effect is defined as the significant adverse biological effect that occurs at the lowest exposure level.

Threshold Approaches—Threshold dose–response relationship characterization includes identification of "no or lowest observed adverse effect levels" (NOAELs or LOAELs). On the dose–response curve illustrated in Figure 4–3, the threshold, indicated as T, represents the dose below which no additional increase in response is observed. The NOAEL is identified as the highest nonstatistically significant dose tested; in this

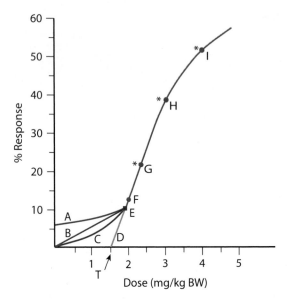

FIGURE 4–3 Dose–response curve. This figure is designed to illustrate a typical dose–response curve with points E to I indicating the biologically determined responses. Statistical significance of these responses is indicated with a "*" symbol. The threshold is shown by T, a dose below which no change in biological response occurs. Point E represents the point of departure (POD), the dose near the lower end of the observed dose–response range, below which extrapolation to lower doses is necessary. Point F is the highest nonstatistical significant response point; hence, it is the "no observed adverse effect level" (NOAEL) for this example. Point G is the "lowest observed adverse effect level" (LOAEL) for this example. Curves A to D show some options for extrapolating the dose–response relationship below the range of biologically observed data points and POD.

example it is point F, at 2 mg/kg body weight. Point G is the LOAEL (~2.3 mg/kg body weight), as it is the lowest dose tested with a statistically significant effect. Lines A to D represent possible extrapolations below the point of departure (POD), which is represented on this figure as a square and is labeled as point E. POD is used to specify the estimated dose near the lower end of the observed dose range, below which extrapolation to lower exposures is necessary.

In general, animal bioassays are constructed with sufficient numbers of animals to biological responses at the 10% response range. *Significance* usually refers to both biological and statistical criteria and is dependent on the number of dose levels tested, the number of animals tested at each dose, and background incidence of the adverse response in the nonexposed control groups. The NOAEL should not be perceived as risk-free.

As described in Chapter 2, approaches for characterizing dose–response relationships include identification of effect levels such as LD_{50} (dose producing 50% lethality), LC_{50} (concentration producing 50% lethality), ED_{10} (dose producing 10% response), as well as NOAELs.

NOAELs have traditionally served as the basis for risk assessment calculations, such as reference doses (RfDs) or acceptable daily intake (ADI) values. RfDs or concentrations (RfCs) are estimates of a daily exposure (oral or inhalation, respectively) to

an agent that is assumed to be without adverse health impact in humans. ADI values may be defined as the daily intake of chemical during an entire lifetime, which appears to be without appreciable risk on the basis of all known facts at that time. RfDs and ADI values typically are calculated from NOAEL values by dividing by uncertainty (UF) and/or modifying factors (MF):

$$RfD = \frac{NOAEL}{UF \times MF}$$

$$ADI = \frac{NOAEL}{UF \times MF}$$

Tolerable daily intakes (TDIs) can be used to describe intakes for chemicals that are not "acceptable" but are "tolerable" as they are below levels thought to cause adverse health effects. These are calculated in a manner similar to ADI. In principle, dividing by these factors allows for interspecies (animal-to-human) and intraspecies (human-to-human) variability with default values of 10 each. An additional UF can be used to account for experimental inadequacies—e.g., to extrapolate from short-exposure-duration studies to a situation more relevant for chronic study or to account for inadequate numbers of animals or other experimental limitations. If only a LOAEL value is available, then an additional 10-fold factor commonly is used to arrive at a value more comparable to a NOAEL. Traditionally, a safety factor of 100 would be used for RfD calculations to extrapolate from a well-conducted animal bioassay (10-fold factor animal-to-human) and to account for human variability in response (10-fold factor human-to-human variability).

MF can be used to adjust the UF if data on mechanisms, pharmacokinetics, or relevance of the animal response to human risk justify such modification.

Recent efforts have focused on using data-derived and chemical-specific adjustment factors to replace the 10-fold UF traditionally used in calculating RfDs and ADIs. Such efforts have included reviewing the human pharmacologic literature from published clinical trials and developing human variability databases for a large range of exposures and clinical conditions. Intra- and interspecies UF have two components: toxicokinetic and toxicodynamic aspects; Figure 4–4 shows these distinctions. This approach provides a structure for incorporating scientific information on specific aspects of the overall toxicologic process into the RfD calculations; thus, relevant data can replace a portion of the overall "uncertainty" surrounding these extrapolations.

NOAEL values have also been utilized for risk assessment by evaluating a "margin of exposure" (MOE), where the ratio of the NOAEL determined in animals and expressed as mg/kg per day is compared with the level to which a human may be exposed. Low values of MOE indicate that the human levels of exposure are close to levels for the NOAEL in animals. Unlike RfD and RfC, there is usually no factor included in this calculation for differences in human or animal susceptibility or animal-to-human extrapolation. Thus, MOE values of less

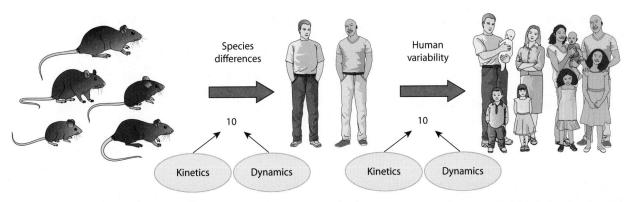

FIGURE 4-4 Toxicokinetic (TK) and toxicodynamic (TD) considerations inherent in interspecies and interindividual extrapolations. *Toxicokinetics* refers to the processes of absorption, distribution, elimination, and metabolism of a toxicant. *Toxicodynamics* refers to the actions and interactions of the toxicant within the organism and describes processes at organ, tissue, cellular, and molecular levels. This figure shows how uncertainty in extrapolation both across and within species can be considered as being due to two key factors: a kinetic component and a dynamic component. Refer to the text for detailed explanations.

than 100 have been used by regulatory agencies as flags for requiring further evaluation.

The NOAEL approach has been criticized on several points, including that (1) the NOAEL must, by definition, be one of the experimental doses tested; and (2) once this is identified, the rest of the dose–response curve is ignored. Because of these limitations, an alternative to the NOAEL approach, the benchmark dose (BMD) method, was proposed. In this approach, the dose–response is modeled and the lower confidence bound for a dose at a specified response level (benchmark response [BMR]) is calculated. The BMR is usually specified at 1%, 5%, or 10%. The BMD_x (with x representing the percent BMR) is used as an alternative to the NOAEL value for reference dose calculations. Thus the RfD would be:

$$RfD = \frac{BMD_x}{UF \times MF}$$

The proposed values to be used for the UF and MF for BMDs can range from the same factors as for the NOAEL to lower values due to increased confidence in the response level and increased recognition of experimental variability owing to use of a lower confidence bound on dose.

Advantages of the BMD approach can include (1) the ability to take into account the full dose–response curve; (2) the inclusion of a measure of variability (confidence limit); and (3) the use of a consistent BMR level for RfD calculations across studies. Obviously, limitations in the animal bioassays in regard to minimal test doses for evaluation, shallow dose–responses, and use of study designs with widely spaced test doses will limit the utility of these assays for any type of quantitative assessments, whether NOAEL- or BMD-based approaches.

Nonthreshold Approaches—As Figure 4–3 shows, numerous dose–response curves can be proposed in the low-dose region of the dose–response curve if a threshold assumption is not made. Because the risk assessor generally needs to extrapolate beyond the region of the dose–response curve for which experimentally observed data are available, the choice of models to generate curves in this region has received lots of attention. For nonthreshold responses, methods for dose-response assessments have also utilized models for extrapolation to de minimus (10^{-4} to 10^{-6}) risk levels at very low doses, far below the biologically observed response range and far below the effect levels evaluated for threshold responses.

Statistical or Probability Distribution Models—Two general types of dose–response models exist: statistical (or probability distribution models) and mechanistic models. The distribution models are based on the assumption that each individual has a tolerance level for a test agent and that this response level is a variable following a specific probability distribution function. These responses can be modeled using a cumulative dose–response function. However, extrapolation of the experimental data from 50% response levels to a "safe," "acceptable," or "de minimus" level of exposure—e.g., one in a million risk above background—illustrates the huge gap between scientific observations and highly protective risk limits (sometimes called *virtually safe doses*, or those corresponding to a 95% upper confidence limit on adverse response rates).

Models Derived from Mechanistic Assumptions—This modeling approach designs a mathematical equation to describe dose–response relationships that are consistent with postulated biological mechanisms of response. These models are based on the idea that a response (toxic effect) in a particular biological unit (animal or human) is the result of the random occurrence of one or more biological events (stochastic events).

Radiation research has spawned a series of "hit models" for cancer modeling, where a hit is defined as a critical cellular event that must occur before a toxic effect is produced. The simplest mechanistic model is the one-hit (one-stage) linear model in which only one hit or critical cellular interaction is required for a cell to be altered. As theories of cancer have grown in complexity, multi-hit models have been developed that can describe hypothesized single-target multi-hit events, as well as multi-target, multi-hit events in carcinogenesis.

Toxicologic Enhancements of the Models—Three exemplary areas of research that have improved the models used in risk extrapolation are time to tumor information, physiologically based toxicokinetic modeling (described in Chapter 7), and biologically based dose–response (BBDR) modeling. The BBDR model aims to make the generalized mechanistic models discussed in the previous section more clearly reflect specific biological processes. Measured rates are incorporated into the mechanistic equations to replace default or computer-generated values.

Development of BBDR models for end points other than cancer is limited; however, several approaches have been explored in developmental toxicity utilizing mode of action information on cell cycle kinetics, enzyme activity, litter effects, and cytotoxicity as critical end points. Approaches have been proposed that link pregnancy-specific toxicokinetic models with temporally sensitive toxicodynamic models for developmental impacts. Unfortunately, the lack of specific, quantitative biological information for most toxicants and for most end points limits study and utilization of these models.

EXPOSURE ASSESSMENT

The primary objectives of exposure assessment are to determine source, type, magnitude, and duration of contact with the agent of interest. Obviously, a critical element of the risk assessment process requires recognition that hazard does not occur in the absence of exposure. However, exposure data are frequently identified as the key area of uncertainty in overall risk determination. The primary goal of using exposure information in quantitative risk assessment is not only to determine the type and amount of total exposure, but also to find out specifically how much may be reaching target tissues. A key step in making an exposure assessment is determining what exposure pathways are relevant for the risk scenario under development. The subsequent steps entail quantitation of each pathway identified as a potentially relevant exposure and then summarizing these pathway-specific exposures for calculation of overall exposure.

Additional considerations for exposure assessments include how time and duration of exposures are evaluated in risk assessments. In general, estimates for cancer risk use averages over a lifetime. In a few cases, short-term exposure limits (STELs) are required and characterization of brief but high levels of exposure is significant. In these cases exposures are not averaged over the lifetime and the effects of high, short-term doses are estimated. With developmental toxicity, a single exposure can be sufficient to produce an adverse developmental effect if exposures occur during a window of developmental susceptibility; thus, daily doses are used, rather than lifetime weighted averages.

RISK CHARACTERIZATION

Variation in Susceptibility

Toxicology has been slow to recognize the marked variation among humans. Generally, assay results and toxicokinetic modeling utilize means and standard deviations to measure variation, or even standard errors of the mean, thereby ignoring variability in response due to differences in age, sex, health status, and genetics.

One key challenge for risk assessment will be interpretation and linking of observations from highly sensitive molecular and genome-based methods with the overall process of toxicity. Biomarkers of early effects, like frank clinical pathology, arise as a function of exposure, response, and time. Early, subtle, and possibly reversible effects can generally be distinguished from irreversible disease states.

The challenge for interpretation of early and highly sensitive response biomarkers is made clear in the analysis of data from gene expression arrays. Because our relatively routine ability to monitor gene responses has grown exponentially in the last decade, the need for toxicologists to interpret such observations for risk assessment and the overall process of toxicity has increased with equal or greater intensity.

Microarray analysis for risk assessment requires sophisticated analyses to arrive at a functional interpretation and linkage to a conventional toxicologic end point. Because of the vast number of measured responses with gene expression arrays, pattern analysis techniques are being used. The extensive databases across chemical classes, pathological conditions, and stages of disease progression that are essential for these analyses are being developed.

INFORMATION RESOURCES

Though numerous information resources are available for risk assessment, a few are listed below in order to provide the reader with examples of risk assessment resources and databases. The Toxicology Data Network (TOXNET) from the National Library of Medicine (http://toxnet.nlm.nih.gov/) provides access to databases on toxicology, hazardous chemicals, and related areas. These information sources vary in the included level of assessment, ranging from just listings of scientific references without comment to extensive peer-reviewed risk assessment information. The World Health Organization (http://who.int/) provides chemical-specific information through the International Programme on Chemical Safety (http://who.int/pcs/IPCS/index.htm) criteria documents and health and safety documents. The International Agency for Research on Cancer (IARC) provides data on specific classes of carcinogens as well as individual agents. The National Institute of Environmental Health Sciences (NIEHS) National Toxicology Program provides technical reports on the compounds tested as a part of this national program (http://ntp.niehs.nih.gov/).

Recently, new toxicogenomic databases that identify and, in some cases, provide characterization of chemicals have become available. The National Center for Biotechnology

Information (NCBI) provides access to an enormous set of biomedical and genomic information which can be valuable for risk assessment, and they have worked to incorporate toxicologically relevant end points. ACToR (http://actor.epa.gov/actor/faces/ACToRHome.jsp), the EPA's online database on chemical toxicity data and potential chemical risks to human health and the environment, is another useful resource for risk assessments. The Comparative Toxicogenomics Database (http://ctd.mdibl.org/) includes data describing cross-species chemical-gene–protein interactions and chemical-gene–disease relationships which illuminate molecular mechanisms underlying variable susceptibility and environmentally induced diseases. Although these databases provide useful hazard identification and mechanistic information, there is little emphasis on exposure data.

RISK PERCEPTION AND COMPARATIVE ANALYSES OF RISK

Individuals respond very differently to information about hazardous situations and products, as do communities and whole societies. Understanding these behavioral responses is critical in stimulating constructive risk communication and evaluating potential risk management options. In a classic study, students, League of Women Voters members, active club members, and scientific experts were asked to rank 30 activities or agents in order of their annual contribution to deaths. Club members ranked pesticides, spray cans, and nuclear power as safer than did other lay persons. Students ranked contraceptives and food preservatives as riskier and mountain climbing as safer than did others. Experts ranked electric power, surgery, swimming, and X-rays as more risky and nuclear power and police work as less risky than did lay persons. There are also group differences in perceptions of risk from chemicals among toxicologists, correlated with their employment in industry, academia, or government.

Psychological factors such as dread, perceived uncontrollability, and involuntary exposure interact with factors that represent the extent to which a hazard is familiar, observable, and "essential" for daily living. Figure 4–5 presents a grid on the parameters controllable/uncontrollable and observable/not observable for a large number of risky activities; for each of the two paired main factors, highly correlated factors are described in the boxes.

Public demand for government regulations often focuses on involuntary exposures (especially in the food supply, drinking

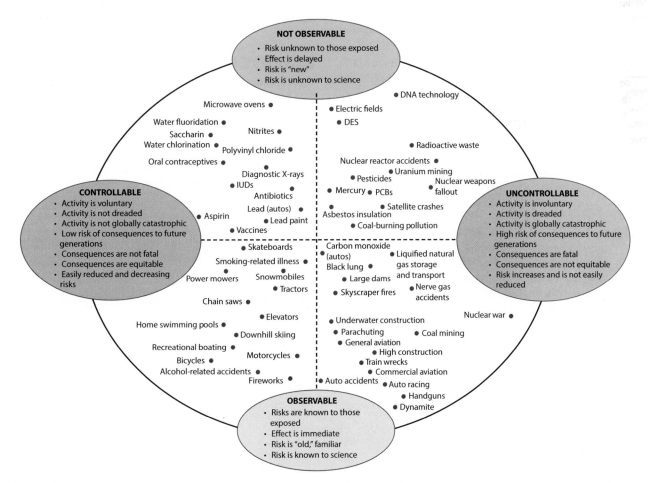

FIGURE 4–5 **Perceptions of risk illustrated using a "risk space" axis diagram.** Risk space has axes that correspond roughly to a hazard's perceived "dreadedness" and to the degree to which it is familiar or observable. Risks in the upper right quadrant of this space are most likely to provoke calls for government regulation.

water, and air) and unfamiliar hazards, such as radioactive waste, electromagnetic fields, asbestos insulation, and genetically modified crops and foods. Many people respond very negatively when they perceive that information about hazards or even about new technologies without reported hazards has been withheld by the manufacturers (genetically modified foods) or by government agencies (HIV-contaminated blood transfusions in the 1980s; extent of hazardous chemical or radioactive wastes).

Most people regularly compare risks of alternative activities—on the job, in recreational pursuits, in interpersonal interactions, and in investments. Determining how best to conduct comparative risk analyses has proved difficult due to the great variety of health and environmental benefits, the gross uncertainties of dollar estimates of benefits and costs, and the different distributions of benefits and costs across the population.

EMERGING CONCEPTS

There is a need to ensure that the risk question(s) is(are) succinctly framed to answer questions in the real world. Environmental health is very dynamic and many divergent emerging environmental challenges such as climate change, energy shortages, and engineered nanoparticles will require an expansion of our context well beyond single-chemical, single-exposure scenarios. In order to accomplish this goal, global and international thinking will be required.

Well-being is increasingly being used to describe human health and the goal of sustainable environmental risk management. Well-being goes beyond "disease-free" existence to freedom from want (including food and water security) and fear (personal safety) and sustainable futures. Recognition that environmental problems are global is essential to how we manage risks and address sustainability. Research and development efforts must examine chemical safety for sustainable and healthy communities with safe and sustainable water, air, and energy resources.

PUBLIC HEALTH RISK MANAGEMENT

Associated with concepts of well-being and sustainability is a public health orientation to use toxicological tests to identify and characterize potential health risks and to prevent the unsafe use of such agents. There are three stages of prevention: *primary*, whose goal is prevention and risk or hazard avoidance; *secondary*, whose goal is mitigation or preparedness including risk or vulnerability reduction and risk transfer; and *tertiary*, where prompt response or recovery is an approach for decreasing residual risk or risk reduction. Figure 4–5 shows an overview of risk assessment and management for public health where

concepts of capacity assessment, vulnerability, and impact assessment are included. In this context, vulnerability assessment would include consideration of exposure and susceptibility as part of the vulnerability assessment. Hazard analysis refers to both hazard identification and probability-based frequency of anticipated events. Capacity assessment has been used for identifying strengths and resiliency of a system to impact.

SUMMARY

Risk assessment objectives vary with the issues, risk management needs, and statutory requirements. Hence, setting the context and problem formation for risk evaluation is essential. The frameworks are sufficiently flexible to address various objectives and to accommodate new knowledge while providing guidance for priority setting in industrial, environmental, governmental, and public health agencies. Risk assessment analyzes the science, identifies uncertainty and provides approaches for decisions. Toxicology, epidemiology, exposure assessment, and clinical observations can be linked with biomarkers, cross-species investigations of mechanisms of effects, and systematic approaches to risk assessment, risk communication, and risk management. Advances in toxicology are certain to improve the quality of risk assessments as scientific findings substitute data for assumptions and help to describe and model uncertainty more credibly.

BIBLIOGRAPHY

Costa L, Eaton D (eds.): *Gene-Environment Interactions: Fundamental of Ecogenetics*. Hoboken, NJ: John Wiley & Sons, 2006.

FDA US: *Critical Path Initiative*. Science & Research. Silver Spring, MD: US Food and Drug Administration; 2011. Available at: http://www.fda.gov/ScienceResearch/SpecialTopics/CriticalPathInitiative/default.htm.

Hood R (ed.): *Developmental and Reproductive Toxicology: A Practical Approach*. 3rd ed. Boca Raton, FL: CRC Press, 2011.

Hsieh A: A nation's genes for a cure to cancer: evolving ethical, social and legal issues regarding population genetic databases. *Columbia J Law Soc Probl* 37:359–411, 2004.

NRC: *Science and Decisions: Advancing Risk Assessment*. Washington, DC: National Academies Press; 2009.

NTP: National Toxicology Program. 2011. Available at: http://ntp.niehs.nih.gov/.

Ryan PB: Exposure assessment, industrial hygiene, and environmental management. In: Frumkin H, ed. *Environmental Health: From Global to Local*. 2nd ed. San Francisco, CA: Jossey-Bass; 2010.

Sahu SC (ed.): *Toxicology and Epigenetics*. New York: John Wiley & Sons; 2012.

US EPA: Ecological Risk Assessments. Pesticides: Environmental Effects. 2011. Available at: http://www.epa.gov/pesticides/ecosystem/ecorisk.htm.

QUESTIONS

1. Which of the following is NOT important in hazard identification?
   a. structure–activity analysis.
   b. in vitro tests.
   c. animal bioassays.
   d. susceptibility.
   e. epidemiology.

2. The probability of an adverse outcome is defined as:
   a. hazard.
   b. exposure ratio.
   c. risk.
   d. susceptibility.
   e. epidemiology.

3. The systematic scientific characterization of adverse health effects resulting from human exposure to hazardous agents is the definition of:
   a. risk.
   b. hazard control.
   c. risk assessment.
   d. risk communication.
   e. risk estimate.

4. Which of the following is not an objective of risk management?
   a. setting target levels for risk.
   b. balancing risks and benefits.
   c. calculating lethal dosages.
   d. setting priorities for manufacturers.
   e. estimating residual risks.

5. Which of the following is NOT a feature in the design of standard cancer bioassays?
   a. more than one species.
   b. both sexes.
   c. near lifetime exposure.
   d. approximately 50 animals per dose group.
   e. same dose level for all groups.

6. Which of the following types of epidemiologic study is always retrospective?
   a. cohort.
   b. cross-sectional.
   c. case–control.
   d. longitudinal.
   e. exploratory.

7. Which of the following is defined as the highest nonstatistically significant dose tested?
   a. ED_{50}
   b. ED_{100}
   c. NOAEL.
   d. ADI.
   e. COAEL.

8. Which of the following represents the dose below which no additional increase in response is observed?
   a. ED_{10}
   b. LD_{10}
   c. RfC.
   d. threshold.
   e. significance level.

9. Which of the following is NOT needed to calculate the reference dose using the BMD method?
   a. MF.
   b. percent benchmark response.
   c. NOAEL.
   d. UF.
   e. benchmark dose.

10. Virtually safe doses are described at which confidence level?
    a. 90%.
    b. 95%.
    c. 99%.
    d. 99.9%.
    e. 99.99%.

C H A P T E R

5

Absorption, Distribution, and Excretion of Toxicants

Lois D. Lehman-McKeeman

INTRODUCTION

The disposition of a chemical or *xenobiotic* is defined as the composite actions of its *absorption, distribution, biotransformation,* and *elimination.* The quantitative characterization of xenobiotic disposition is termed *pharmacokinetics* or *toxicokinetics* (see Chapter 7).

The toxicity of a substance depends on the dose. The concentration of a chemical at the site of action is usually proportional to the dose, but the same dose of two or more chemicals may lead to vastly different concentrations in a particular target organ of toxicity owing to differences in the disposition of the chemicals. Various factors affecting disposition are depicted in Figure 5–1, such as (1) if the fraction absorbed or the rate of absorption is low, a chemical may never attain a sufficiently high concentration at a potential site of action to cause toxicity; (2) the distribution of a toxicant may be such that it is concentrated in a tissue other than the target organ, thus decreasing toxicity; (3) biotransformation of a chemical may result in the formation of less toxic or more toxic metabolites at a fast or

slow rate with obvious consequences for the concentration and, thus, the toxicity at the target site; and (4) the more rapidly a chemical is eliminated from an organism, the lower will be its concentration and hence its toxicity in target tissues. If a chemical is distributed to and stored in fat, its elimination is likely to be slow because very low plasma levels preclude rapid renal clearance or other clearances.

The skin, lungs, and alimentary canal are the main barriers that separate higher organisms from an environment containing a large number of chemicals. Toxicants must cross one or several of these incomplete barriers to exert deleterious effects. Only chemicals that are caustic and corrosive agents (acids, bases, salts, and oxidizers) and act topically at the point of contact are exceptions. A chemical absorbed into the bloodstream through any of these three barriers is distributed throughout the body, including the site where it produces damage, the *target organ* or *target tissue.* A chemical may have one or several target organs, and, in turn, several chemicals may have the same target organ(s). Because several factors other than the concentration influence the susceptibility of organs to toxicants, the

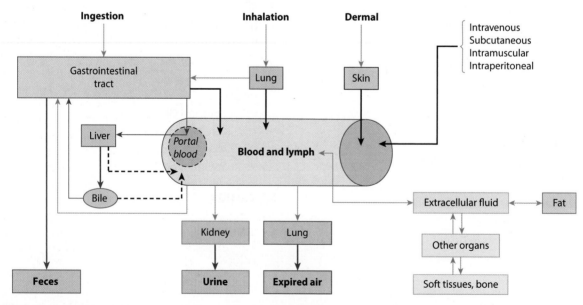

FIGURE 5–1 Routes of absorption, distribution, and excretion of toxicants in the body. Black lines represent routes of absorption into the blood stream; blue lines designate distribution; green lines identify pathways of final excretion; red lines show enterohepatic circulation.

organ or tissue with the highest concentration of a toxicant is not necessarily the site of toxicity. It is important to note that the processes comprising xenobiotic disposition are interrelated and influence each other (Figure 5–1).

CELL MEMBRANES

All processes of toxicant distribution involve passage across biological membranes. Toxicants usually pass through the membranes of a number of cells, such as the stratified epithelium of skin, the thin cell layers of lungs or gastrointestinal tract, the capillary endothelium, and the cells of the target organ or tissue; the plasma membranes surrounding all these cells are remarkably similar.

The basic unit of the cell membrane is a lipid bilayer, composed primarily of phospholipids, glycolipids, and cholesterol. Phospholipids are amphiphilic, consisting of a hydrophilic polar head and a hydrophobic lipid tail. In membranes, the polar head groups are oriented toward the outer and inner surfaces of the membrane, whereas the hydrophobic tails are oriented inward and face each other to form a continuous hydrophobic inner space. Hydrophobic interaction between these fatty acids is the major driving force for the formation of membrane lipid bilayers. Numerous proteins are inserted or embedded in the bilayer, and some transmembrane proteins traverse the entire lipid bilayer, functioning as important biological receptors or allowing the formation of aqueous pores, ion channels, and transporters (Figure 5–2). Fatty acids of the phospholipids and glycolipids do not have a rigid crystalline structure, but are semifluid at physiological temperatures. Many factors influence this fluid character, including degree of unsaturation (lack of double bonds), the presence of cholesterol, and temperature.

A key characteristic of plasma membranes is their ability to be differentially permeable, which regulates what enters into or exits from cells. A toxicant may pass through a membrane by either (1) passive transport, in which the cell expends no energy or (2) specialized transport, in which the cell provides energy to translocate the toxicant across its membrane.

Passive Transport

Simple Diffusion—Most toxicants cross membranes by simple diffusion, following the principles of Fick's law, which establishes that chemicals move from regions of higher concentration to regions of lower concentration without any energy expenditure. Small hydrophilic molecules (up to a molecular weight of about 600 daltons [Da]) permeate membranes through aqueous pores, in a process termed *paracellular diffusion*. In contrast, hydrophobic molecules diffuse across the lipid domain of membranes, in a process called transcellular diffusion. The smaller a hydrophilic molecule is, the more readily it traverses membranes by simple diffusion, and, consequently, a small water-soluble compound such as ethanol is rabidly absorbed and distributed.

For larger organic molecules with differing degrees of lipid solubility, the rate of transport across membranes correlates with lipophilicity. Their rate of transport across membranes correlates with their lipid solubility, which is determined by the octanol/water partition coefficient, P, which is defined as the ratio of the concentration of neutral compound in organic and aqueous phases under equilibrium conditions. The octanol/water partition coefficient is usually expressed in log form, and is an informative physicochemical parameter relative to assessing potential membrane permeability, with positive values associated with high lipid solubility.

Many chemicals are weak organic acids or bases, which are ionized in solution according to Arrhenius' theory. The ionized form of weak organic acids or bases usually has low lipid solubility and does not permeate readily through the lipid domain of a membrane. In contrast, the nonionized form is more lipid soluble and diffuses across membranes at a rate that is proportional to its lipid solubility. The pH at which a weak organic acid or base is 50% ionized is called its pK_a or pK_b. Values for pK_a relay the relative strength or weakness of the acid such that low values indicate a strong acid and high values indicate a weak acid; the opposite is true for bases. Both pK_a and pK_b are defined as the negative logarithm of the ionization constant of a weak organic acid or base. Knowing pK_b, one can calculate pK_a for weak organic bases with the equation $pK_a = 14 - pK_b$. Knowledge of the chemical structure is required to distinguish between organic acids and bases, as the numerical value of pK_a does not indicate this characteristic.

The degree of ionization of a chemical depends on its pK_a and on the pH of the solution. The relationship between pK_a and pH is described by the Henderson–Hasselbalch equations:

$$\text{For acids: } pK_a - pH = \log\frac{[\text{nonionized}]}{[\text{ionized}]}$$

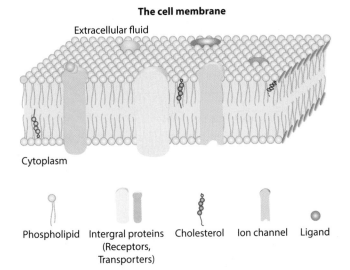

The cell membrane

Extracellular fluid

Cytoplasm

Phospholipid | Intergral proteins (Receptors, Transporters) | Cholesterol | Ion channel | Ligand

FIGURE 5–2 Schematic model of a biological membrane.

$$\text{For bases } pK_a - pH = \log \frac{[\text{ionized}]}{[\text{nonionized}]}$$

The effect of pH on the degree of ionization of an organic acid (benzoic acid) and an organic base (aniline) is illustrated in Figure 5–3. According to Brönsted–Lowry acid-base theory, an acid is a proton (H^+) donor and a base is a proton acceptor. Thus, the ionized and nonionized forms of an organic acid represent an acid–base pair, with the nonionized moiety being the acid and the ionized moiety being the base.

Filtration—When water flows in bulk across a porous membrane, any solute small enough to pass through the pores flows with it. Passage through these channels is called *filtration*. One of the main differences between various membranes is the size of these channels. In the renal glomeruli, a primary site of blood filtration and subsequent urine formation, these pores are relatively large and allow molecules smaller than albumin (approximately 60 kDa) to pass through. The channels in most cells are much smaller, permitting substantial passage of molecules with molecular weights of no more than a few hundred daltons.

Special Transport

There are numerous compounds whose movement across membranes cannot be explained by simple diffusion or filtration. Some compounds are too large to pass through aqueous pores or too lipid-insoluble to diffuse across the lipid domain of plasma membranes. Nevertheless, these molecules are still transported, often very rapidly, across plasma membranes and even against concentration gradients. Specialized transport systems have been identified to explain these phenomena, and identifying such transporters and their dysfunctions is a developing area of toxicology.

Facilitated Diffusion—Facilitated diffusion is carrier-mediated transport that exhibits the properties of active transport except that the substrate is not moved against an electrochemical or concentration gradient and the transport process does not require the input of energy. Because this process is energy-independent, metabolic poisons do not interfere with this type of transport, as they would with active transport.

Active Transport—Active transport is characterized by (1) movement of chemicals against electrochemical or concentration gradients, (2) saturability at high substrate concentrations, thus exhibiting a transport maximum (T_m), (3) selectivity for certain structural features of chemicals, (4) competitive inhibition by chemical antagonists or compounds that are carried by the same transporter, and (5) requirement for expenditure of energy (often in the form of ATP), so that metabolic inhibitors block the transport process.

Xenobiotic Transporters—Around 5% of all human genes are transporter related, indicating the importance of transport function in normal biological and toxicological outcomes. Transporters mediate the influx (uptake) and efflux of xenobiotics and can be divided into two categories determined by whether they employ active transport or facilitative diffusion (Tables 5–1 and 5–2).

Energy-dependent xenobiotic transporters are part of a large superfamily known as ATP-binding cassette (ABC) transporters, and seven subfamilies (classified A to G) have been now identified. Many of these transporters play key roles in the homeostasis of numerous endogenous substances, including absorption from the GI tract and maintenance of the blood-brain barrier (BBB); mutations can lead to multidrug resistance (MDR). A notable example is from the B subfamily, called MDR1 (ABCB1) that, in cancerous cells, exudes cytotoxic drugs out of the tumor cells thereby protecting the cell from drug-mediated destruction. The C subfamily of ABC transporters is also known as the multidrug resistance-associated protein (MRP) family, and they are also involved in efflux of chemicals from cells.

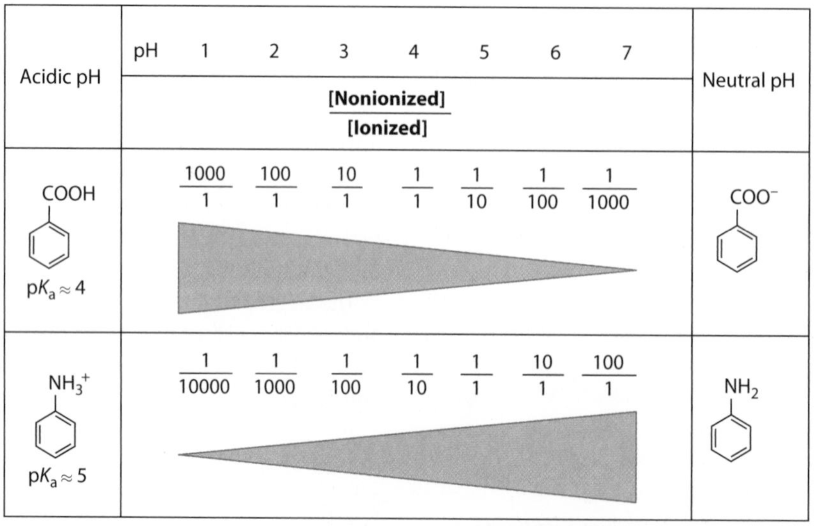

FIGURE 5–3 Effect of pH on the ionization of benzoic acid ($pK_a = 4$) and aniline ($pK_a = 5$).

DISTRIBUTION

After gaining entry into the bloodstream, regardless of route of exposure, a toxicant may distribute to tissues throughout the body. The rate of distribution to organs or tissues is determined primarily by blood flow and the rate of diffusion out of the capillary bed into the cells of a particular organ or tissue. The final distribution depends largely on the affinity of a xenobiotic for various tissues.

Volume of Distribution

A key concept in understanding the disposition of a toxicant is its *volume of distribution (Vd)*, which is defined as the volume in which the amount of drug would need to be uniformly dissolved in order to produce the observed blood concentration. The total water in one's body accounts for approximately 60% of body weight and is partitioned into two main compartments: (1) intracellular water and (2) extracellular water. Extracellular water is further divided into interstitial water and plasma water. If a chemical distributes only to the plasma compartment (no tissue distribution), it has a high plasma concentration and a low Vd. In contrast, if a chemical distributes throughout the body (into both compartments), it has a low plasma concentration and a high Vd. The distribution of toxicants is more complex than this, however, and strongly influenced by factors such as binding to and/or dissolution in fat, liver, and bone.

Some toxicants do not readily cross cell membranes and therefore have restricted distribution, whereas other toxicants rapidly pass through cell membranes and are distributed throughout the body. Some toxicants selectively accumulate in certain parts of the body as a result of protein binding, active transport, or high solubility in fat. The target organ for toxicity may be the site of accumulation of a toxicant, but this is not always the case. If a toxicant accumulates at a site other than the target organ or tissue, the accumulation may be viewed as a protective process in that plasma levels and consequently the concentration of a toxicant at the site of action are diminished. However, because any chemical in a storage depot is in equilibrium with the free fraction (unbound) of toxicant in plasma, it is released into the circulation as the unbound fraction of toxicant is eliminated.

Storage of Toxicants in Tissues

Since only the free fraction (unbound) of a chemical is in equilibrium throughout the body, binding to or dissolving in certain body constituents greatly alters the distribution of a xenobiotic. Toxicants are often concentrated in a specific tissue, called a storage depot, which may or may not be their site of toxic action. Toxicants in storage depots are always in equilibrium with the free fraction in plasma, so that as a chemical is biotransformed or excreted from the body, more is released from the storage site. As a result, the biological half-life of stored compounds can be very long.

Plasma Proteins as Storage Depot—Several plasma proteins bind xenobiotics as well as some endogenous constituents of the body. As depicted in Figure 5–6, albumin is the major protein in plasma and it binds many different compounds compared to other proteins, such as globulins, lipoproteins, and glycoproteins.

Protein–ligand interactions occur primarily as a result of hydrophobic forces, hydrogen bonding, and van der Waals forces. Because of their high molecular weight, plasma proteins and the toxicants bound to them cannot cross capillary walls. Consequently, the fraction of toxicant bound to plasma proteins is not immediately available for distribution into the extravascular space or filtration by the kidneys. However, the interaction of a chemical with plasma proteins is a reversible process. As unbound chemical diffuses out of capillaries, bound chemical dissociates from the protein until the free fraction reaches equilibrium between the vascular space and the extravascular space. In turn, diffusion in the extravascular space to sites more distant from the capillaries continues, and the resulting concentration gradient causes continued dissociation of the bound fraction in plasma.

The binding of toxicants to plasma proteins is an important concept in toxicology for two reasons. First, toxicity is typically manifested by the amount of a xenobiotic that is unbound. Therefore, a compound with a high degree of plasma protein binding may not show toxicity when compared to one that is less extensively bound to plasma proteins. Severe toxic reactions can occur if a toxicant is displaced from plasma proteins by another agent, increasing the free fraction of the toxicant in plasma. This will result in an increased equilibrium concentration of the toxicant in the target organ, with the potential for toxicity. Xenobiotics can also compete with and displace endogenous compounds that are bound to plasma proteins, which can allow the endogenous compound to exert a toxic effect.

Plasma protein binding can also give rise to observed species differences in the disposition of toxicants. Factors that

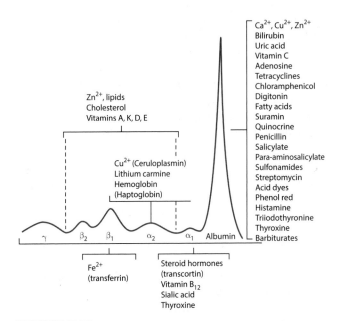

FIGURE 5–6 **Ligand interactions with plasma proteins.**

influence plasma protein binding across species include differences in the concentration of albumin, binding affinity, and/or competitive binding of endogenous substances.

Liver and Kidney as Storage Depots—The liver and kidney have a high capacity for binding a multitude of chemicals. These two organs probably concentrate more toxicants than do all the other organs combined. In most cases, binding to tissue components is likely to be involved.

Fat as Storage Depot—Many highly lipophilic toxicants with a high lipid/water partition coefficient are distributed and concentrated in body fat. Storage lowers the concentration of the toxicant in the target organ; therefore, the toxicity of such a compound can be expected to be less severe in an obese person than in a lean individual. However, the possibility of a sudden increase in the concentration of a chemical in the blood and thus in the target organ of toxicity when rapid mobilization of fat occurs must be considered. Several studies have shown that signs of intoxication can be produced by short-term starvation of experimental animals that were previously exposed to persistent organochlorine insecticides.

Bone as Storage Depot—Skeletal uptake of xenobiotics is essentially a surface chemistry phenomenon, with exchange taking place between the bone surface of hydroxyapatite crystals and the extracellular fluid in contact with it. Deposition and reversible storage of toxicants in bone is dynamic and may or may not be detrimental. For instance, lead is not toxic to bone, but the chronic effects of fluoride deposition (skeletal fluorosis) and radioactive strontium (osteosarcoma and other neoplasms) are well documented.

Blood–Brain Barrier

Access to the brain is restricted by the presence of two barriers: the blood–brain barrier (BBB) and the blood–cerebrospinal fluid barrier (BCSFB). Although neither represents an absolute barrier to the passage of toxic chemicals into the central nervous system (CNS), many toxicants do not enter the brain in appreciable quantities compared to other body tissues.

There are four major anatomical and physiologic reasons why some toxicants do not readily enter the CNS. First, the capillary endothelial cells of the CNS are tightly joined, leaving few or no pores between the cells, which prevents diffusion of polar compounds through paracellular pathways. Second, the capillaries in the CNS are to a large extent surrounded by glial cell processes (astrocytes), which secrete chemical factors that modulate endothelial permeability. Third, the protein concentration in the interstitial fluid of the CNS is much lower than that in other body fluids, limiting the movement of water-insoluble compounds by paracellular transport, which is possible in a largely aqueous medium only when such compounds are bound to proteins. Fourth, ATP-dependent transporters include members of both ABC and SLC families (Tables 5–1 and 5–2). Efflux transporters MDR1, BCRP, and MRP1, 2, 4,

and 5 are located on the blood side of the capillary endothelium function to move xenobiotics back into the blood and hence limit their distribution into the brain.

The blood cerebrospinal fluid (CSF) barrier is found between the circulating blood and the circulating CSF in the brain. Certain areas (the choroid plexus, the arachnoid membrane, and the area postrema) are more permeable on the blood side, whereas the epithelium on the CSF side is a barrier. In addition, efflux transporters contribute to xenobiotic removal from the CSF thereby protecting against toxicant distribution into the CNS.

In general, only the free unbound toxicant equilibrates rapidly with the brain. Lipid solubility and the degree of ionization are important determinants of the rate of entry of a compound into the CNS. Increased lipid solubility enhances the rate of penetration of toxicants into the CNS, whereas ionization greatly diminishes it. A few xenobiotics appear to enter the brain by carrier-mediated processes. Some lipophilic compounds may enter the brain, but are so efficiently removed by these transporters that they never reach appreciable concentrations.

The BBB is not fully developed at birth, and this is one reason why some chemicals are more toxic to newborns than to adults.

Passage of Toxicants across the Placenta

The term "placental barrier" has been associated with the concept that the main function of the placenta is to protect the fetus against the passage of noxious substances from the mother. However, the placenta is a multifunctional organ that also provides nutrition, exchanges maternal and fetal blood gases, disposes of fetal excretory material, and maintains pregnancy through complex hormonal regulation. Placental structure and function show more species differences than any other mammalian organ.

Most vital nutrients for fetal development, including vitamins, amino acids, essential sugars, iron, and calcium, are transported by active transport systems from mother to fetus. Many foreign substances can cross the placenta, and the same factors that dictate the passage of xenobiotics across other biological membranes are important determinants of placental transfer. These include previously discussed attributes including the degree of ionization, lipophilicity, protein binding, molecular weight, blood flow, and the concentration gradient across the placenta. Among the substances that cross the placenta by passive diffusion, more lipid-soluble substances attain a maternal–fetal equilibrium more rapidly. Under steady-state conditions, the concentrations of a toxic compound in the plasma of the mother and fetus are usually the same. The concentration in the various tissues of the fetus depends on the ability of fetal tissue to concentrate a toxicant. Differential body composition between mother and fetus may be another reason for an apparent placental barrier. For example, fetuses have very little fat; hence, they do not accumulate highly lipophilic chemicals.

Besides chemicals, viruses (e.g., rubella virus), cellular pathogens (e.g., syphilis spirochetes), and globulin antibodies can traverse the placenta. In this regard, the placental barrier is not as precise an anatomical unit as the BBB. Anatomically, the placental barrier consists of a number of cell layers—at most six—interposed between the fetal and maternal circulations. Active transport systems and biotransformation enzymes are differentially expressed through the cell layers. These help protect the fetus from some xenobiotics while regulating the movement of essential nutrients.

Redistribution of Toxicants

The most critical factors that affect the distribution of xenobiotics are the organ blood flow and its affinity for a xenobiotic. The initial phase of distribution is determined primarily by blood flow to the various parts of the body. Therefore, a well-perfused organ such as the liver may attain high initial concentrations of a xenobiotic. However, chemicals may have a high affinity for a binding site (e.g., intracellular protein or bone matrix) or to a cellular constituent (e.g., fat), and, with time, will redistribute to these high-affinity sites.

EXCRETION

Toxicants are eliminated from the body by several routes. Many xenobiotics, though, have to be biotransformed to more water-soluble products before they can be excreted into urine (Chapter 6). All body secretions appear to have the ability to excrete chemicals; toxicants have been found in sweat, saliva, tears, and milk.

Urinary Excretion

Toxic compounds are excreted into urine by the same mechanisms the kidney uses to remove end products of intermediary metabolism from the body: glomerular filtration, tubular excretion by passive diffusion, and active tubular secretion. (See Chapter 14 for greater discussion of renal anatomy and physiology). Compounds up to a molecular weight of about 60 kDa are filtered at the glomeruli. The degree of plasma protein binding affects the rate of filtration, because protein–xenobiotic complexes are too large to pass through the pores of the glomeruli.

A toxicant filtered at the glomeruli may remain in the tubular lumen and be excreted with urine or may be reabsorbed across the tubular cells of the nephron back into the bloodstream. Toxicants with a high lipid/water partition coefficient are reabsorbed efficiently, whereas polar compounds and ions are excreted with urine. The pH of urine may vary but is usually slightly acidic (~6.0 to 6.5). Just as the Henderson–Hasselbalch calculations determine the absorption of nonionized compounds from the GI tract, they also determine urinary excretion. In this case, urinary excretion of the ionized moiety is favored, such that bases are excreted to a greater extent at lower pH whereas excretion of acids predominates at higher urinary pH.

Toxic agents can also be excreted from plasma into urine by passive diffusion through the tubule. This process is probably of minor significance because filtration is much faster than excretion by passive diffusion through the tubules, providing a favorable concentration gradient for reabsorption rather than excretion.

Xenobiotics can also be excreted into urine by active secretion. This process involves the uptake of toxicants from blood into the cells of the renal proximal tubule, with subsequent efflux from the cell into the tubular fluid from which urine is formed. Figure 5–7 illustrates the various families of transporters expressed in the human kidney that are directly involved in xenobiotic disposition. There are numerous other transporters such as specific glucose transporters or nucleotide transporters

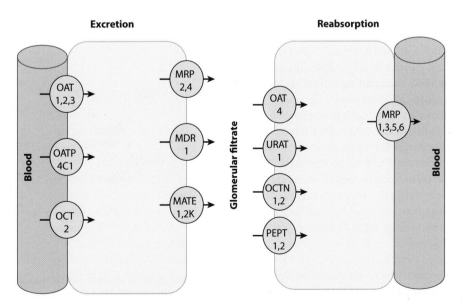

FIGURE 5–7 **Schematic model showing the transport systems in the proximal tubule of the kidney.** The families of transporters are organic-anion transporters (OAT), organic-cation transporters (OCT), multidrug-resistant protein (MDR), multidrug resistance-associated protein (MRP), peptide transporters (PEP), and urate transporter (URAT).

that play a role predominantly in the flux of endogenous substances that are not presented here. Transporters may be expressed on the apical cell membrane where efflux pumps contribute to tubular secretion and influx pumps are important for reabsorption. Transporters localized to the basolateral membranes serve to transport xenobiotics to and from the systemic circulation or the renal tubular cells and also contribute to reabsorptive and excretory processes. Specific transporters expressed on the basolateral side of renal tubules in humans include OATs, OCTs, OATP4C1, and a subset of MRPs. Brush border transporters include MRPs, MDRs, MATEs, URATs, PEPTs, and OAT4.

Because many functions of the kidney are incompletely developed at birth, some xenobiotics are eliminated more slowly in newborns than in adults and therefore may be more toxic to newborns. For example, the clearance of penicillin by premature infants is only about 20% of that observed in older children. The renal proximal tubule reabsorbs small plasma proteins that are filtered at the glomerulus. A toxicant binding those small proteins can be carried into the proximal tubule cells and exert toxicity.

Species differences in urinary excretion can be explained by variance in the pH urine, differences in plasma protein binding, and xenobiotic transporter expression, regulation, and function.

Fecal Excretion

Fecal excretion is the second major pathway for the elimination of xenobiotics from the body. Many chemicals in feces directly transfer from blood into the intestinal contents by passive diffusion. In some instances, rapid exfoliation of intestinal cells may contribute to the fecal excretion of some compounds. Intestinal excretion is a relatively slow process that is a major pathway of elimination only for compounds that have low rates of biotransformation and/or low renal or biliary clearance.

Nonabsorbed Ingesta—In addition to indigestible material, varying proportions of nutrients and xenobiotics that are present in food or are ingested voluntarily (drugs) pass through the alimentary canal unabsorbed, contributing to fecal excretion.

Mucosal biotransformation and reexcretion into the intestinal lumen occur with many compounds. It has been estimated that 30% to 42% of fecal dry matter originates from bacteria. Moreover, a considerable proportion of fecally excreted xenobiotic is associated with excreted bacteria. However, chemicals may be profoundly altered by bacteria before excretion with feces. It seems that biotransformation by intestinal flora favors reabsorption rather than excretion. Nevertheless, there is evidence that in many instances xenobiotics found in feces derive from bacterial biotransformation.

Biliary Excretion—The biliary route of elimination is perhaps the most important contributing source to the fecal excretion of xenobiotics and their metabolites. Hepatic anatomy and physiology and bile formation are discussed in greater detail in Chapter 13. To summarize, nutrients and xenobiotics in portal venous blood from the GI tract are available for uptake by the liver or passage into the systemic circulation. The liver can extract compounds from blood and prevent their distribution to other parts of the body. Furthermore, the liver is the main site of biotransformation of toxicants, and the metabolites thus formed may be excreted directly into bile or into the hepatic venous blood for systemic distribution. Xenobiotics and/or their metabolites entering the intestine with bile may be excreted with feces or undergo an enterohepatic circulation.

Figure 5–8 illustrates the many transporters localized on hepatic parenchymal cells that move foreign substances from plasma into liver and from liver into bile. Biliary excretion is regulated predominantly by xenobiotic transporters present on the canalicular membrane. Sodium-dependent taurocholate peptide (ntcp) present on the sinusoidal side of the parenchymal cell transports bile acids such as taurocholate into the liver, whereas the bile salt excretory protein (bsep) transports bile acids out of the liver cell into the bile canaliculi. The sinusoidal membrane of the hepatocyte has a number of transporters including organic-anion transporting polypeptide (oatp) 1 and 2, and oct that move xenobiotics into the liver. Once inside the hepatocyte, the xenobiotic itself can be transported into the blood or bile, or be biotransformed by phase I and II drug-metabolizing enzymes to more water-soluble products that are then transported into the bile or back into the blood. Multidrug-resistant protein one (mdr1) and multidrug resistance–associated protein two (mrp2) are responsible for transporting xenobiotics into bile, whereas mrp3 and mrp6 transport xenobiotics back into the blood.

An important concept relating to biliary excretion is the phenomenon of enterohepatic circulation. Once a compound is excreted into bile and enters the intestine, it can be reabsorbed or eliminated with feces. Many organic compounds are conjugated before excretion into bile. Such polar metabolites are not sufficiently lipid soluble to be reabsorbed. However,

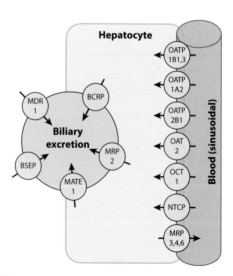

FIGURE 5–8 Schematic model showing the transport systems in the liver. OATP = organic-anion transporting polypeptide, OCT = organic-cation transporter, BSEP = bile salt excretory protein, MDR = multidrug-resistant protein, MRP = multidrug resistance-associated protein, BCRP = breast cancer resistance protein, and NTCP = sodium-dependent taurocholate peptide.

intestinal microflora may hydrolyze glucuronide and sulfate conjugates, making them sufficiently lipophilic for reabsorption and enterohepatic cycling. This principle has been utilized in the treatment of dimethylmercury poisoning; ingestion of a polythiol resin binds the mercury and thus prevents its reabsorption and cycling.

Exhalation

Substances that exist predominantly in the gas phase at body temperature and volatile liquids are eliminated mainly by the lungs. Because volatile liquids are in equilibrium with their gas phase in the alveoli, they may also be excreted via the lungs. The amount of liquid eliminated via the lungs is proportional to its vapor pressure. A practical application of this principle is seen in the breath analyzer test for determining the amount of ethanol in the body.

No specialized transport systems have been described for the excretion of toxic substances by the lungs. Some xenobiotic transporters, including MRP1 and MDR1, have been identified in the lung, but overall, compounds seem to be eliminated by simple diffusion. Elimination of gases is roughly inversely proportional to the rate of their absorption. The rate of elimination of a gas with low solubility in blood is perfusion-limited, whereas that of a gas with high solubility in blood is ventilation-limited.

Other Routes of Elimination

Cerebrospinal Fluid—All compounds can leave the CNS with the bulk flow of cerebrospinal fluid (CSF) through arachnoid villi, which allow fluid to flow from CSF to the venous system. In addition, lipid-soluble toxicants also can exit at the site of the BBB. Active transport using the transport systems present in the BCSFB can also remove toxicants.

Milk—The secretion of toxic compounds into milk is extremely important because (1) a toxicant may be passed with milk from the mother to the nursing offspring and (2) compounds can be passed from cows to humans by way of dairy products. Toxic agents are excreted into milk by simple diffusion. Because milk is more acidic (pH ≈ 6.5) than plasma, basic compounds may be concentrated in milk, whereas acidic compounds may attain lower concentrations in milk than in plasma. About 3% to 4% of milk consists of lipids, and the lipid content of milk after parturition is even higher. Importantly, lipid-soluble xenobiotics diffuse along with fats from plasma into the mammary gland and are excreted with milk during lactation.

Sweat and Saliva—The excretion of toxic agents in sweat and saliva is quantitatively of minor importance. Again, excretion depends on the diffusion of the nonionized, lipid-soluble form of an agent. Toxic compounds excreted into sweat may produce dermatitis (inflammation of the skin). Substances excreted in saliva enter the mouth, where they are usually swallowed to become available for GI absorption.

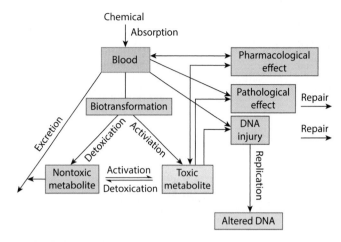

FIGURE 5–9 Schematic representation of the disposition and toxic effects of chemicals.

CONCLUSION

Humans are in continuous contact with toxic agents. Depending on their physical and chemical properties, toxicants may be absorbed by the GI tract, the lungs, and/or the skin. The body has the ability to biotransform and excrete these compounds into urine, feces, and air. However, when the rate of absorption exceeds the rate of elimination, toxic compounds may accumulate, reaching a critical concentration at a target site, and toxicity may ensue (Figure 5–9). Whether a chemical elicits toxicity depends not only on its inherent potency and site specificity, but also on how an organism can dispose of that toxicant.

Many chemicals have very low inherent toxicity but have to be activated by biotransformation into toxic metabolites and the toxic response depends on the rate of production of toxic metabolites. Alternatively, a very potent toxicant may be detoxified rapidly by biotransformation. The fundamental and overarching concept is that adverse toxic effects are related to the unbound concentration of "toxic chemical" at the site of action (in the target organ), whether a chemical is administered or generated by biotransformation in the target tissue or at a distant site. Accordingly, the toxic response exerted by chemicals is critically influenced by the rates of absorption, distribution, biotransformation, and excretion.

BIBLIOGRAPHY

Anzai N, Kanai Y, Endou H: Organic anion transporter family: current knowledge. *J Pharmacol Sci* 100:411–426, 2006.

Goodman J: *Goodman and Gilman's The Pharmacological Basis of Therapeutics*, 12th ed. New York: McGraw-Hill, 2011.

Klaassen CD, Aleksunes LM: Xenobiotic, bile acid, and cholesterol transporters: function and regulation. *Pharmacol Rev* 62:1–96, 2010.

Lin JH: Tissue distribution and pharmacodynamics: a complicated relationship. *Curr Drug Metab* 7:39–65, 2006.

Myllynen P, Pasanen M, Pelkonen O: Human placenta: a human organ for developmental toxicology research and biomonitoring. *Placenta* 26:361–371, 2005.

Zhai H, Wilhelm KP, Maibach HI (eds.): *Marzulli and Maibach's Dermatotoxicology*, 7th ed. Boca Raton, FL: CRC Press, 2008.

QUESTIONS

1. Biotransformation is vital in removing toxins from the circulation. All of the following statements regarding biotransformation are true EXCEPT:
   a. Many toxins must be biotransformed into a more lipid-soluble form before they can be excreted from the body.
   b. The liver is the most active organ in the biotransformation of toxins.
   c. Water solubility is required in order for many toxins to be excreted by the kidney.
   d. The kidney plays a major role in eliminating toxicants from the body.
   e. The lungs play a minor role in ridding the body of certain types of toxins.

2. Which of the following statements about active transport across cell membranes is FALSE?
   a. Unlike simple or facilitated diffusion, active transport pumps chemicals against an electrochemical or concentration gradient.
   b. Unlike simple diffusion, there is a rate at which active transport becomes saturated and cannot move chemicals any faster.
   c. Active transport requires the expenditure of ATP in order to move chemicals against electrochemical or concentration gradients.
   d. Active transport exhibits a high level of specificity for the compounds that are being moved.
   e. Metabolic inhibitors do not affect the ability to perform active transport.

3. Which of the following might increase the toxicity of a toxin administered orally?
   a. increased activity of the mdr transporter (*p*-glycoprotein).
   b. increased biotransformation of the toxin by gastrointestinal cells.
   c. increased excretion of the toxin by the liver into bile.
   d. increased dilution of the toxin dose.
   e. increased intestinal motility.

4. Which of the following most correctly describes the first-pass effect?
   a. The body is most sensitive to a toxin the first time that it passes through the circulation.
   b. Orally administered toxins are partially removed by the GI tract before they reach the systemic circulation.
   c. It only results from increased absorption of toxin by GI cells.
   d. It is often referred to as "postsystemic elimination."
   e. A majority of the toxin is excreted after the first time the blood is filtered by the kidneys.

5. Which of the following is an important mechanism of removing particulate matter from the alveoli?
   a. coughing.
   b. sneezing.
   c. blowing one's nose.
   d. absorption into the bloodstream, followed by excretion via the kidneys.
   e. swallowing.

6. For a toxin to be absorbed through the skin, it must pass through multiple layers in order to reach the systemic circulation. Which of the following layers is the most important in slowing the rate of toxin absorption through the skin?
   a. stratum granulosum.
   b. stratum spinosum.
   c. stratum corneum.
   d. stratum basale.
   e. dermis.

7. A toxin is selectively toxic to the lungs. Which of the following modes of toxin delivery would most likely cause the LEAST damage to the lungs?
   a. intravenous.
   b. intramuscular.
   c. intraperitoneal.
   d. subcutaneous.
   e. inhalation.

8. Which of the following is NOT an important site of toxicant storage in the body?
    a. adipose tissue.
    b. bone.
    c. plasma proteins.
    d. muscle.
    e. liver.

9. Which of the following regarding the blood–brain barrier is TRUE:
    a. The brains of adults and newborns are equally susceptible to harmful blood-borne chemicals.
    b. The degree of lipid solubility is a primary determinant in whether or not a substance can cross the blood–brain barrier.
    c. Astrocytes play a role in increasing the permeability of the blood–brain barrier.
    d. Active transport processes increase the concentration of xenobiotics in the brain.
    e. The capillary endothelial cells of the CNS possess large fenestrations in their basement membranes.

10. Which of the following will result in DECREASED excretion of toxic compounds by the kidneys?
    a. a toxic compound with a molecular weight of 25,000 Da.
    b. increased activity of the multidrug-resistance (mdr) protein.
    c. increased activity of the multiresistant drug protein (mrp).
    d. increased activity of the organic cation transporter.
    e. increased hydrophilicity of the toxic compound.

Biotransformation of Xenobiotics

6

Andrew Parkinson, Brian W. Ogilvie, David B. Buckley, Faraz Kazmi, Maciej Czerwinski, and Oliver Parkinson

GENERAL PRINCIPLES

HYDROLYSIS, REDUCTION, AND OXIDATION

Hydrolysis

Carboxylesterases, Cholinesterases, and Paraoxonase

Prodrugs and Alkaline Phosphatase

Peptidases

Epoxide Hydrolase

Reduction

Azo- and Nitro-reduction

Carbonyl Reduction

Disulfide Reduction

Sulfoxide and *N*-Oxide Reduction

Quinone Reduction

Dehalogenation

Oxidation

Alcohol Dehydrogenase

Aldehyde Dehydrogenase

Dihydrodiol Dehydrogenase

Molybdenum Hydroxylases

Xanthine Oxidoreductase

Aldehyde Oxidase

Monoamine Oxidase

Peroxidase-dependent Cooxidation

Flavin Monooxygenases

Cytochrome P450

Activation of Xenobiotics by Cytochrome P450

Inhibition of Cytochrome P450

Induction of Cytochrome P450

CONJUGATION

Glucuronidation

Sulfonation

Methylation

Acetylation

Amino Acid Conjugation

Glutathione Conjugation

KEY POINTS

- *Biotransformation* is the metabolic conversion of endogenous and xenobiotic chemicals to more water-soluble compounds.
- Xenobiotic biotransformation is accomplished by a limited number of enzymes with broad substrate specificities.
- Phase I reactions involve hydrolysis, reduction, and oxidation. These reactions expose or introduce a functional group ($-OH$, $-NH_2$, $-SH$, or $-COOH$), and usually result in only a small increase in hydrophilicity.
- Phase II biotransformation reactions include glucuronidation, sulfonation (more commonly called sulfation), acetylation, methylation, and conjugation with glutathione (mercapturic acid synthesis), which usually result in increased hydrophilicity and elimination.

The enzymes that catalyze xenobiotic biotransformation are often called drug-metabolizing enzymes. The acronym ADME stands for *a*bsorption, *d*istribution, *m*etabolism, and *e*limination. This acronym is widely used in the pharmaceutical industry to describe the four main processes governing drug disposition. The acronym is sometimes extended to include drug transport (AMDET) or drug toxicity (ADME-Tox). This chapter describes some fundamental principles of xenobiotic biotransformation, and describes the major enzyme systems involved in the biotransformation (or metabolism) of drugs and other xenobiotics.

GENERAL PRINCIPLES

The following points, which might be considered principles or rules, apply in the majority of cases:

Point 1 Xenobiotic biotransformation or drug metabolism is the process of converting lipophilic (fat-soluble) chemicals, which are readily absorbed from the gastrointestinal tract and other sites, into hydrophilic (water-soluble) chemicals, which are readily excreted in urine or bile. There are exceptions even to this most basic rule. For example, acetylation and methylation are biotransformation reactions that can actually decrease the water solubility of certain xenobiotics.

Point 2 The biotransformation of xenobiotics is catalyzed by various enzyme systems that can be divided into four categories based on the reaction they catalyze: (1) hydrolysis (e.g., carboxylesterase); (2) reduction (e.g., carbonyl reductase); (3) oxidation (e.g., cytochrome P450 [CYP]); and (4) conjugation (e.g., UDP-glucuronosyltransferase [UGT]). The mammalian enzymes involved in the hydrolysis, reduction, oxidation, and conjugation of xenobiotics are listed in Table 6–1, together with their principal subcellular location.

Point 3 In general, individual xenobiotic-biotransforming enzymes are located in a single organelle. In Table 6–1, some enzymes are listed with two or more subcellular locations.

Point 4 In general, xenobiotic biotransformation is accomplished by a limited number of enzymes with broad substrate specificities. In humans, e.g., 2 CYP enzymes—namely, CYP2D6 and CYP3A4—metabolize over half the orally effective drugs in current use. Many of the enzymes involved in xenobiotic biotransformation are arranged in families and subfamilies and named according to nomenclature systems based on the primary amino acid sequence of the individual enzymes. The convention of using italic and regular letters to distinguish between the gene and gene products (mRNA and protein), respectively, and the convention of using lower case letters to designate mouse genes and gene products is not followed in this chapter.

The structure (i.e., amino acid sequence) of a given xenobiotic-biotransforming enzyme may differ among individuals, which can give rise to differences in rates of drug metabolism. The broad substrate specificity of xenobiotic-biotransforming enzymes makes them catalytically versatile but slow compared with most other enzymes (with the exception of hydrolytic reactions). The sequential oxidation, conjugation, and transport of a xenobiotic tend to proceed quicker at each subsequent step, which prevents the accumulation of intracellular metabolites. Were it not for the low catalytic turnover of CYP (one molecule of which may take several seconds or minutes to oxidize a single drug molecule), it would not be possible to achieve the once-a-day dosing characteristic of a large number of drugs.

Point 5 Hydrolysis, reduction, and oxidation expose or introduce a functional group (such as $-OH$, $-NH_2$, $-SH$, or $-COOH$) that can be converted to a water-soluble conjugate. The functional group introduced or exposed by hydrolysis, reduction, or oxidation must be nucleophilic (in the case of glucuronidation, sulfonation, methylation, acetylation, and conjugation with glycine or taurine) or electrophilic (in the case of glutathionylation). The first three reactions (hydrolysis, reduction, and oxidation) are often called Phase 1 reactions, and the conjugation reactions are often called Phase 2 reactions.

Point 6 Oxidation, reduction, hydrolysis, methylation, and acetylation generally cause a modest increase in the water solubility of a xenobiotic, whereas glucuronidation, sulfonation, glutathionylation, and amino acid conjugation generally cause a marked increase in hydrophilicity.

Point 7 Xenobiotics can undergo biotransformation both by enzymes that normally participate in intermediary (endobiotic) metabolism and by enzymes within gut microflora.

Point 8 Just as some xenobiotics are biotransformed by the so-called endobiotic-metabolizing enzymes (Point 7), certain endobiotics are biotransformed by the so-called xenobiotic-metabolizing enzymes. For example, the same CYP enzymes implicated in xenobiotic biotransformation also contribute to the hepatic catabolism of steroid hormones, and the same UGTs that conjugate xenobiotics also glucuronidate bilirubin, thyroid hormones, and steroid hormones. On a case-by-case basis, there is often no clear-cut distinction between endobiotic- and xenobiotic-biotransforming enzymes.

Point 9 Several xenobiotic-biotransforming enzymes are inducible, meaning their expression can be increased (upregulated) usually in response to exposure to high concentrations of xenobiotics. Xenobiotics can act as ligands for certain receptors (so-called xenosensors). Activated xenosensors (i.e., those bound to xenobiotics) interact with DNA-binding proteins which upregulate the transcription of various genes encoding for xenobiotic-biotransforming enzymes. The major xenosensors are aryl hydrocarbon receptor (AhR), which induces CYP1 enzymes, the constitutive androstane receptor (CAR) and the pregnane X receptor (PXR), which induce CYP2B, 2C, and 3A enzymes, and the peroxisome proliferator–activated receptor-α (PPARα), which induces CYP4 enzymes.

Certain xenosensors are activated by endogenous ligands (e.g., bilirubin, bile acids, and fatty acids activate CAR, PXR, and PPARα, respectively). Induction is a reversible, adaptive response to xenobiotic exposure. Induction is also a pleiotropic response: activation of AhR, CAR, PXR, PPARα, and Nrf2 all results in alterations in the expression of numerous genes.

TABLE 6–1 General pathways of xenobiotic biotransformation and their major subcellular location.

Reaction	Enzyme or Specific Reaction	Localization
Hydrolysis	Carboxylesterase	Microsomes, cytosol, lysosomes, blood
	Butyrylcholinesterase	Plasma and most tissues
	Acetylcholinesterase	Erythrocytes and most tissues
	Paraoxonases	Plasma, microsomes, inner mitochondrial membrane
	Alkaline phosphatase	Plasma membrane
	Peptidase	Blood, lysosomes
	β-Glucuronidase	Microsomes, lysosomes, microflora
	Epoxide hydrolase	Microsomes, cytosol
Reduction	Azo- and nitro-reduction	Microflora
	Carbonyl (aldo-keto) reduction	Cytosol, microsomes, blood
	Disulfide reduction	Cytosol
	Sulfoxide reduction	Cytosol
	Quinone reduction	Cytosol, microsomes
	Dihydropyrimidine dehydrogenase	Cytosol
	Reductive dehalogenation	Microsomes
	Dehydroxylation (mARC)*	Mitochondria
	Dehydroxylation (aldehyde oxidase)	Cytosol
Oxidation	Alcohol dehydrogenase	Cytosol
	Aldehyde dehydrogenase	Mitochondria, cytosol
	Aldehyde oxidase	Cytosol
	Xanthine oxidase	Cytosol
	Class I amine oxidases	
	Monoamine oxidase-A and B	Inner mitochondrial membrane, platelets
	Class II amine oxidases (CuAOs)	
	Diamine oxidase	Microsomes, extracellular matrix
	Peroxidase	Microsomes, lysosomes, saliva
	Flavin-monooxygenases	Microsomes
	Cytochrome P450	Microsomes, mitochondria
Conjugation	UDP-glucuronosyltransferase	Microsomes
	Sulfotransferase	Cytosol
	Glutathione transferase	Cytosol, microsomes, mitochondria
	Amino acid transferase	Mitochondria, microsomes
	N-Acetyltransferase	Mitochondria, cytosol
	Methyltransferase	Cytosol, microsomes, blood

*mARC, mitochondrial amidoxime-reducing component.

Suppression (down-regulation) of drug-metabolizing enzymes is often associated with inflammatory diseases (such as arthritis), cancer, infectious diseases (both bacterial and viral), vaccination, and treatment with certain proinflammatory biologics (therapeutic proteins). These disease processes activate nuclear factor-kappa B (NF-κB) and other nuclear receptors, which suppress the expression and induction of CYP and other xenobiotic-metabolizing enzymes. This is because activated NF-κB suppresses all four xenosensors (AhR, CAR, PXR, and PPARα) as well as several other nuclear receptors. By reversing the disease process—such as lessening the inflammation associated with rheumatoid arthritis—some biologics (large drug molecules such as monoclonal antibodies and other types of therapeutic proteins) can reverse the suppression of drug-metabolizing enzymes and restore their activity to normal (pre-disease) levels.

Point 10 Xenobiotic biotransformation can alter the biological properties of a xenobiotic. The biotransformation of drugs can result in (1) a loss of pharmacological activity, (2) no change in pharmacological activity, or (3) an increase in pharmacological activity.

Point 11 The toxicity and potential carcinogenicity of electrophilic metabolites produced by CYP and other xenobiotic-biotransforming enzymes is reduced and often altogether eliminated by their conjugation with reduced glutathione (GSH).

Point 12 The biotransformation of some xenobiotics results in the production of reactive oxygen species (ROS), which can cause cell toxicity (including DNA damage) through oxidative stress and lipid peroxidation. GSH, GSTs, and glutathione peroxidases (GPXs) all limit the toxic effects of ROS just as they limit the toxicity of reactive metabolites formed directly from xenobiotics. Oxidative stress and the formation of electrophilic metabolites reduce GSH levels and thus result in the concurrent oxidation of KEAP-1, which then releases Nrf2, which in turn upregulates the expression of enzymes that detoxify electrophilic metabolites (e.g., epoxides) and those metabolites that generate ROS (e.g., quinones).

Point 13 The balance between activation and detoxication by xenobiotic-biotransforming enzymes is often a key determinant of chemical toxicity, and is often the basis for organ or species differences in toxicity.

Point 14 Exposure to xenobiotics (especially drugs) is largely through oral ingestion, and the small intestine and liver are highly developed to limit systemic exposure to orally ingested xenobiotics, a process known as *first-pass elimination* (or *presystemic elimination*). The enterocytes at the tips of the small intestinal villi express the efflux transporters P-glycoprotein (ABCB1 or MDR1) and BCRP (ABCG2), which serve to limit xenobiotic absorption. Enterocytes and hepatocytes express high levels of certain CYP and UGT enzymes, which biotransform a wide variety of xenobiotics.

Point 15 Although the small intestine and liver contain the highest concentrations, xenobiotic-biotransforming enzymes are nevertheless widely distributed throughout the body.

Point 16 Species differences in xenobiotic-biotransforming enzymes are often the basis for species differences in both the qualitative and quantitative aspects of xenobiotic biotransformation and toxicity.

Point 17 In sexually mature rats and, to a lesser extent, mice there are marked gender differences in the expression of certain xenobiotic-biotransforming enzymes (both oxidative and conjugating enzymes). In other species, including humans, gender differences either do not exist or generally represent less than a twofold difference.

Point 18 Large interindividual differences in pharmacokinetic parameters upon administration or exposure to a chemical can reflect genetically determined differences in the activity of xenobiotic-biotransforming enzymes or transporters (genetic polymorphisms) or environmental factors, such as drug–drug interactions. The study of the causes, prevalence, and impact of heritable differences in xenobiotic-biotransforming enzymes is known as *pharmacogenetics*.

Point 19 Stereochemical aspects can play an important role in the interaction between a xenobiotic and its biotransforming enzyme (from both a substrate and an inhibitor perspective), and xenobiotic-biotransforming enzymes can play a key role in converting one stereoisomer to another, a process known as *mutarotation* or *inversion of configuration*.

Point 20 Mass spectrometry is widely used to characterize the structure of metabolites. Certain xenobiotic reactions are associated with discrete changes in mass: the loss of 2 atomic mass units (amu) signifies dehydrogenation, whereas the loss of 14 amu usually signifies demethylation ($-CH_2$). Several reactions result in an increase in mass, including reduction (+2 amu = 2H), methylation (+14 amu = CH_2), oxidation (+16 amu = O), hydration (+18 amu = H_2O), acetylation (+42 amu = C_2H_2O), sulfonation (+80 amu = SO_3), glucuronidation (+176 amu = $C_6H_8O_6$), carbamoyl glucuronidation (+220 amu = $C_7H_8O_8$), and conjugation with GSH (+305 amu = $C_{10}H_{15}N_3O_6S$). Conjugation of acidic drugs with CoA (to form acyl-CoA thioesters) increases mass by 749 amu, but these conjugates are not transported out of cells and, hence, are not detected in blood, bile, or urine.

HYDROLYSIS, REDUCTION, AND OXIDATION

Hydrolysis

Carboxylesterases, Cholinesterases, and Paraoxonase—
The hydrolysis of carboxylic acid esters, amides, and thioesters is largely catalyzed by carboxylesterases and by two cholinesterases: true acetylcholinesterase in erythrocyte membranes and pseudocholinesterase, which is also known as butyrylcholinesterase and is located in serum. Phosphoric acid esters are hydrolyzed by paraoxonase, a serum enzyme also known as aryldialkylphosphatase. Phosphoric acid anhydrides are hydrolyzed by a related organophosphatase.

Carboxylesterases in serum and tissues and serum cholinesterase collectively determine the duration and site of action of certain drugs. The hydrolysis of xenobiotic esters and amides

endoplasmic reticulum, which facilitates their interaction. As shown in Figure 6–4, the first part of the catalytic cycle involves the activation of oxygen, and the final part involves substrate oxidation, which entails the abstraction of a hydrogen atom or an electron from the substrate followed by oxygen rebound (radical recombination). Following the binding of substrate to the CYP enzyme, the heme iron is reduced from the ferric (Fe^{3+}) to the ferrous (Fe^{2+}) state by the addition of a single electron from NADPH–cytochrome P450 reductase. Release of the oxidized substrate returns cytochrome P450 to its initial state. If the catalytic cycle is interrupted, oxygen is released as superoxide anion (O_2^{-}) or hydrogen peroxide (H_2O_2).

Cytochrome P450 catalyzes the following types of oxidation reactions:

1. hydroxylation of an aliphatic or aromatic carbon
2. epoxidation of a double bond
3. heteroatom (*S-*, *N-*, and *I-*) oxygenation and *N*-hydroxylation
4. heteroatom (*O-*, *S-*, *N-*, and *Si-*) dealkylation
5. oxidative group transfer
6. cleavage of esters
7. dehydrogenation

Liver microsomes from all mammalian species contain numerous P450 enzymes, each with the potential to catalyze the various reactions shown in Figures 6–5 to 6–12. In general,

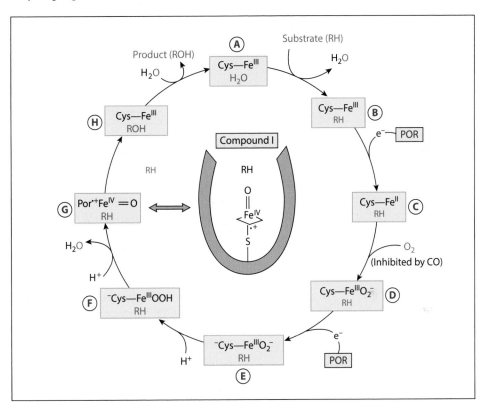

Other reactions

One-electron reduction	**C** ($Cys\text{—}Fe^{II}RH$)	→ **A** ($Cys\text{—}Fe^{III} + RH^{-}$)
Superoxide anion production	**D** ($Cys\text{—}Fe^{III}O_2^{-} RH$)	→ **B** ($Cys\text{—}Fe^{III} RH$) + O_2^{-}
Hydrogen peroxide production	**E** ($^{-}Cys\text{—}Fe^{III}O_2^{-} RH$) + $2H^{+}$	→ **B** ($Cys\text{—}Fe^{III} RH$) + H_2O_2
Hydrogen peroxide shunt	**B** ($Cys\text{—}Fe^{III} RH$) + H_2O_2	→ **F** ($^{-}Cys\text{—}Fe^{III}OOH RH$) + H^{+}
Peroxide shunt to form Compound I	**B** ($Cys\text{—}Fe^{III} RH$) + XOOH	→ **G** ($Por^{\cdot+}Fe^{IV}=O$ RH) + XOH

FIGURE 6–4 Catalytic cycle of cytochrome P450. Cytochrome P450 is represented as Cys-Fe^{III}, where Cys represents the fifth ligand (a cysteine thiolate) to the ferric heme iron. RH and ROH represent the substrate and product (hydroxylated metabolite), respectively. The intermediates in the catalytic cycle are as follows: A, ferric resting state; B, substrate bound; C, ferrous intermediate; D, ferrisuperoxo anion intermediate; E, ferriperoxo intermediate with an electron delocalized over the Cys thiolate bond; F, ferrihydroperoxy intermediate (with a negative charge on the Cys thiolate bond); G, compound I, an iron^{IV}-oxo porphyrin cation, which is responsible for most substrate oxidation reactions; H, enzyme in its resting state prior to the release of product formed by hydrogen abstraction followed by oxygen rebound. Fe^{II}, Fe^{III}, Fe^{IV}, and Fe^{V} refer to iron in the ferrous, ferric, ferryl, and perferryl state, respectively. It should be noted that although it is written as por$^{\cdot+}Fe^{IV}=O$, compound I is in the highly oxidized perferryl (Fe^{V}) state when the oxidation state of the porphyrin ring is also taken into account.

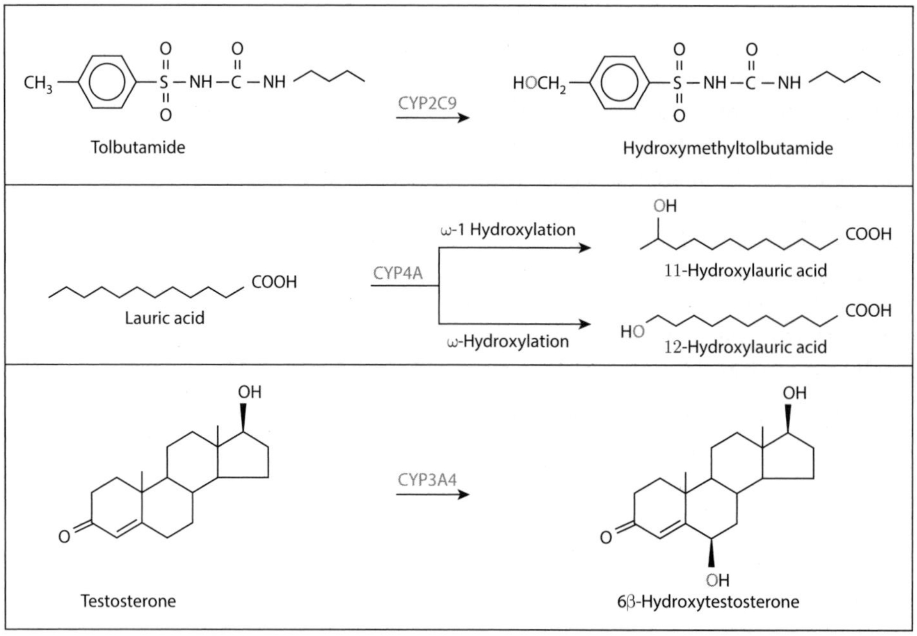

FIGURE 6–5 Examples of reactions catalyzed by cytochrome P450: hydroxylation of aliphatic carbon.

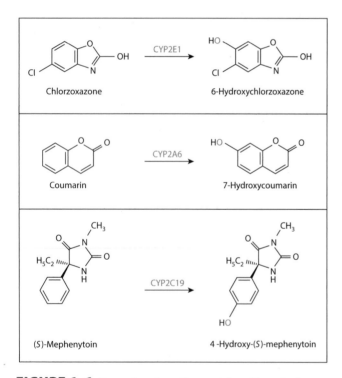

FIGURE 6–6 Examples of reactions catalyzed by cytochrome P450: hydroxylation of aromatic carbon.

The levels and activity of each CYP enzyme vary from one individual to the next, due to environmental and/or genetic factors. Decreased CYP enzyme activity can result from (1) a genetic mutation that either blocks the synthesis of a CYP enzyme or leads to the synthesis of a catalytically compromised, inactive, or unstable enzyme, which gives rise to the poor and intermediate metabolizer genotypes; (2) exposure to an environmental factor (such as an infectious disease or an inflammatory process) that suppresses CYP enzyme expression; or (3) exposure to a xenobiotic that inhibits or inactivates a preexisting CYP enzyme. By inhibiting cytochrome P450, one drug can impair the biotransformation of another, which may lead to an exaggerated pharmacologic or toxicologic response to the second drug. Increased CYP enzyme activity can result from (1) gene duplication leading to overexpression of a CYP enzyme, (2) exposure to drugs and other xenobiotics that induce the synthesis of cytochrome P450, or (3) stimulation of preexisting enzyme by a xenobiotic.

Induction of cytochrome P450 by xenobiotics increases CYP enzyme activity. By inducing cytochrome P450, one drug can stimulate the metabolism of a second drug and thereby decrease or ameliorate its therapeutic effect. Allelic variants, which arise by point mutations in the wild-type gene, are another source of interindividual variation in CYP activity. Environmental factors known to affect CYP levels include medications, foods, social habits (e.g., alcohol consumption and cigarette smoking), and disease status (diabetes, inflammation, viral and bacterial infection, hyperthyroidism, and hypothyroidism). When environmental factors influence CYP enzyme levels, considerable variation may be observed during repeated measures of xenobiotic biotransformation (e.g., drug metabolism) in the same individual. Due to their broad substrate specificity, it is possible that two or more CYP enzymes can contribute to the metabolism of a single compound.

CYP enzymes are classified into subfamilies based on amino acid sequence identity.

The function and regulation of CYP1A1, CYP1A2, CYP1B1, CYP2E1, CYP2R1, CYP2S1, CYP2U1, and CYYP2W1 are highly conserved among mammalian species and these proteins have the same names in all mammalian species. In most other cases, the CYP enzymes are named in a species-specific manner.

The pharmacologic or toxic effects of certain drugs are exaggerated in a significant percentage of the population due to a heritable deficiency in a CYP enzyme. Inasmuch as the biotransformation of a xenobiotic in humans is frequently dominated by a single CYP enzyme, the considerable effort in identifying which CYP enzyme or enzymes are involved in eliminating the drug is known as *reaction phenotyping* or *enzyme mapping*. Four approaches to reaction phenotyping are as follows:

1. *Correlation analysis* involves measuring the rate of xenobiotic metabolism by several samples of human liver microsomes and correlating reaction rates with the variation in the level or activity of the individual P450 enzymes in the same microsomal samples.

2. *Chemical inhibition* evaluates the effects of known CYP enzyme inhibitors on the metabolism of a xenobiotic by human liver microsomes. Inhibitors of cytochrome CYP must be used cautiously because most of them can inhibit more than one CYP enzyme.

3. *Antibody inhibition* determines the effects of inhibitory antibodies against selected CYP enzymes on the biotransformation of a xenobiotic by human liver microsomes. This method alone can potentially establish which human CYP enzyme is responsible for biotransforming a xenobiotic.

4. *Biotransformation by purified or recombinant human CYP enzymes* establishes whether a particular CYP enzyme can or cannot biotransform a xenobiotic, but it does not address whether that CYP enzyme contributes substantially to reactions catalyzed by human liver microsomes.

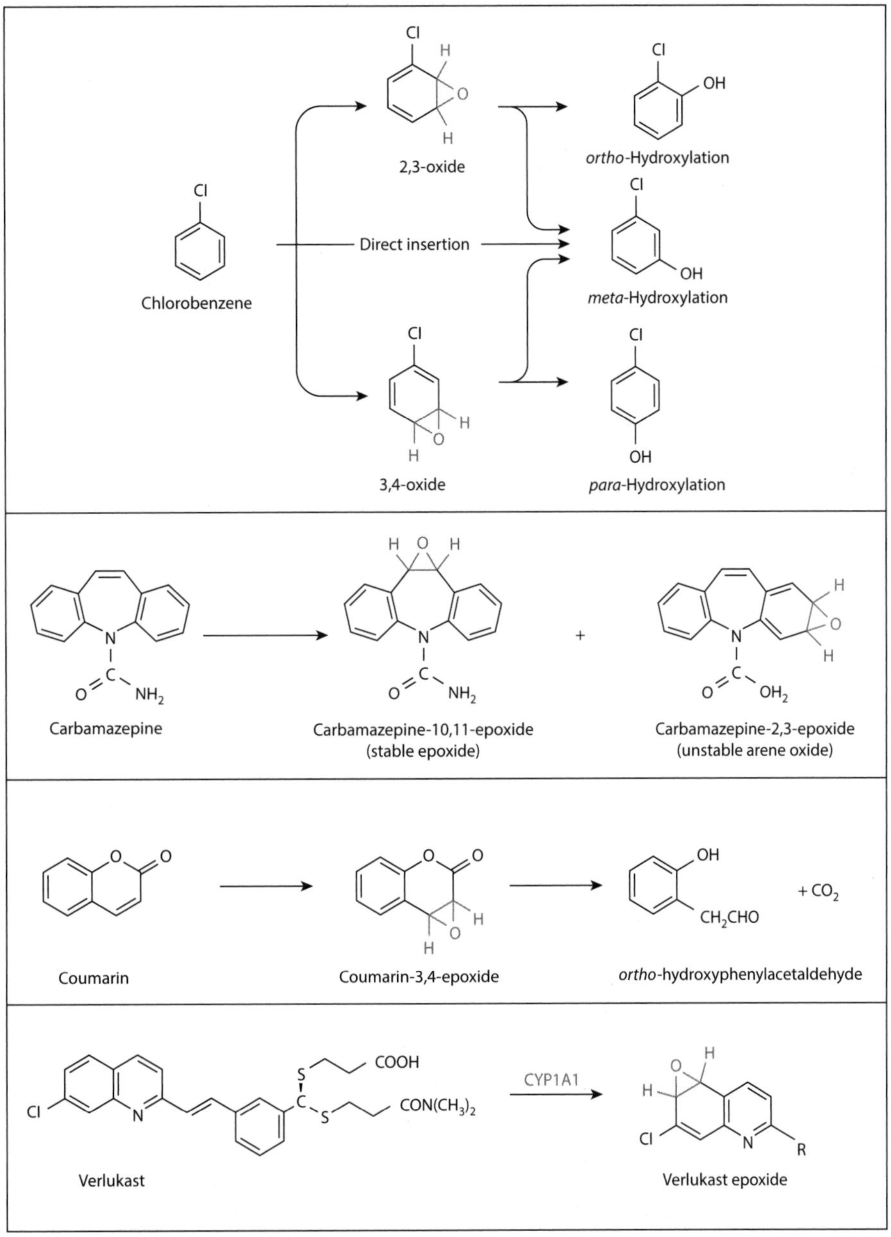

FIGURE 6-7 Examples of reactions catalyzed by cytochrome P450: epoxidation.

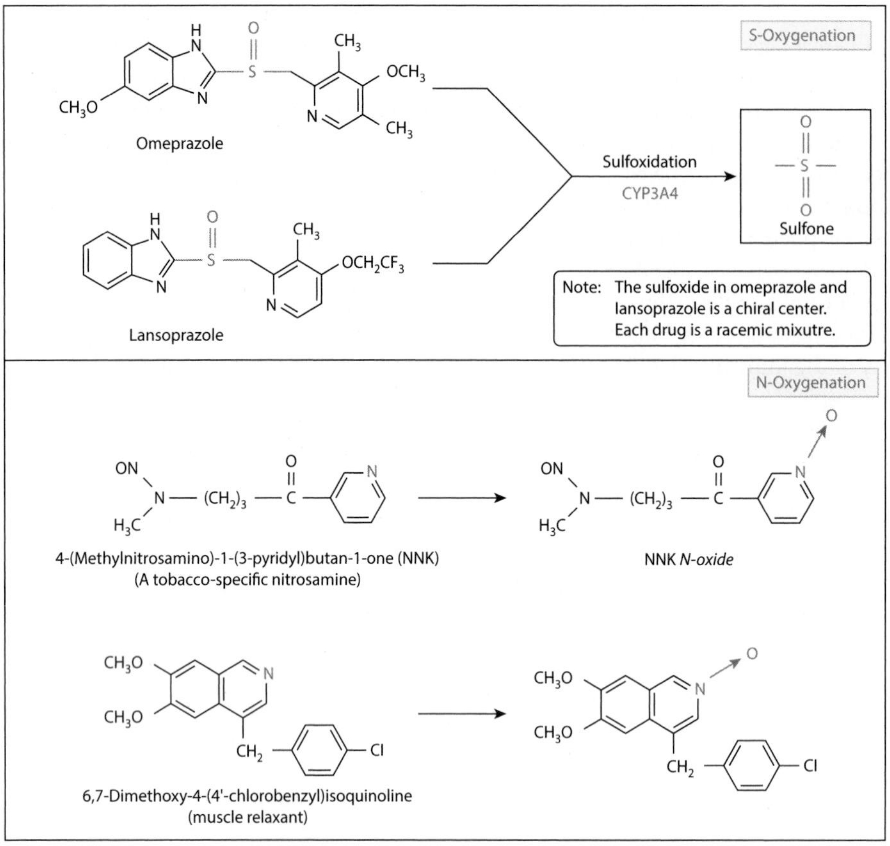

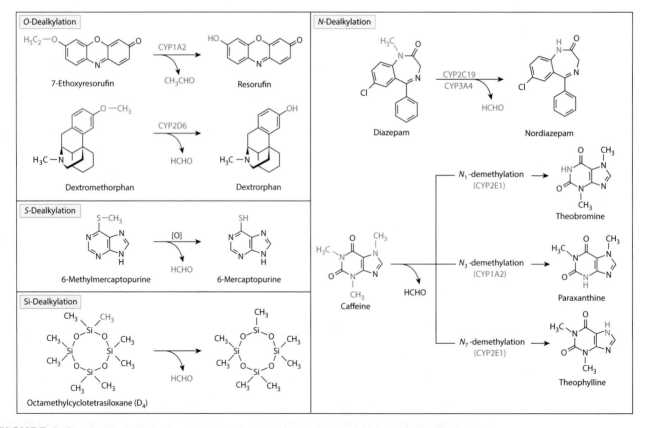

FIGURE 6–8 Examples of reactions catalyzed by cytochrome P450: heteroatom oxygenation.

FIGURE 6–9 Examples of reactions catalyzed by cytochrome P450: heteroatom dealkylation.

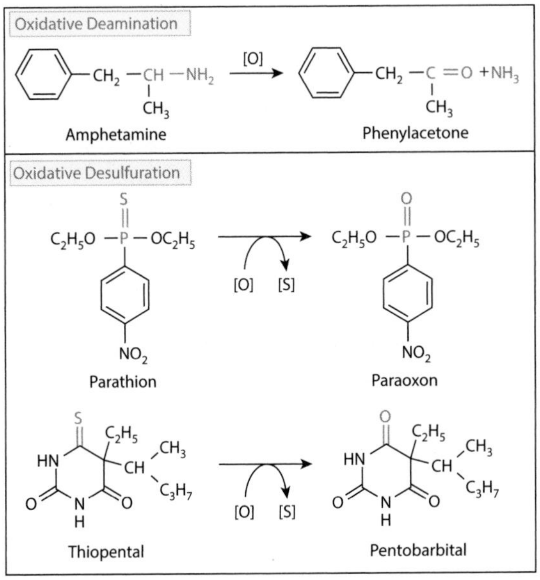

FIGURE 6–10 Examples of reactions catalyzed by cytochrome P450: oxidative group transfer.

Examples of substrates, inhibitors, and inducers for each CYP enzyme in human liver microsomes are given in Table 6–2. Because reaction phenotyping in vitro is not always carried out with toxicologically relevant substrate concentrations, the CYP enzyme that appears responsible for biotransforming the drug in vitro may not be the CYP enzyme responsible for biotransforming the drug in vivo.

Activation of Xenobiotics by Cytochrome P450—The role of human CYP enzymes in the activation of procarcinogens and protoxicants and some cytochrome P450–dependent reactions are summarized in Table 6–3. Many of the chemicals listed in Table 6–3 are also detoxified by cytochrome P450 by conversion to less toxic metabolites. In some cases, the same CYP enzyme catalyzes both activation and detoxication reactions. For example, CYP3A4 activates aflatoxin B_1 to the hepatotoxic and tumorigenic 8,9-epoxide, but it also detoxifies aflatoxin B_1 by 3-hydroxylation to aflatoxin Q_1. Complex factors determine the balance between xenobiotic activation and detoxication.

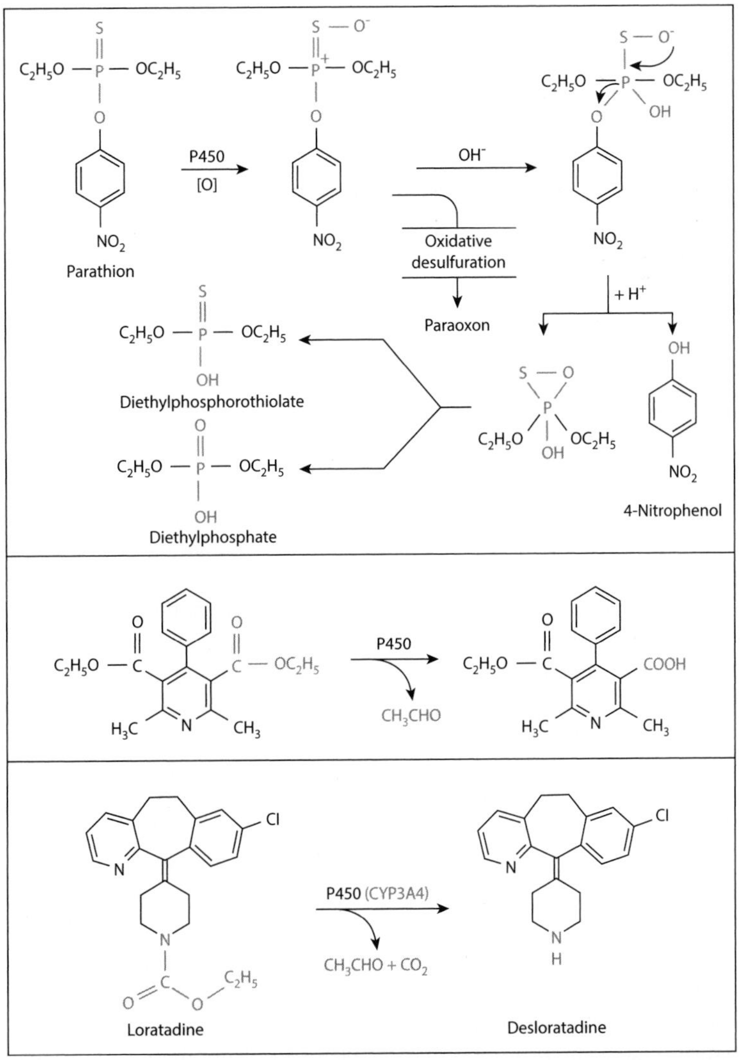

FIGURE 6–11 Examples of reactions catalyzed by cytochrome P450 that resemble hydrolytic reactions: cleavage of a thiophosphate (parathion), a carboxylic acid ester (2,6-dimethyl-4-phenyl-3,5-pyridinecarboxylic acid diethyl ester), and a carbamate (loratadine).

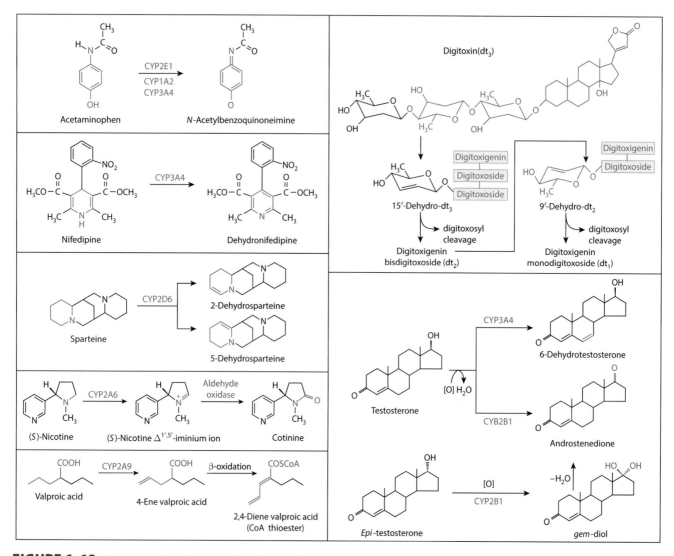

FIGURE 6–12 Examples of reactions catalyzed by cytochrome P450: dehydrogenation.

Inhibition of Cytochrome P450—Inhibition of CYP is a major cause of drug–drug interactions and may cause the withdrawal of regulatory approval. The magnitude of the drug–drug interaction depends on the degree of CYP inhibition by the perpetrator drug (those xenobiotics that inhibit or induce the enzyme that is responsible for clearing a victim drug) and the fractional metabolism of the victim drug (xenobiotic whose clearance is largely determined by a single route of elimination, such as a single CYP) by the affected enzyme. Inhibitory drug interactions generally fall into two categories: direct inhibition (which can be competitive, noncompetitive, and uncompetitive) and metabolism-dependent inhibition (which can be irreversible or quasi-irreversible). Direct inhibition can be subdivided into two types. The first involves competition between two drugs that are metabolized by the same CYP enzyme. The second is also competitive in nature, but the inhibitor is not a substrate for the affected CYP enzyme. Metabolism-dependent inhibition occurs when cytochrome P450 converts a xenobiotic to a metabolite that is a more potent inhibitor, either reversible or irreversible, than the parent compound.

Induction of Cytochrome P450—Xenosensors The induction (upregulation) of xenobiotic-biotransforming enzymes and transporters is a receptor-mediated, adaptive process that augments xenobiotic elimination during periods of high xenobiotic exposure. It is not a toxicological or pathological response, but enzyme induction is often associated with liver enlargement (due to both hepatocellular hypertrophy and hyperplasia), and it may be associated with toxicological and pharmacological consequences, especially for the safety evaluation of drug candidates in laboratory animals and for clinical practice in humans. In animals and humans, enzyme induction may be associated with pharmacokinetic tolerance, whereby the xenobiotic induces its own elimination.

Inducers of cytochrome P450 increase the rate of xenobiotic biotransformation. Some of the CYP enzymes in human liver microsomes are inducible (Table 6–2). P450 induction typically lowers blood levels, which compromises the therapeutic goal of drug therapy but does not cause an exaggerated response to the drug.

TABLE 6–2 Examples of clinically relevant substrates, inhibitors, and inducers of the major human liver microsomal P450 enzymes involved in xenobiotic biotransformation.

	CYP1A2	CYP2A6	CYP2B6	CYP2C8	CYP2C9	CYP2C19	CYP2E1
Substrates	Alosetron	Coumarin	Bupropion	Amodiaquine	Diclofenac	Fluoxetine	Aniline
	Caffeine	Nicotine	Efavirenz	Cerivastatin	Fluoxetine	S-Mephenytoin	Chlorzoxazone
	Duloxetine		Propofol	Paclitaxel	Flurbiprofen	Lansoprazole	Lauric acid
	7-Ethoxyresorufin		S-Mephenytoin	Rosiglitazone	Phenytoin	Moclobemide	4-Nitrophenol
	Phenacetin		Cyclophosphamide	Repaglinide	Tolbutamide	Omeprazole	
	Tacrine		Ketamine		S-Warfarin	Pantoprazole	
	Tizanidine		Meperidine				
	Theophylline		Nevirapine				
Inhibitors	Acyclovir	Methoxsalen	Clopidogrel	Gemfibrozil	Amiodarone	Fluvoxamine	Clomethiazole
	Cimetidine	Pilocarpine	3-Isopropenyl-3-methyl diamantane	Montelukast	Capecitabine	Moclobemide	Diallyldisulfide
	Ciprofloxacin	Tranylcypromine	2-Isopropenyl-2-methyladamantane	Quercetin	Fluconazole	Nootkatone	Diethyldithiocarbamate
	Famotidine	Tryptamine	Phencyclidine	Rosiglitazone	Fluoxetine	Omeprazole	Disulfiram
	Fluvoxamine		Sertraline	Rosuvastatin	Fluvoxamine	Ticlopidine	
	Furafylline		Thio-TEPA	Trimethoprim	Oxandrolone		
	Mexiletine		Ticlopidine		Sulfaphenazole		
	α-Naphthoflavone		Phenylethylpiperidine		Sulfinpyrazone		
	Norfloxacin				Tienilic acid		
	Propafenone						
	Verapamil						
	Zileuton						
Inducers	3-Methylcholanthrene	Dexamethasone	Phenobarbital	Phenobarbital	Phenobarbital	Phenobarbital	Ethanol
	β-Naphthoflavone	Pyrazole	Phenytoin	Rifampin	Rifampin	Rifampin	Isoniazid
	Omeprazole		Rifampin				
	Lansoprazole						
	TCDD						

	CYP2AD6			CYP3A4			
Substrates	Atomoxetine	(R)-Metoprolol		Alfentanil	Clopidogrel	Fentanyl	Midazolam	Saquinavir
	Amitriptyline	Methylphenidate		Alfuzosin	Cyclosporine	Fluticasone	Mifepristone	Sildenafil
	Aripiprazole	Mexiletine		Alprazolam	Depsipeptide	Gallopamil	Mosapride	Sibutramine
	Brofaromine	Morphine		Amlodipine	Dexamethasone	Gefitinib	Nicardipine	Simvastatin

(Continued)

TABLE 6–2 Examples of clinically relevant substrates, inhibitors, and inducers of the major human liver microsomal P450 enzymes involved in xenobiotic biotransformation. (Continued)

	CYP2AD6	CYP3A4
Substrates	(±)-Bufuralol, (S)-Chlorpheniramine, Chlorpromazine, Clomipramine, Codeine, Debrisoquine, Desipramine, Dextromethorphan, Dolasetron, Duloxetine, Fentanyl, Haloperidol (reduced), Imipramine, Loperamide, Nortriptyline, Ondansetron, Paroxetine, Perhexiline, Pimozide, Propafenone, (+)-Propranolol, Sparteine, Tamoxifen, Thioridazine, Timolol, Tramadol, (R)-Venlafaxine	Amprenavir, Aprepitant, Artemether, Astemizole, Atazanavir, Atorvastatin, Azithromycin, Barnidipine, Bexarotene, Bortezomib, Brotizolam, Budesonide, Buspirone, Capravirine, Carbamazepine, Cibenzoline, Cilastazol, Cisapride, Clarithromycin, Clindamycin, Dextromethorphan, Diergotamine, α-Dihydroergocriptine, Disopyramide, Docetaxel, Domperidone, Dutasteride, Ebastine, Eletriptan, Eplerenone, Ergotamine, Erlotinib, Erythromycin, Eplerenone, Ethosuximide, Etoperidone, Everolimus, Ethinyl estradiol, Etoricoxib, Felodipine, Gepirone, Granisetron, Gestodene, Halofantrine, Laquinimod, Imatinib, Indinavir, Isradipine, Itraconazole, Karenitecin, Ketamine, Levomethadyl, Lonafarnib, Lopinavir, Loperamide, Lumefantrine, Lovastatin, Medroxyprogesterone, Methylprednisolone, Mexazolam, Nifedipine, Nimoldipine, Nisoldipine, Nitrendipine, Norethindrone, Oxatomide, Oxybutynin, Perospirone, Pimozide, Pranidipine, Praziquantel, Quetiapine, Quinidine, Quinine, Reboxetine, Rifabutin, Ritonavir, Rosuvastatin, Ruboxistaurin, Salmetrol, Sirolimus, Sunitinib, Tacrolimus, Tadalafil, Telithromycin, Terfenadine, Testosterone, Tiagabine, Tipranavir, Tirilazad, Tofisopam, Triazolam, Trimetrexate, Vardenafil, Vinblastine, Vincristine, Vinorelbine, Ziprasidone, Zonisamide
Inhibitors	Amiodarone, Buproprion, Chlorpheniramine, Cimetidine, Clomipramine, Duloxetine, Haloperidol, Fluoxetine, Methadone, Mibefradil, Paroxetine, Quinidine, Sertraline, Terbinafine	Amiodarone, Amprenavir, Aprepitant, Atazanavir, Azamulin, Bosentan, Amprenavir, Cimetidine, Clarithromycin, Diltiazem, Erythromycin, Felbamate, Fluconazole, Efavirenz, Fluvoxamine, Fosamprenavir, Gestodene, Grapefruit juice, Ketoconazole, Indinavir, Nifedipine, Itraconazole, Mibefradil, Nefazodone, Nelfinavir, Ritonavir, Roxithromycin, Rifampin, Saquinavir, St. John's wort, Telithromycin, Troleandomycin, Verapamil, Troglitazone
Inducers	NA	Avasimibe, Bosentan, Carbamazepine, Clotrimazole, Cyproterone acetate, Dexamethasone, Etoposide, Guggulsterone, Hyperforin, Lovastatin, Mifepristone, Nelfinavir, Omeprazole, Paclitaxel, PCBs, Phenobarbital, Phenytoin, Rifabutin, Rifapentine, Ritonavir, Simvastatin, Spironolactone, Sulfinpyrazone, Topotecan, Troleandomycin, Vitamin E, Vitamin K2, Yin zhi wuang

TABLE 6–3 Examples of xenobiotics activated by human P450.

CYP1A2	**CYP2D6**	**CYP2E1**
Acetaminophen	**NNK**	Acetaminophen
2-Acetylaminofluorene		Acrylonitrile
4-Aminobiphenyl	**CYP2F1**	Benzene
2-Aminofluorene	3-Methylindole	Carbon tetrachloride
2-Naphthylamine	Acetaminophen	Chloroform
NNK	Valproic acid	Dichloromethane
Amino acid pyrolysis products (DiMeQx, MeIQ, MeIQx, Glu P-2, IQ, PhIP, Trp P-1, Trp P-2)	**CYP1A1 and 1B1**	1,2-Dichloropropane
	Benzo[a]pyrene and other polycyclic aromatic hydrocarbons	Ethylene dibromide
Tacrine		Ethylene dichloride
		Ethyl carbamate
CYP2A6 and 2A13	**CYP3A4**	Halothane
NNK and bulky nitrosamines	Acetaminophen	N-Nitrosodimethylamine
N-Nitrosodiethylamine	Aflatoxin B1 and G1	Styrene
Aflatoxin B1	6-Aminochrysene	Trichloroethylene
	Benzo[a]pyrene 7,8-dihydrodiol	Vinyl chloride
CYP2B6	Cyclophosphamide	
6-Aminochrysene	Ifosfamide	**CYP4B1**
Cyclophosphamide	1-Nitropyrene	Ipomeanol
Ifosfamide	Sterigmatocystin	3-Methylindole
	Senecionine	2-Aminofluorene
CYP2C8, 9, 18, 19	Tris(2,3-dibromopropyl) phosphate	
Tienilic acid		
Phenytoin		
Valproic acid		

NNK, 4-(methylnitrosamino)-1-(3-pyridyl)-1-butanone, a tobacco-specific nitrosamine.
Data from Guengerich FP, Shimada T: Oxidation of toxic and carcinogenic chemicals by human cytochrome P-450 enzymes. *Chem Res Toxicol*, 1991 Jul-Aug;4(4):391–407.

Although induction of cytochrome P450 may increase the activation of procarcinogens to DNA-reactive metabolites, there is little evidence from either human epidemiologic studies or animal experimentation that P450 induction enhances the incidence or multiplicity of tumors caused by known chemical carcinogens. In fact, most evidence points to a protective role of enzyme induction against chemical-induced neoplasia. Cytochrome P450 induction can cause pharmacokinetic tolerance whereby larger drug doses must be administered to achieve therapeutic blood levels due to increased drug bio-transformation.

CYP induction is mediated by four ligand-activated receptors, namely, AhR, CAR, PXR, and PPARα (Table 6–4). These so-called xenosensors resemble other nuclear receptors, such as steroid and thyroid hormone receptors, with cross-talk among xenosensors and cross-talk between xenosensors and other nuclear receptors. Xenosensors have a ligand-binding domain (LBD) and a DNA-binding domain (DBD). In general, CYP induction involves the following steps (with steps 2 and 3 reversed in the case of AhR): (1) binding of ligand (xenobiotic) to the receptor, which triggers conformational changes that promote its dissociation from accessory proteins (such as corepressors, chaperones, and cytoplasm retention proteins) and promote its association with coactivators; (2) dimerization of the ligand-bound receptor with a partner protein to form a DNA-binding heterodimer (which is analogous to the two halves of a clothes peg coming together to form a functional unit); (3) translocation of the functional receptor heterodimer from the cytoplasm to the nucleus; (4) binding of the functional receptor heterodimer to discrete regions of DNA (response elements) that are typically located in the 5′-promoter region of the gene (which is analogous to a clothes peg being fastened to a clothes line); (5) recruitment of other transcription factors and coactivators (such as histone and RNA methyltransferases, histone and chromatin deacetylases, and histone remodeling helicases) and RNA polymerase to form a transcription complex; and (6) gene transcription, which leads to increased levels of CYP mRNA and protein (as well as other xenobiotic-biotransforming enzymes and transporters). As is the case with all nuclear receptors, the details of the process of activating a xenosensor to its transcriptionally active form are complex and multifaceted.

CONJUGATION

Conjugation reactions include glucuronidation, sulfonation (often called sulfation), acetylation, methylation, conjugation with glutathione (mercapturic acid synthesis), and conjugation with amino acids (such as glycine, taurine, and glutamic acid). The cosubstrates for these reactions, which are shown in Figure 6–13, react with functional groups that are either present

TABLE 6–4 Receptors mediating the induction (or suppression) of cytochrome P450 enzymes and other xenobiotic-biotransforming enzymes and transporters.

Nuclear Receptor	Response Element(s)	Receptor Activators	Regulated Genes*
AhR	XRE	PAHs, TCDD (other PHAHs), β-naphthoflavone, indigoids, tryptophan metabolites, omeprazole, lansoprazole	CYP1A1, 1A2, 1B1, 2S1, UGT1A1, UGT1A6, AKR1A1, AKR1C1-4
CAR	DR-3 DR-4 ER-6	Phenobarbital, phenytoin, carbamazepine, CITCO (human), TCPOBOP (mouse), clotrimazole, (Many PXR agonists are also CAR agonists, and vice versa)	CYP2A6, 2B6, 2C8, 2C9, 2C19, 3A4, UGT1A1, SULT1A1, AKR1D1, ALAS, MRP2, MRP3, MRP4
PXR	DR-3 DR-4 ER-6 ER-8	Amprenavir, avasimibe, bosentan, bile acids, carbamazepine, clindamycin, clotrimazole, cortisol, cyproterone acetate, dicloxacillin, efavirenz, etoposide, dexamethasone, griseofulvin, guggulsterone, hyperforin (SJW), indinavir, lovastatin, mifepristone, nafcillin, nelfinavir, nifedipine, omeprazole, paclitaxel, PCBs, phenobarbital, phthalate monoesters, 5β-pregnane-3,20-dione, rifabutin, rifampin, ritonavir, saquinavir, simvastatin, spironolactone, sulfinpyrazone, TAO, tetracycline, topotecan, transnonachlor, troglitazone, verapamil, vitamin E, vitamin K_2	CYP2A6, 2B6, 2C8, 2C9, 2C19, 3A4, 3A7, 4F12, 7A1↓, CES2, SULT2A1, UGT1A1, 1A3, 1A4, 1A6, GSTA1, AKR1D1, PAPSS2, ALAS, MDR1, MRP2, AhR
PPARα	DR-1	Fibrates, WY-14643, perfluorodecanoic acid	CYP4A, UGT1A9, 2B4
Nrf2	ARE	β-Naphthoflavone, oltipraz, phenolic antioxidants (e.g., BHA and BHT), phenylisothiocyanate, diethyl maleate, phorone	NQO1, mEH, AKR7A, UGTs, GSTA1, γ-GCL, MRP1
GR	GRE	Glucocorticoids (e.g., dexamethasone)	CYP2C9, 2B6, 3A4, 3A5, CAR, PXR
FXR	IR-1	Bile acids, GW4064, AGN29, AGN31	BSEP, I-BABP, MDR3, UGT2B4, SULT2A1, OATP1B3, PPARα, SHP
LXRα	DR-4	GW3965, T0901317, paxiline, F_3methylIAA,† acetylpodocarpic dimer (APD)	LRH1, SHP, CYP7A, LXRα, CYP3A4 ↓↓, 2B6 ↓
VDR	DR-3 ER-6 IR-0	1α,25-Dihydroxyvitamin D_3, lithocholate	CYP2B6, 2C9, 3A4, SULT2A1
HNF1α‡			OATP1B1, OATP1B3, CYP7A1, UGT1A6, 1A8, 1A9, 1A10, HNF4α, PXR, kidney-specific expression of OAT1, OAT3, URAT1
HNF4α	DR		CYP2A6, 2B6, 2C9, 2D6, 3A4, DD4, MDR1, PXR, CAR, FXR, PPARα, HNF1α
LRH-1	DR-4		CYP7A, ASBT
SHP	None		Targets of PPARα ↓, AhR ↓, PXR ↓, CAR ↓, LRH-1 ↓, HNF4α ↓, LXRα ↓, GR ↓

A downward arrow indicates downregulation (suppression). All others are upregulated (induced).

†*[3-Chloro-4-(3-(7-propyl-3-trifluoromethyl-6-(4,5)-isoxazolyl)propylthio)-phenylacetic acid].*

‡*The HNF1α consensus sequence is GTTTAATNATTAAC.*

on the xenobiotic or are introduced or exposed during oxidation, reduction, or hydrolysis. With the exception of methylation and acetylation, conjugations result in a large increase in xenobiotic hydrophilicity, which greatly facilitates excretion of foreign chemicals. Glucuronidation, sulfation, acetylation, and methylation involve reactions with activated or "high-energy" cosubstrates, whereas conjugation with amino

acids or glutathione involves reactions with activated xenobiotics. Except for the glucuronosyltransferases, most conjugation enzymes are mainly located in the cytosol (Table 6–1).

Glucuronidation

Glucuronidation requires the cosubstrate uridine diphosphate-glucuronic acid (UDP-glucuronic acid), and the reaction is

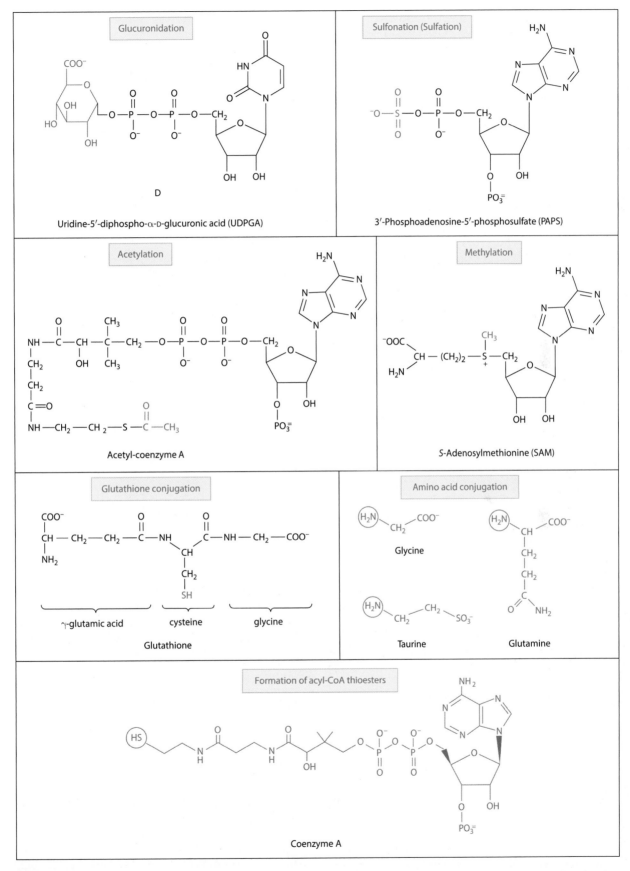

FIGURE 6–13 Structures of cofactors for phase II biotransformation. The functional group that reacts with or is transferred to the xenobiotic is shown in red.

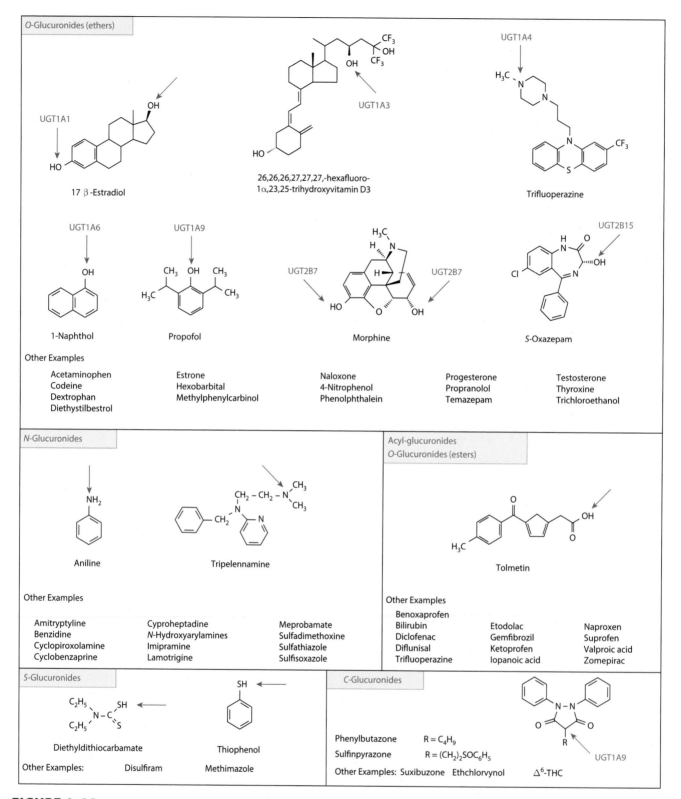

FIGURE 6–14   Examples of xenobiotics and endogenous substrates that are glucuronidated. The arrow indicates the site of glucuronidation, with the UGT enzyme if selective.

catalyzed by UDP-glucuronosyltransferases (UGTs). Examples of xenobiotics that are glucuronidated are shown in Figure 6–14. The site of glucuronidation is generally an electron-rich nucleophilic heteroatom (O, N, or S) as found in aliphatic alcohols and phenols, carboxylic acids, primary and secondary aromatic and aliphatic amines, and free sulfhydryl groups. Endogenous substrates for glucuronidation include bilirubin, steroid hormones, and thyroid hormones.

Glucuronide conjugates of xenobiotics and endogenous compounds are polar, water-soluble metabolites. Whether glucuronides are excreted from the body in bile or urine depends on the size of the aglycone (parent compound or unconjugated metabolite). The carboxylic acid moiety of glucuronic acid, which is ionized at physiologic pH, promotes excretion because (1) it increases the aqueous solubility of the xenobiotic and (2) it is recognized by the biliary and renal organic anion transport systems, which enables glucuronides to be secreted into urine and bile. Glucuronides of xenobiotics are substrates for β-glucuronidase present in the intestinal microflora. The intestinal enzyme can release the aglycone, which undergoes *enterohepatic circulation* delaying elimination of the xenobiotic.

Cofactor availability can limit the rate of glucuronidation of drugs that are administered in high doses and are conjugated extensively, such as aspirin and acetaminophen.

Sulfonation

Many xenobiotics and endogenous substrates undergo sulfonation. Sulfate conjugation is catalyzed by sulfotransferases, a multigene family of enzymes that generally produces a highly water-soluble sulfuric acid ester. The cosubstrate for the reaction is 3′-phosphoadenosine-5′-phosphosulfate (PAPS; see Figure 6–13).

Sulfate conjugation involves the transfer of sulfonate, not sulfate (i.e., SO_3^-, not SO_4^-) from PAPS to the xenobiotic. (The commonly used terms *sulfation* and *sulfate conjugation* are used here, even though *sulfonation* and *sulfonate conjugation* are more appropriate descriptors.) Table 6–4 lists examples of xenobiotics and endogenous compounds that are sulfonated without prior biotransformation by oxidation enzymes. An even greater number of xenobiotics are sulfated after a hydroxyl group is exposed or introduced during oxidative or hydrolytic biotransformation.

Sulfate conjugates of xenobiotics are excreted mainly in urine. Sulfatases present in the endoplasmic reticulum and lysosomes primarily hydrolyze sulfates of endogenous compounds. Some sulfate conjugates are substrates for further biotransformation.

PAPS is synthesized from inorganic sulfate (SO_4^{2-}) and ATP in a two-step reaction. The major source of sulfate required for the synthesis of PAPS appears to be derived from cysteine through a complex oxidation sequence. The low cellular concentration of PAPS (~75 μM versus ~350 μM UDP-glucuronic acid and ~10 mM glutathione) limits the capacity for xenobiotic sulfonation.

Multiple sulfotransferases have been identified in all mammalian species examined. There are two major enzyme classes: membrane-bound enzymes are found in the Golgi apparatus and soluble enzymes are located in the cytoplasm. Sulfotransferases are arranged into gene families (SULT1 to SULT5) that share at least 45% amino acid sequence identity, and are further subdivided into several subfamilies. Each family appears to work on a specific functional group (i.e., phenols, alcohols, and amines) (Table 6–5).

In general, sulfonation is an effective means of decreasing the pharmacologic and toxicologic activity of xenobiotics. However, as shown in Figure 6–15, sulfonation has a role in the activation of aromatic amines, methyl-substituted polycyclic aromatic hydrocarbons, and safrole to tumorigenic metabolites.

Methylation

Methylation, a minor pathway of biotransformation, generally decreases the water solubility of xenobiotics and masks functional groups that might otherwise be conjugated by other enzymes. Methylation can also lead to increased toxicity. The cosubstrate for methylation is *S*-adenosylmethionine (SAM) (Figure 6–13). The methyl group bound to the sulfonium ion in SAM is transferred to xenobiotics and endogenous substrates by nucleophilic attack from an electron-rich heteroatom (*O*, *N*, or *S*) leaving *S*-adenosylhomocysteine. Examples of xenobiotics and endogenous substrates that undergo *O*-, *N*-, or *S*-methylation are shown in Figure 6–16.

The *O*-methylation of phenols and catechols is catalyzed by two different enzymes known as phenol *O*-methyltransferase (POMT) in microsomes and catechol-*O*-methyltransferase (COMT) in cytosol and microsomes. In rats and humans, COMT is encoded by a single gene with two different promoters and transcription initiation sites. Transcription at one site produces a cytosolic form of COMT, whereas transcription from the other site produces a membrane-bound form by adding a 50-amino acid segment that targets COMT to the endoplasmic reticulum. Substrates for COMT include several catecholamine neurotransmitters and catechol drugs, such as L-DOPA and methyldopa.

Several *N*-methyltransferases have been described in humans and other mammals. Phenylethanolamine *N*-methyltransferase catalyzes the *N*-methylation of the neurotransmitter norepinephrine to form epinephrine in the adrenal medulla and in certain regions of the brain, and is of minimal significance in xenobiotic biotransformation. However, histamine and nicotine *N*-methyltransferases expressed in liver, intestine, and/or kidney do methylate xenobiotics.

S-Methylation is an important pathway in the biotransformation of sulfhydryl-containing xenobiotics. In humans, *S*-methylation is catalyzed by thiopurine methyltransferase in cytosol and thiol methyltransferase in microsomes.

Acetylation

N-Acetylation is a major route of biotransformation for xenobiotics containing an aromatic amine (R—NH_2) or a hydrazine group (R—NH—NH_2), which are converted to aromatic amides (R—NH—$COCH_3$) and hydrazides (R—NH—NH—$COCH_3$), respectively. *N*-Acetylation masks an amine with a nonionizable group, so that many *N*-acetylated metabolites are less water soluble than the parent compound. Nevertheless, *N*-acetylation of certain xenobiotics, such as isoniazid, facilitates their urinary excretion.

Xenobiotic *N*-acetylation catalyzed by cytosolic *N*-acetyltransferases requires the cosubstrate acetyl-coenzyme A (acetyl-CoA; Figure 6–13). The two-step reaction involves (1) transfer of the acetyl group from acetyl-CoA to an active site cysteine residue within the enzyme with release of coenzyme A and (2) subsequent transfer of the acetyl group from the acylated enzyme to the amino group of the substrate with regeneration of the enzyme.

NAT1 and NAT2, the two acetyltransferases existing in humans, are 79% to 95% identical in amino acid sequence with

TABLE 6–5 Properties of the human cytosolic sulfotransferases (SULTs).

Human Sult	Polymorphic?	Tissue Distribution	Major Substrates[†]
SULT1A1	Yes *1–*4	Liver (very high), platelets. placenta, adrenals, endometrium, colon, jejunum, leukocytes, brain (cerebellum, occipital and frontal lobes)	4-Nitrophenol, 4-ethylphenol, 4-cresol, 2-naphthol, other phenols, acetaminophen, minoxidil, N-hydroxy-PhIP, T2, T3, 17β-estradiol (and other phenolic steroids), dopamine, benzylic alcohols, 2-nitropropane, aromatic amines, hydroxylamines, hydroxamic acids, apomorphine, troglitazone, genestein, epinephrine
SULT1A2	Yes *1–*6	Liver, kidney, brain, GI tract, bladder tumors	4-Nitrophenol, N-hydroxy-2-acetylaminofluorene, 2-naphthol, various aromatic hydroxylamines and hydroxamic acids
SULT1A3	Yes *1–*4	Jejunum and colon mucosa (very high), liver (low), platelets, placenta, brain (superior temporal gyrus, hippocampus, and temporal lobe), leukocytes, fetal liver	Dopamine, 4-nitrophenol, 1-hydroxymethylpyrene, norepinephrine, salbutamol, dobutamine, vanillin, albuterol
SULT1A4		Liver, pancreas, colon, brain	Not characterized. Likely similar to SULT1A3
SULT1B1		Colon (highest), liver, leukocytes, small intestine	4-Nitrophenol, T2, T3, r-T3, T4, dopamine, benzylic alcohols
SULT1C2	Yes *1–*5	Fetal lung and kidney, kidney, stomach, thyroid gland	4-Nitrophenol, N-hydroxy-2-AAF, aromatic hydroxylamines, thyroid hormones
SULT1C4		Kidney, ovary, spinal cord, fetal kidney, fetal lung (highest)	4-Nitrophenol, N-hydroxy-2-AAF, 17β-estrone, bisphenol-A, 4-octylphenol, nonylphenol, diethylstilbestrol, 1-hydroxymethylpyrene
SULT1E1		Liver (highest), endometrium, jejunum, adrenals, mammary epithelial cells, fetal liver, fetal lung, fetal kidney	17β-Estradiol, estrone, ethinyl estradiol, 17β-estrone, equilenin, 2-hydroxy-estrone, 2-hydroxy-estradiol, 4-hydroxy-estrone, 4-hydroxy-estradiol, diethylstilbestrol, tamoxifen, thyroid hormones, 4-hydroxylonazolac, pregnenolone, dehydroepiandrosterone, 1-naphthol, naringenin
SULT2A1	Yes *1–*3	Liver (highest), adrenals, ovaries, prostate, jejunum, kidney, brain	Dehydroepiandrosterone (DHEA), 1-hydroxymethylpyrene, 6-hydroxymethylbenzo[a]-pyrene, hycanthone, bile acids, pregnenolone, testosterone, androgens, estrone, 17β-estradiol, other hydroxysteroids, budesonide
SULT2B1a (SULT2B_v1)		Placenta (highest), prostate, trachea, skin	Dehydroepiandrosterone, pregnenolone, oxysterols, other hydroxysteroids
SULT2B1b (SULT2B_v2)		Lung, spleen, thymus, kidney, prostate, ovary, adrenal gland, liver (low), GI tract (low)	Cholesterol, pregnenolone, dehydroepiandrosterone, other hydroxysteroids
SULT4A1a (SULT4A_v1)		Brain: cortex, globus pallidus, islands of Calleja, septum, thalamus, red nucleus, substantia nigra and pituitary	Endogenous: 4 unidentified compounds from mouse brain homogenate Other: T3, T4, estrone, 4-nitrophenol, 2-naphthylamine, 2-naphthol
SULT4A1b (SULT4A_v2)			
SULT6B1		Testis	

[†]T4 is thyroxine. T2 and T3 are diiodothyronine and triiodothyronine. r-T3 is reverse triiodothyronine.

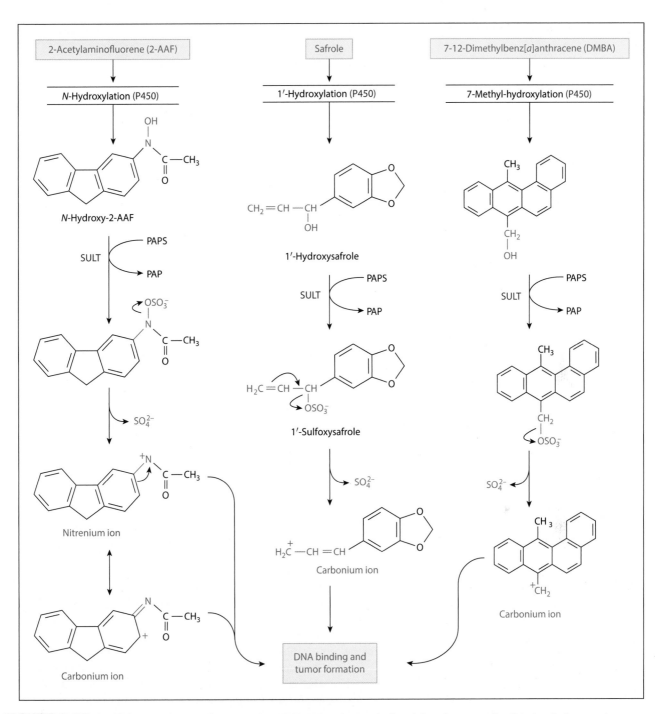

FIGURE 6–15 Role of sulfonation in the generation of tumorigenic metabolites (nitrenium or carbonium ions) of 2-acetylaminofluorene, safrole, and 7,12-dimethylbenz[a]anthracene (DMBA).

an active site cysteine residue in the N-terminal region. Although encoded by genes on the same chromosome, NAT1 is expressed in most tissues of the body, whereas NAT2 is mainly expressed only in liver and intestine. Most (but not all) of the tissues that express NAT1 also appear to express low levels of NAT2, at least at the level of mRNA. NAT1 and NAT2 also have different but overlapping substrate specificities. Examples of drugs that are N-acetylated by NAT1 and NAT2 are shown in Figure 6–17.

Genetic polymorphisms for N-acetylation have been documented in humans, hamsters, rabbits, and mice. Polymorphisms in NAT2 have a number of pharmacologic and toxicologic consequences: slow NAT2 acetylators are predisposed to drug toxicities, including excessive hypotension from hydralazine, peripheral neuropathy from isoniazid and dapsone, systemic lupus erythematosus from hydralazine and procainamide, and the toxic effects of coadministration of the anticonvulsant phenytoin with isoniazid.

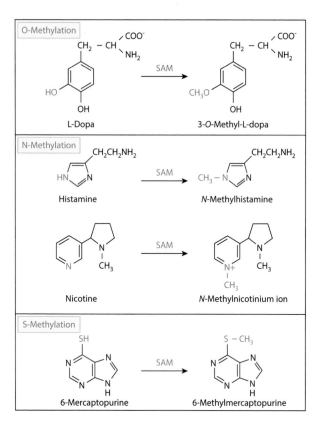

FIGURE 6–16 Examples of compounds that undergo *O-*, *N-*, or *S*-methylation.

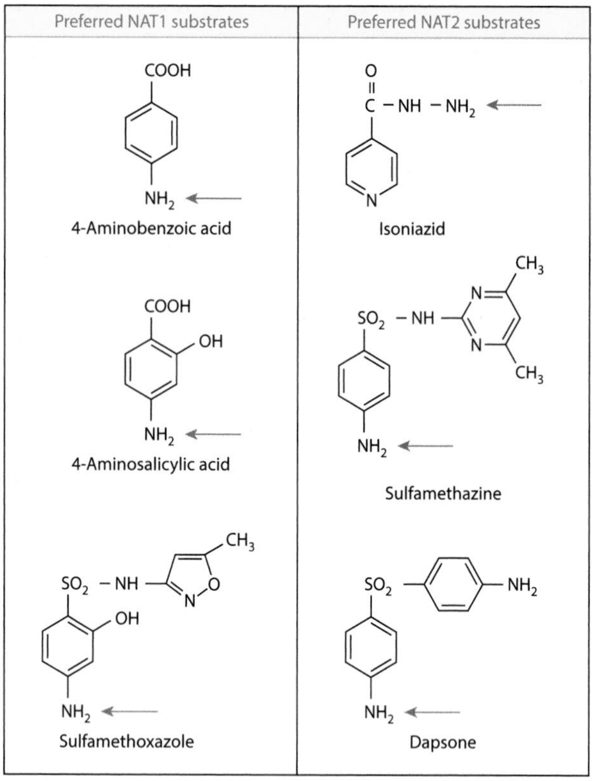

FIGURE 6–17 Examples of substrates for human *N*-acetyltransferases, NAT1, and the highly polymorphic NAT2.

The *N*-acetyltransferases detoxify aromatic amines by converting them to the corresponding amides that are less likely to be activated to DNA-reactive metabolites. However, *N*-acetyltransferases can activate aromatic amines if they are first *N*-hydroxylated by cytochrome P450. The acetoxy esters of *N*-hydroxyaromatic amines, like the corresponding sulfonate esters (Figure 6–15), can break down to form highly reactive nitrenium and carbonium ions that bind to DNA. Whether fast acetylators are protected from or predisposed to the cancer-causing effects of aromatic amines depends on the nature of the aromatic amine and other risk modifiers.

Amino Acid Conjugation

Two principal pathways by which xenobiotics are conjugated with amino acids are illustrated in Figure 6–18. The first involves conjugation of xenobiotics containing a carboxylic acid group with the amino group of amino acids such as glycine, glutamine, and taurine (see Figure 6–13). After activation of the xenobiotic by conjugation with CoA, the acyl-CoA thioether reacts with the *amino group* of an amino acid to form an amide linkage. The second pathway involves conjugation of xenobiotics containing an aromatic hydroxylamine with the *carboxylic acid group* of such amino acids as serine and proline. This pathway involves activation of an amino acid by aminoacyl-tRNA synthetase, which reacts with an aromatic hydroxylamine to form a reactive *N*-ester.

Substrates for amino acid conjugation are restricted to certain aliphatic, aromatic, heteroaromatic, cinnamic, and arylacetic acids. The ability of xenobiotics to undergo amino acid conjugation depends on steric hindrance around the carboxylic acid group, and by substituents on the aromatic ring or aliphatic side chain. Amino acid conjugates of xenobiotics are eliminated primarily in urine. The acceptor amino acid used for conjugation is both species- and xenobiotic-dependent.

Amino acid conjugation of *N*-hydroxy aromatic amines (hydroxylamines) is an activation reaction producing *N*-esters that can degrade to form electrophilic nitrenium and carbonium ions. Conjugation of hydroxylamines with amino acids is catalyzed by cytosolic aminoacyl-tRNA synthetases and requires ATP (Figure 6–18).

Glutathione Conjugation

Conjugation of xenobiotics with glutathione includes an enormous array of electrophilic xenobiotics, or xenobiotics that can be biotransformed to electrophiles. The tripeptide glutathione comprises glycine, cysteine, and glutamic acid (Figure 6–13). Glutathione conjugates are thioethers, which form by nucleophilic attack of glutathione thiolate anion (GS⁻) with an electrophilic carbon, oxygen, nitrogen, or sulfur atom in the xenobiotic. This conjugation reaction is catalyzed by a family

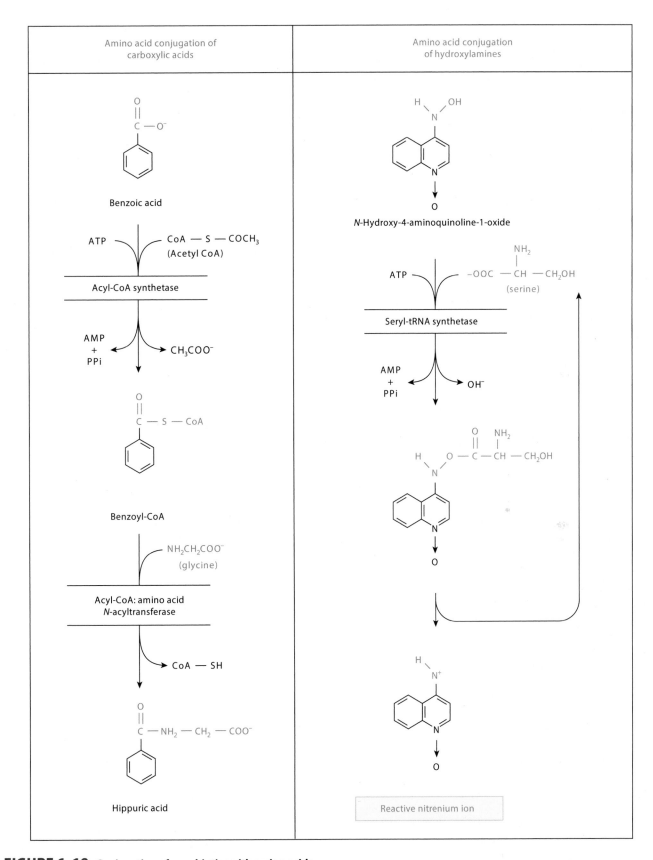

FIGURE 6–18 Conjugation of xenobiotics with amino acids.

of glutathione *S*-transferases that are present in most tissues, where they are localized in the cytoplasm (>95%) and endoplasmic reticulum (<5%).

Substrates for glutathione *S*-transferase are commonly hydrophobic, contain an electrophilic atom, and react nonenzymatically with glutathione at some measurable rate. The mechanism by which glutathione *S*-transferase increases the rate of glutathione conjugation involves deprotonation of GSH to GS$^-$. The concentration of glutathione in liver is extremely high (~5 to 10 mM); hence, the nonenzymatic conjugation of certain xenobiotics with glutathione can be significant. However, some xenobiotics are conjugated with glutathione stereoselectively, indicating that the reaction is largely catalyzed by glutathione *S*-transferase. Like glutathione, the glutathione *S*-transferases are themselves abundant cellular components, accounting for up to 10% of the total cellular protein. These enzymes bind, store, and/or transport a number of compounds that are not substrates for glutathione conjugation. The cytoplasmic protein formerly known as ligandin, which binds heme, bilirubin, steroids, azo-dyes, polycyclic aromatic hydrocarbons, and thyroid hormones, is an alpha-class GST.

As shown in Figure 6–19, substrates for glutathione conjugation can be divided into two groups: those sufficiently electrophilic to be conjugated directly and those that must first be biotransformed to an electrophilic metabolite prior to conjugation. The conjugation reactions themselves can be divided into two types: *displacement reactions,* in which glutathione displaces an electron-withdrawing group, and *addition reactions,* in which glutathione is added to an activated double bond or strained ring system.

The displacement of an electron-withdrawing group by glutathione typically occurs when the substrate contains halide, sulfate, sulfonate, phosphate, or a nitro group (i.e., good *leaving groups*) attached to an allylic or benzylic carbon atom.

The addition of glutathione to a carbon–carbon double bond is also facilitated by the presence of a nearby electron-withdrawing group; hence, substrates for this reaction typically contain a double bond attached to —CN, —CHO, —COOR, or —COR.

Glutathione can also conjugate xenobiotics with an electrophilic heteroatom (*O, N,* and *S*). In each of the examples shown in Figure 6–20, the initial conjugate formed between

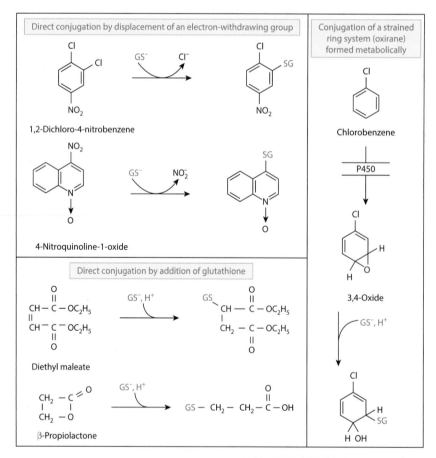

FIGURE 6–19 **Examples of glutathione conjugation of xenobiotics with an electrophilic carbon.** GS$^-$ represents the anionic form of glutathione.

glutathione and the heteroatom is cleaved by a second molecule of glutathione to form oxidized glutathione (GSSG). The initial reactions are catalyzed by glutathione S-transferase, whereas the second reaction (which leads to GSSG formation) generally occurs nonenzymatically.

Glutathione conjugates formed in the liver can be effluxed into bile and blood, and they can be converted to mercapturic acids in the kidney and excreted in urine. As shown in Figure 6–21, the conversion of glutathione conjugates to mercapturic acids involves the sequential cleavage of glutamic acid and glycine from the glutathione moiety, followed by N-acetylation of the resulting cysteine conjugate.

Glutathione S-transferases are dimers composed of identical subunits, although some forms are heterodimers. Each subunit contains 199 to 244 amino acids and one catalytic site. Numerous subunits have been cloned and sequenced and differ in substrate specificity, tissue location, and cellular location. Conjugation with glutathione represents an important detoxication reaction because electrophiles are potentially toxic species that can bind to critical nucleophiles, such as proteins and nucleic acids, causing cellular damage and genetic mutations (see Chapter 8 for more information). Glutathione is also a cofactor for glutathione peroxidase, which is important in protecting cells against lipid and hemoglobin peroxidation.

In some cases, conjugation with glutathione enhances the toxicity of a xenobiotic. Glutathione conjugates of various compounds can activate xenobiotics to become toxic by releasing a toxic metabolite, being inherently toxic itself, or being degraded to a toxic metabolite.

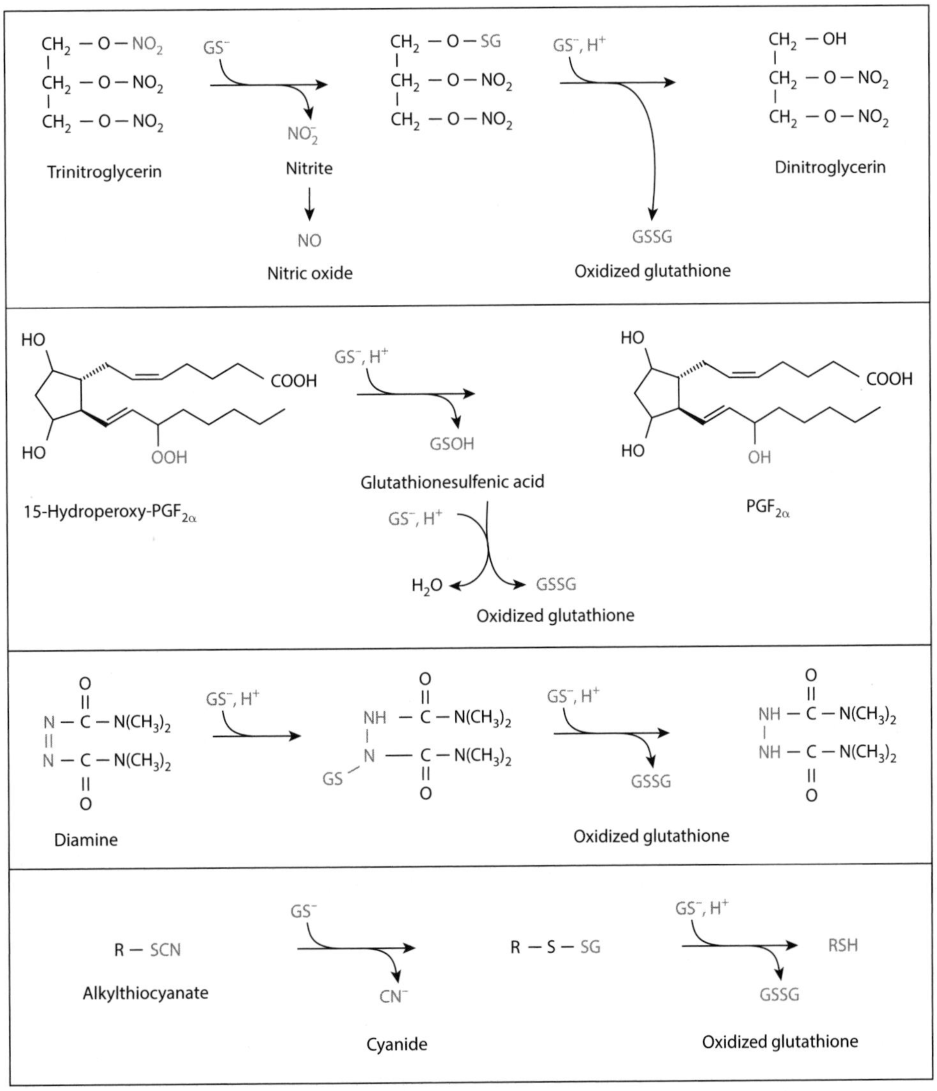

FIGURE 6–20 Examples of glutathione conjugation of electrophilic heteroatoms.

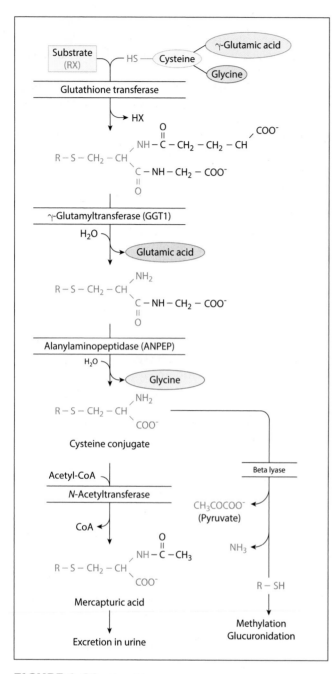

FIGURE 6–21 **Glutathione conjugation and mercapturic acid biosynthesis.**

BIBLIOGRAPHY

Coleman MD: *Human Drug Metabolism: An Introduction,* 2nd ed. Hoboken, NJ: Wiley-Blackwell, 2010.

Lee PW, Aizawa H, Gan L, Prakash C, Zhong D (eds.): *Handbook of Metabolic Pathways of Xenobiotics.* Hoboken, NJ: John Wiley & Sons, 2014.

Nassar AF: *Biotransformation and Metabolite Elucidation of Xenobiotics: Characterization and Identification.* Hoboken, NJ: John Wiley & Sons, 2010.

Yan Q: *Pharmacogenomics in Drug Discovery and Development,* 2nd ed. Totowa, NJ: Humana Press, 2014.

QUESTIONS

1. Xenobiotic biotransformation is performed by multiple enzymes in multiple subcellular locations. Where would one of these enzymes most likely NOT be located?
   a. cytosol.
   b. Golgi apparatus.
   c. lysosome.
   d. mitochondria.
   e. microsome.

2. All of the following statements regarding hydrolysis, reduction, and oxidation biotransformations are true EXCEPT:
   a. The xenobiotic can be hydrolyzed.
   b. The xenobiotic can be reduced.
   c. There is a large increase in hydrophilicity.
   d. The reactions introduce a functional group to the molecule.
   e. The xenobiotic can be oxidized.

3. Which of the following is often conjugated to xenobiotics during phase II biotransformations?
   a. alcohol group.
   b. sulfhydryl group.
   c. sulfate group.
   d. aldehyde group.
   e. carbonyl group.

4. Which of the following is a true statement about the biotransformation of ethanol?
   a. Alcohol dehydrogenase is only present in the liver.
   b. Ethanol is reduced to acetaldehyde by alcohol dehydrogenase.
   c. Ethanol and hydrogen peroxide combine to form acetaldehyde with the aid of catalase.
   d. In spite of its catalytic versatility, cytochrome P450 does not aid in ethanol oxidation.
   e. Acetaldehyde is oxidized to acetic acid in the mitochondria by aldehyde dehydrogenase.

5. Which of the following enzymes is responsible for the biotransformation and elimination of serotonin?
   a. cytochrome P450.
   b. monoamine oxidase.
   c. flavin monooxygenase.
   d. xanthine oxidase.
   e. paraoxonase.

6. Which of the following reactions would likely NOT be catalyzed by cytochrome P450?
   a. dehydrogenation.
   b. oxidative group transfer.
   c. epoxidation.
   d. reductive dehalogenation.
   e. ester cleavage.

7. All of the following statements regarding cytochrome P450 are true EXCEPT:
   a. Poor metabolism or biotransformation of xenobiotics is often due to a genetic deficiency in cytochrome P450.
   b. Cytochrome P450 can be inhibited by both competitive and noncompetitive inhibitors.
   c. Certain cytochrome P450 enzymes can be induced by one's diet.
   d. Increased activity of cytochrome P450 always slows the rate of xenobiotic activation.
   e. Induction of cytochrome P450 can lead to increased drug tolerance.

8. Which of the following statements regarding phase II biotransformation (conjugation) reactions is true?
   a. Phase II reactions greatly increase the hydrophilicity of the xenobiotic.
   b. Phase II reactions are usually the rate-determining step in the biotransformation and excretion of xenobiotics.
   c. Carboxyl groups are very common additions of phase II reactions.
   d. Most phase II reactions occur spontaneously.
   e. Increased phase II reactions result in increased xenobiotic storage in adipocytes.

9. Where do most phase II biotransformations take place?
   a. mitochondria.
   b. ER.
   c. blood.
   d. nucleus.
   e. cytoplasm.

10. Which of the following is not an important cosubstrate for phase II biotransformation reactions?
    a. UDP-glucuronic acid.
    b. 3′-phosphoadenosine-5′-phosphosulfate (PAPS).
    c. S-adenosylmethionine (SAM).
    d. N-nitrosodiethylamine.
    e. acetyl CoA.

Toxicokinetics

Danny D. Shen

KEY POINTS

- *Toxicokinetics* is the study of the modeling and mathematical description of the time course of disposition (absorption, distribution, biotransformation, and excretion) of xenobiotics in the whole organism.

- The apparent volume of distribution (V_d) is the space into which an amount of chemical is distributed in the body to result in a given plasma concentration.

- Clearance describes the rate of chemical elimination from the body in terms of volume of fluid containing chemical that is cleared per unit of time.

- The half-life of elimination ($T_{1/2}$) is the time required for the blood or plasma chemical concentration to decrease by one-half.

INTRODUCTION

Toxicokinetics is the study of the modeling and mathematical description of the time course of disposition (absorption, distribution, biotransformation, and excretion) of xenobiotics in the whole organism. In the *classic model,* chemicals are said to move throughout the body as if there were one or more compartments that may have no apparent physiologic or anatomical reality. An alternate and newer approach, physiologically based toxicokinetic modeling, attempts to portray the body as an elaborate system of discrete tissue or organ compartments that are interconnected via the circulatory system. There is no inherent contradiction between the classic and physiologically based approaches, yet certain assumptions differ between the two models. Ideally, physiologic models can predict tissue concentrations, whereas classic models cannot.

CLASSIC TOXICOKINETICS

The least invasive and simplest method to gather information on absorption, distribution, metabolism, and elimination of a compound is by sampling blood or plasma over time. Assuming that the concentration of a compound in blood or plasma is in equilibrium with concentrations in tissues, then changes in plasma toxicant concentrations should reflect changes in tissue toxicant concentrations. Compartmental pharmacokinetic models consist of a central compartment representing plasma and tissues that rapidly equilibrate with chemical, connected to one or more peripheral compartments that represent tissues that more slowly equilibrate with the chemical (Figure 7–1). Chemical is administered into the central compartment and distributes between central and peripheral compartments. Chemical elimination occurs from the central compartment, which is assumed to contain rapidly perfused tissues capable of eliminating the chemical (e.g., kidneys, lungs, and liver). Compartmental pharmacokinetic models require no information on tissue physiology or anatomical structure, and they are valuable in predicting the plasma chemical concentrations at different doses, establishing

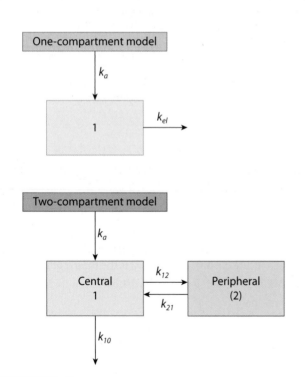

FIGURE 7–1 Compartmental pharmacokinetic models. k_a is the first-order extravascular absorption rate constant into the central compartment (1), k_{el} is the first-order elimination rate constant from the central compartment (1), and k_{12} and k_{21} are the first-order rate constants for distribution of chemical into and out of the peripheral compartment (2) in a two-compartment model, whereas k_{10} is the first-order elimination rate constant from the central compartment in a two compartment model.

the time course of chemical in plasma and tissues and the extent of chemical accumulation with multiple doses, and determining effective dose and dose regimens in toxicity studies.

One-compartment Model

The simplest toxicokinetic analysis entails measurement of the plasma concentrations of a xenobiotic at several time points after the administration of a bolus intravenous injection. If the data obtained yield a straight line when they are plotted as the logarithm of plasma concentrations versus time, the kinetics of the xenobiotic can be described with a one-compartment model (Figure 7–2). Compounds whose toxicokinetics can be described with a one-compartment model rapidly equilibrate, or mix uniformly, between blood and the various tissues relative to the rate of elimination. The one-compartment model depicts the body as a homogeneous unit. This does not mean that the concentration of a compound is the same throughout the body, but it does assume that the changes that occur in the plasma concentration reflect proportional changes in tissue chemical concentrations.

In the simplest case, a curve of this type can be described by the following expression:

$$C = C_0 e^{-k_{el}t}$$

where C is the blood or plasma chemical concentration over time t, C_0 the initial blood concentration at time $t = 0$, and k_{el} the first-order elimination rate constant with dimensions of reciprocal time (e.g., t^{-1}). k_{el} represents the overall elimination of the chemical, which includes biotransformation, exhalation, and/or excretion pathways.

Two-compartment Model

After the rapid intravenous administration of some chemicals, the semilogarithmic plot of plasma concentration versus time yields a curve rather than a straight line, which implies that there is more than one dispositional phase. In these instances, the chemical requires a longer time for tissue concentrations to reach equilibrium with the concentration in plasma, and a multicompartmental analysis of the results is necessary (Figure 7–2). A multiexponential mathematical equation then best characterizes the elimination of the xenobiotic from the plasma.

Generally, a curve of this type can be resolved into two monoexponential terms (a two-compartment model) and is described by:

$$C = Ae^{-\alpha t} + Be^{-\beta t}$$

where A and B are proportionality constants and α and β the first-order distribution and elimination rate constants, respectively (Figure 7–2). During the distribution (α) phase, concentrations of the chemical in the plasma decrease more rapidly than they do in the postdistributional elimination (β) phase. The distribution phase may last for only a few minutes or for

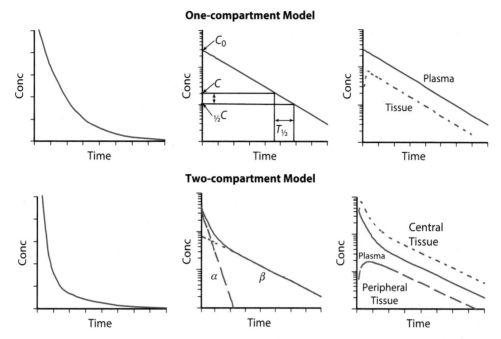

FIGURE 7–2 **Plasma concentration versus time curves of toxicants exhibiting kinetic behavior conforming to a one-compartment model (top row) and a two-compartment model (bottom row) following intravenous bolus injection.** Left and middle panels show the plots on a rectilinear and semilogarithmic scale, respectively. Right panels illustrate the relationship between tissue (*dashed lines*) and plasma (*solid line*) concentration over time. The right panel for the one-compartment model shows a typical tissue with a higher concentration than plasma. Note that tissue concentration can be higher, nearly the same, or lower than plasma concentration. Tissue concentration peaks almost immediately, and thereafter declines in parallel with plasma concentration. The right panel for the two-compartment model shows typical tissues associated with the central (1) and peripheral (2) compartments as represented by short-and-long dash lines, respectively. For tissues associated with the central compartment, their concentrations decline in parallel with plasma. For tissues associated with peripheral compartment, toxicant concentration rises, while plasma concentration declines rapidly during the initial phase; it then reaches a peak and eventually declines in parallel with plasma in the terminal phase. Elimination rate constant k_{el} for one-compartment model and the terminal exponential rate constant β are determined from the slope of the log-linear concentration versus time curve. Half-life ($T_{1/2}$) is the time required for plasma toxicant concentration to decrease by one-half. C_0 is the concentration of a toxicant for a one-compartment model at $t = 0$ determined by extrapolating the log-linear concentration time curve to the Y-axis.

hours or days. The equivalent of k_{el} in a one-compartment model is β in a two-compartment model.

Elimination

Elimination includes biotransformation, exhalation, and excretion. The elimination of a chemical from the body whose disposition is described by a one-compartment model usually occurs through a first-order process; that is, the rate of elimination at any time is proportional to the amount of the chemical in the body at that time. First-order reactions occur at chemical concentrations that are not sufficiently high to saturate elimination processes.

The equation for a monoexponential model, $C = C_0 e^{-k_{el}t}$, can be transformed to a logarithmic equation that has the general form of a straight line, $y = mx + b$:

$$\log C = \left(\frac{k_{el}}{2.303}\right)t + \log C_0$$

where $\log C_0$ represents the y-intercept or initial concentration and ($k_{el}/2.303$) the slope of the line. The first-order

elimination rate constant (k_{el}) can be determined from the slope of the log C versus time plot (i.e., $k_{el} = 2.303 \times$ slope). The first-order elimination rate constants, k_{el} and β, have units of reciprocal time (e.g., min^{-1} and h^{-1}) and are independent of dose.

Mathematically, the fraction of dose remaining in the body over time (C/C_0) is calculated using the elimination rate constant by rearranging the equation for the monoexponential function and taking the antilog to yield:

$$\frac{C}{C_0} = \text{Antilog}\left[\left(\frac{-k_{el}}{2.303}\right)t\right]$$

Apparent Volume of Distribution

In a one-compartment model, all chemical is assumed to distribute and equilibrate into plasma and tissues instantaneously. The apparent volume of distribution (V_d) is a proportionality constant that relates the total amount of chemical in the body to its concentration in plasma, and typically has units of liters or liters per kilogram of body weight. V_d is the apparent space into which an amount of chemical is distributed in the body to result in a given plasma concentration. The apparent volume of distribution of a chemical in the body is determined after intravenous bolus administration, and is mathematically defined as the quotient of the amount of chemical in the body and its plasma concentration. V_d is calculated as follows:

$$V_d = \frac{\text{Dose}_{iv}}{\beta \times \text{AUC}_0^\infty}$$

where Dose_{iv} is the intravenous dose or known amount of chemical in body at time zero, β the elimination rate constant, and AUC_0^∞ the area under the chemical concentration versus time curve from time zero to infinity. The product, $\beta \times \text{AUC}_0^\infty$, is the concentration of xenobiotic in plasma.

For a one-compartment model, V_d can be simplified by the following equation:

$$V_d = \frac{\text{Dose}_{iv}}{C_0}$$

where C_0 is the concentration of chemical in plasma at time zero. C_0 is determined by extrapolating the plasma disappearance curve after intravenous injection to the zero time point (Figure 7–2). V_d is called the *apparent volume of distribution*. The magnitude of the V_d term is chemical-specific and represents the extent of distribution of chemical out of plasma and into other body tissues. Thus, a chemical with high affinity for tissues will also have a large volume of distribution. Alternatively, a chemical that predominantly remains in the plasma will have a low V_d that approximates the volume of plasma. Once the V_d for a chemical is known, it can be used to estimate the amount of chemical remaining in the body at any time if the plasma concentration at that time is also known by the relationship $X_c = V_d C_p$, where X_c is the amount of chemical in the body and C_p the plasma chemical concentration.

Clearance

Clearance describes the rate of chemical elimination from the body in terms of volume of fluid containing chemical that is cleared per unit of time. Thus, clearance has the units of flow (mL/min). A clearance of 100 mL/min means that 100 mL of blood or plasma containing xenobiotic is completely cleared of the substance each minute.

The overall efficiency of the removal of a chemical from the body can be characterized by clearance. High values of clearance indicate efficient and generally rapid removal, whereas low clearance values indicate slow and less efficient removal of a xenobiotic from the body. *Total body clearance* is defined as the sum of clearances by individual eliminating organs:

$$\text{Cl} = \text{Cl}_{\text{renal}} + \text{Cl}_{\text{hepatic}} + \text{Cl}_{\text{intestinal}} + \cdots$$

Each organ clearance is determined by blood perfusion flow through the organ and the fraction of toxicant in the arterial inflow that is irreversibly removed. After bolus intravenous administration, total body clearance is defined as:

$$\text{Cl} = \frac{\text{Dose}_{iv}}{\text{AUC}_0^\infty}$$

Clearance can also be calculated if the volume of distribution and elimination rate constants are known, and can be defined as $\text{Cl} = V_d k_{el}$ for a one-compartment model and $\text{Cl} = V_d \beta$ for a two-compartment model.

Relationship of Elimination Half-life to Clearance and Volume

The half-life of elimination ($T_{1/2}$) is the time required for the blood or plasma chemical concentration to decrease by one-half, and is dependent on both volume of distribution and clearance. $T_{1/2}$ can be calculated from V_d and Cl:

$$T_{1/2} = \frac{0.693\, V_d}{\text{Cl}}$$

Because of the relationship $T_{1/2} = 0.693 k_{el}$, the half-life of a compound can be calculated after k_{el} (or β) has been determined from the slope of the line that designates the elimination phase on the log C versus time plot. The $T_{1/2}$ can also be determined by means of visual inspection of the log C versus time plot, as shown in Figure 7–2. For compounds eliminated by first-order kinetics, the time required for the plasma concentration to decrease by one-half is constant. After seven half-lives, 99.2% of a chemical is eliminated, which can be practically viewed as complete elimination. The half-life of a chemical obeying first-order elimination kinetics is independent of the dose, and does not change with increasing dose.

Absorption, Bioavailability, and Metabolite Kinetics

For most chemicals in toxicology, exposure occurs by extravascular routes (inhalation, dermal, or oral), and absorption is often incomplete. The extent of absorption of a xenobiotic can be experimentally determined by comparing the plasma AUC_0^∞ after intravenous and extravascular dosing. The resulting index quantifies the fraction of dose absorbed systemically and is called *bioavailability* (F). Bioavailability can be determined by using different doses, provided that the compound does not display dose-dependent or saturable kinetics. Pharmacokinetic data following intravenous administration are used as the reference from which to compare extravascular absorption because all of the chemical is delivered to the systemic circulation (100% bioavailable). For example, bioavailability following an oral exposure can be determined as follows:

$$F = \frac{\text{AUC}_{po}/\text{Dose}_{po}}{\text{Dose}_{iv}/\text{AUC}_{iv}}$$

where AUC_{po}, AUC_{iv}, $Dose_{po}$, and $Dose_{iv}$ are the respective area under the plasma concentration versus time curves and doses for oral and intravenous administration. Bioavailabilities for various chemicals range in values between 0 and 1. Complete availability of chemical to systemic circulation is demonstrated by $F = 1$. When $F < 1$, less than 100% of the dose reaches systemic circulation. The fraction of a chemical that reaches the systemic circulation is of critical importance in determining toxicity. Several factors can greatly alter this systemic availability, including (1) limited absorption after oral dosing, (2) intestinal first-pass effect, (3) hepatic first-pass effect, and (4) mode of formulation, which affects, e.g., dissolution rate or incorporation into micelles (for lipid-soluble compounds).

The toxicity of a chemical is in some cases attributed to its biotransformation product(s). Hence, the formation and disposition kinetics of a toxic metabolite is of considerable interest. As expected, the plasma concentration of a metabolite rises as the parent drug is transformed into the metabolite. A biologically active metabolite assumes toxicologic significance when it is the major metabolic product and is cleared much less efficiently than the parent compound.

Saturation Toxicokinetics

As the dose of a compound increases, its volume of distribution or its rate of elimination may change, owing to saturation kinetics. Biotransformation, active transport processes, and protein binding have finite capacities and can be saturated. When the concentration of a chemical in the body is higher than the K_m (chemical concentration at one-half V_{max}, the maximum metabolic capacity), the rate of elimination is no longer proportional to the dose. The transition from first-order to saturation kinetics is important in toxicology because it can lead to prolonged residency time of a compound in the body or increased concentration at the target site of action, which may result in increased toxicity.

Nonlinear toxicokinetics are indicated by the following: (1) the decline in the levels of the chemical in the body is not exponential, (2) AUC_0^∞ is not proportional to the dose, (3) V_d, Cl, k_{el} (or β), or $T_{1/2}$ changes with increasing dose, (4) the composition of excretory products changes quantitatively or qualitatively with the dose, and (5) dose–response curves show a nonproportional change in response to an increasing dose, starting at the dose level at which saturation effects become evident.

Important characteristics of zero-order processes are as follows: (1) an arithmetic plot of plasma concentration versus time yields a straight line, (2) the rate or amount of chemical eliminated at any time is constant and is independent of the amount of chemical in the body, and (3) a true $T_{1/2}$ or k_{el} does not exist, but differs depending on dose.

By comparison, the important characteristics of first-order elimination are (1) the rate at which a chemical is eliminated at any time is directly proportional to the amount of that chemical in the body at that time; (2) a semilogarithmic plot of plasma concentration versus time yields a single straight line; (3) the elimination rate constant (k_{el} or β), apparent volume of

distribution (V_d), clearance (Cl), and half-life ($T_{1/2}$) are independent of dose; and (4) the concentration of the chemical in plasma and other tissues decreases similarly by some constant fraction per unit of time, the elimination rate constant (k_{el} or β).

Accumulation during Continuous or Intermittent Exposure

Chronic exposure to a chemical leads to its cumulative intake and accumulation in the body. At a fixed level of continuous exposure, accumulation of a toxicant in the body eventually reaches a point when the intake rate of the toxicant equals its elimination rate, the steady state.

Accumulation can also occur with intermittent exposure. For a chemical with a relatively short half-life compared with the interval between episodes of exposure, little accumulation is expected. In contrast, for a chemical with an elimination half-life approaching or exceeding the between-exposure interval, progressive accumulation is expected over the intervals.

Conclusion

For many chemicals, blood or plasma chemical concentration versus time data can be adequately described by a one- or two-compartment, classic pharmacokinetic model when basic assumptions are made (e.g., instantaneous mixing within compartments and first-order kinetics). In some instances, more sophisticated models with increased numbers of compartments will be needed to describe blood or plasma toxicokinetic data. Knowledge of toxicokinetic data and compartmental modeling are useful in deciding what dose or dosing regimen of chemical to use in the planning of toxicology studies (e.g., targeting a toxic level of exposure), in choosing appropriate sampling times for biological monitoring, and in seeking an understanding of the dynamics of a toxic event (e.g., what blood or plasma concentrations are achieved to produce a specific response, how accumulation of a chemical controls the onset and degree of toxicity, and the persistence of toxic effects following termination of exposure).

PHYSIOLOGIC TOXICOKINETICS

In classic kinetics, the rate constants are defined by the data and these models are often referred to as *data-based*. In *physiologically based* models, the rate constants represent known or hypothesized biological processes. The advantages of physiologically based models are that (1) these models can provide the time course of distribution of xenobiotics to any organ or tissue, (2) they allow estimation of the effects of changing physiologic parameters on tissue concentrations, (3) the same model can predict the toxicokinetics of chemicals across species by allometric scaling, and (4) complex dosing regimens and saturable processes such as metabolism and binding are easily accommodated.

The disadvantages are that (1) much more information is needed to implement these models compared with classic models, (2) the mathematics can be difficult for many toxicologists to handle, and (3) values for parameters are often poorly defined in various species and pathophysiologic states. Nevertheless, physiologically based toxicokinetic models are conceptually sound and are potentially useful tools for gaining rich insight into the kinetics of toxicants beyond what classic toxicokinetic models can provide.

Basic Model Structure

Physiologic models often look like a number of classic one-compartment models that are linked together by the circulatory system. The actual model *structure,* or *how* the compartments are linked together, depends on both the chemical and the organism being studied. It is important to realize that there is no generic physiologic model. Models are simplifications of reality and ideally should contain elements believed to be important in describing a chemical's disposition.

Physiologic modeling has enormous potential predictive power compared with classic compartmental modeling. Because the kinetic constants in physiologic models represent measurable biological or chemical processes, the resultant physiologic models have the potential for extrapolation from observed data to predicted situations.

One of the best illustrations of the predictive power of physiologic models is their ability to extrapolate kinetic behavior from laboratory animals to humans. *Simulations* are the outcomes or results (such as a chemical's concentration in blood or tissue) of numerically integrating model equations over a simulated time period, using a set of initial conditions (such as intravenous dose) and parameter values (such as organ weights and blood flow). Whereas the model structures for the kinetics of chemicals in rodents and humans may be identical, the parameter values, such as organ weight, heart beat rate, and respiration rate, for rodents and humans are different. Other parameters, such as solubility in tissues, are similar in the rodent and human models because the composition of tissues in different species is similar. Because the parameters underlying the model structure represent measurable biological and chemical determinants, the appropriate values for those parameters can be chosen for each species, forming the basis for successful interspecies extrapolation. Because physiologic models represent real, measurable values, such as blood flows and ventilation rates, the same model structure can resolve such disparate kinetic behaviors among species.

Compartments

The basic unit of the physiologic model is the lumped compartment (Figure 7–3), which is a single region of the body with a uniform xenobiotic concentration. A compartment may be a particular functional or anatomical portion of an organ, a single blood vessel with surrounding tissue, an entire discrete organ such as the liver or kidney, or a widely distributed tissue type such as fat or skin. Compartments consist of three individual well-mixed phases, or subcompartments. These subcompartments are

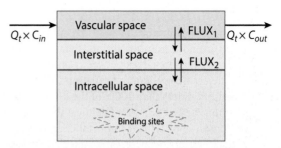

FIGURE 7–3   Schematic representation of a lumped compartment in a physiologic model. The blood capillary and cell membranes separating the vascular, interstitial, and intracellular subcompartments are depicted in black. The vascular and interstitial subcompartments are often combined into a single extracellular subcompartment. Q_t is blood flow, C_{in} is chemical concentration into the compartment, and C_{out} is chemical concentration out of the compartment.

(1) the *vascular* space through which the compartment is perfused with blood, (2) the *interstitial* space that surrounds the cells, and (3) the *intracellular* space consisting of the cells in the tissue.

As shown in Figure 7–3, the toxicant enters the vascular subcompartment at a certain rate in mass per unit of time (e.g., mg/h). The rate of entry is a product of the blood flow rate to the tissue (Q_t, L/h) and the concentration of the toxicant in the blood entering the tissue (C_{in}, mg/L). Within the compartment, the toxicant moves from the vascular space to the interstitial space at a certain net rate (Flux$_1$) and from the interstitial space to the intracellular space at a different net rate (Flux$_2$). Some toxicants can bind to cell components; thus, within a compartment there may be both free and bound toxicants. The toxicant leaves the vascular space at a certain venous concentration (C_{out}). C_{out} is equal to the concentration of the toxicant in the vascular space.

Parameters

The most common types of parameters, or information required, in physiologic models are *anatomical, physiologic, thermodynamic,* and *transport.*

Anatomical—Anatomical parameters are used to physically describe the various compartments. The size of each of the compartments in the physiologic model must be known. The size is generally specified as a volume (milliliters or liters) because a unit density is assumed even though weights are most frequently obtained experimentally. If a compartment contains subcompartments such as those in Figure 7–3, those volumes also must be known. Volumes of compartments often can be obtained from the literature or from specific toxicokinetic experiments.

Physiologic—Physiologic parameters encompass various processes including blood flow, ventilation, and elimination. The blood flow rate (Q_t, in volume per unit time, such as mL/min or L/h) to individual compartments must be known.

Additionally, information on the total blood flow rate or cardiac output (Q_c) is necessary. If inhalation is the route for exposure to the xenobiotic or is a route of elimination, the alveolar ventilation rate (Q_p) also must be known. Blood flow rates and ventilation rates can be taken from the literature or obtained experimentally. Parameters for renal excretion and hepatic metabolism are another subset of physiologic parameters that are required if these processes are important in describing the elimination of a xenobiotic.

Thermodynamic—Thermodynamic parameters relate the *total* concentration of a xenobiotic in a tissue (C_t) to the concentration of *free* xenobiotic in that tissue (C_f). Two important assumptions are that (1) total and free concentrations are in equilibrium with each other and (2) only free xenobiotic can be exchanged between the tissue subcompartments. Whereas total concentration is measured experimentally, it is the free concentration that is available for binding, metabolism, or removal from the tissue by blood. The extent to which a xenobiotic partitions into a tissue is directly dependent on the composition of the tissue and independent of the concentration of the xenobiotic. Thus, the relationship between free and total concentration becomes one of proportionality: total = free × partition coefficient, or $C_t = C_f P_t$. Knowledge of the value of P_t, a *partition* or *distribution* coefficient, permits an indirect calculation of the free concentration of xenobiotic or $C_f = C_t / P_t$.

Table 7–1 compares the partition coefficients for a number of toxic volatile organic chemicals. The larger values for the fat/blood partition coefficients compared with those for other tissues suggest that these chemicals distribute into fat to a greater extent than they distribute into other tissues.

A more complex relationship between the free concentration and the total concentration of a chemical in tissues occurs when the chemical may bind to saturable binding sites on tissue components. In these cases, nonlinear functions relating the free concentration in the tissue to the total concentration are necessary.

Transport—The passage of a chemical across a biological membrane is complex and may occur by passive diffusion, carrier-mediated transport, facilitated transport, or a combination of processes. The simplest of these processes—passive diffusion—is a first-order process described by Fick's law. Diffusion of xenobiotics can occur across the blood capillary endothelium (Flux₁ in

Figure 7–3) or across the cell membrane (Flux₂ in Figure 7–3). Flux refers to the rate of transfer of a chemical across a boundary. For simple diffusion, the net flux (mg/h) from one side of a membrane to the other is described as Flux = permeability coefficient × driving force, or:

$$\text{Flux} = [PA](C_1 - C_2) = [PA]C_1 - [PA]C_2$$

The term *PA* is often called the *permeability–area product* for the membrane or cellular barrier in flow units (e.g., L/h), and is a product of the barrier permeability coefficient (P in velocity units, e.g., μm/h) for the toxicant and the total barrier surface area (A, in μm²). The permeability constant takes into account the rate of diffusion of the specific xenobiotic and the thickness of the cell membrane. C_1 and C_2 are the *free* concentrations of xenobiotic on each side of the membrane.

For any given xenobiotic, thin membranes, large surface areas, and large concentration differences enhance diffusion. Membrane transporters offer an additional route of entry into cells, and allow more effective tissue penetration for toxicants that have limited passive permeability. Alternately, the presence of efflux transporters at epithelial or endothelial barriers can limit toxicant penetration into critical organs, even for highly permeable toxicants. There are two limiting conditions for the uptake of a toxicant into tissues: perfusion-limited and diffusion-limited.

Perfusion-limited Compartments

A perfusion-limited compartment is also referred to as *blood flow–limited,* or simply *flow-limited.* A flow-limited compartment can be developed if the cell membrane permeability coefficient [PA] for a particular xenobiotic is much greater than the blood flow rate to the tissue (Q_t). In this case, uptake of xenobiotic by tissue subcompartments is limited by the rate at which the blood containing a xenobiotic arrives at the tissue and not by the rate at which the xenobiotic crosses the cell membranes. In most tissues, transport across vascular cell membranes is perfusion-limited. In the generalized tissue compartment in Figure 7–3, this means that transport of the xenobiotic through the loosely knit blood capillary walls of most tissues is rapid compared with delivery of the xenobiotic to the tissue by the blood. As a result, the vascular blood is in equilibrium with the interstitial subcompartment and the two subcompartments are usually lumped together as a single compartment that is often called the *extracellular space.*

As indicated in Figure 7–3, the cell membrane separates the extracellular compartment from the intracellular compartment. The cell membrane is the most important diffusional barrier in a tissue. Nonetheless, for molecules that are very small (molecular weight < 100) or lipophilic, cellular permeability generally does not limit the rate at which a molecule moves across cell membranes. For these molecules, flux across the cell membrane is fast compared with the tissue perfusion rate ($PA_2 \gg Q_t$), and the molecules rapidly distribute throughout the subcompartments. In this case, free toxicant in the

TABLE 7–1 Partition coefficients for four volatile organic chemicals in several tissues.

Chemical	Blood/Air	Muscle/Blood	Fat/Blood
Isoprene	3	0.67	24
Benzene	18	0.61	28
Styrene	40	1	50
Methanol	1,350	3	11

intracellular compartment is always in equilibrium with the extracellular compartment, and these tissue subcompartments can be lumped as a single compartment. This flow-limited tissue compartment is shown in Figure 7–4. Movement into and out of the entire tissue compartment can be described by a single equation:

$$V_t \frac{dC_t}{dt} = Q_t(C_{in} - C_{out})$$

where V_t is the volume of the tissue compartment, C_t the concentration of free xenobiotic in the compartment (V_tC_t equals the amount of xenobiotic in the compartment), $V_t(dC_t/dt)$ the change in the amount of xenobiotic in the compartment with time expressed as mass per unit of time, Q_t the blood flow to the tissue, C_{in} the xenobiotic concentration entering the compartment, and C_{out} the xenobiotic concentration leaving the compartment. Equations of this type are called mass-balance differential equations. Differential refers to the term dC_t/dt. Mass balance refers to the requirement that the rate of change in the amount of toxicant in a compartment equals the difference in the rate of entry via arterial inflow and the rate of departure via venous outflow.

In the perfusion-limited case, the concentration of toxicant in the venous drainage from the tissue is equal to the concentration of toxicant in the tissue when the toxicant is not bound to blood constituents (i.e., $C_{out} = C_t = C_f$). As was noted previously, when there is binding of toxicant to tissue constituents, C_f (or C_{out}) can be related to the total concentration of toxicant in the tissue through a simple linear partition coefficient, $C_{out} = C_f = C_t/P_t$. In this case, the differential equation describing the rate of change in the amount of a toxicant in a tissue becomes:

$$V_t \frac{dC_t}{dt} = Q_t\left(C_{in} - \frac{C_t}{P_t}\right)$$

In a flow-limited compartment, the assumption is that the concentrations of a xenobiotic in all parts of the tissue are in equilibrium. Additionally, estimates of flux are not required to develop the mass balance differential equation for the compartment. Given the challenges in measuring flux across the vascular endothelium and cell membrane, this is a simplifying assumption that significantly reduces the number of parameters required in the physiologic model.

Diffusion-limited Compartments

When uptake of a toxicant into a compartment is governed by its diffusion or transport across cell membrane barriers, the model is said to be diffusion-limited or barrier-limited. Diffusion-limited uptake or release occurs when the flux, or the transport of a toxicant across cell barriers, is slow compared with blood flow to the tissue. In this case, the permeability–area product is small compared with blood flow, that is, $PA \ll Q_t$. Figure 7–5 shows the structure of such a compartment. The toxicant concentrations in the vascular and interstitial spaces are in equilibrium and make up the extracellular subcompartment, where uptake from the incoming blood is flow-limited. The rate of toxicant uptake across the cell membrane from the extracellular space into the intracellular space is limited by membrane permeability. Two mass-balance differential equations are necessary to describe the events in these two subcompartments:

1. Extracellular space:

$$V_{t1} \frac{dC_{t1}}{dt} = Q_t(C_{in} - C_{out}) - PA_t\left(\frac{C_{t1}}{P_{t1}}\right) + PA_t\left(\frac{C_{t2}}{P_{t2}}\right)$$

2. Intracellular space:

$$V_{t2} \frac{dC_{t2}}{dt} = PA_t\left(\frac{C_{t1}}{P_{t1}}\right) - PA_t\left(\frac{C_{t2}}{P_{t2}}\right)$$

Here, Q_t is blood flow and C the *free* xenobiotic concentration in entering blood (in), exiting blood (out), extracellular space (1), or intracellular space (2). Both equations contain terms for flux, or transfer across the cell membrane $[PA](C_1 - C_2)$.

Specialized Compartments

Lung—The inclusion of a lung compartment in a physiologic model is an important consideration because inhalation is a common route of exposure to many toxic chemicals. The

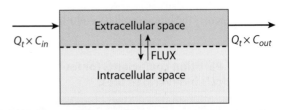

FIGURE 7–5 **Schematic representation of a compartment that is membrane-limited.** Perfusion of blood into and out of the extracellular compartment is depicted by thick arrows. Transmembrane transport (flux) from the extracellular to the intracellular subcompartment is depicted by thin double arrows. Q_t is blood flow, C_{in} is chemical concentration into the compartment, and C_{out} is chemical concentration out of the compartment.

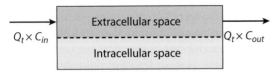

FIGURE 7–4 **Schematic representation of a compartment that is blood flow–limited.** Rapid exchange between the extracellular space (*salmon*) and intracellular space (*bisque*) maintains the equilibrium between them as symbolized by the dashed line. Q_t is blood flow, C_{in} is chemical concentration into the compartment, and C_{out} is chemical concentration out of the compartment.

assumptions inherent in this compartment description are as follows: (1) ventilation is continuous, not cyclic; (2) conducting airways (nasal passages, larynx, trachea, bronchi, and bronchioles) function as inert tubes, carrying the vapor to the alveoli where gas exchange occurs; (3) diffusion of vapor across the alveolar epithelium and capillary walls is rapid compared with blood flow through the alveolar region; (4) all chemicals disappearing from the inspired air appears in the arterial blood (i.e., there is no hold-up of chemical in the lung tissue and insignificant lung mass); and (5) vapor in the alveolar air and arterial blood within the lung compartment are in rapid equilibrium.

In the lung compartment depicted in Figure 7–6, the rate of inhalation of xenobiotic is controlled by the ventilation rate (Q_p) and the inhaled concentration (C_{inh}). The rate of exhalation of a xenobiotic is a product of the ventilation rate and the xenobiotic concentration in the alveoli (C_{alv}). Xenobiotic also can enter the lung compartment via venous blood returning from the heart, represented by the product of cardiac output (Q_c) and the concentration of xenobiotic in venous blood (C_{ven}). Xenobiotic leaving the lungs via the blood is a function of both cardiac output and the concentration of xenobiotic in arterial blood (C_{art}). Putting these four processes together, a mass balance differential equation can be written for the rate of change in the amount of xenobiotic in the lung compartment (L):

$$\frac{dL}{dt} = Q_p(C_{inh} - C_{alv}) + Q_c(C_{ven} - C_{art})$$

During continuous exposure at steady state, the rate of change in the amount of xenobiotic in the lung compartment becomes equal to zero ($dL/dt = 0$). C_{alv} can be replaced by $C_{art}/P_{b/a}$, and the differential equation can be solved for the arterial blood concentration:

$$C_{art} = \frac{Q_p C_{inh} + Q_c C_{ven}}{Q_c + (Q_p/P_{b/a})}$$

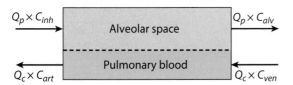

FIGURE 7–6 Simple model of gas exchange in the alveolar region of the respiratory tract. Rapid exchange in the lumped lung compartment between the alveolar gas (*blue*) and the pulmonary blood (*salmon*) maintains the equilibrium between them as symbolized by the dashed line. Q_p is alveolar ventilation (L/h); Q_c is cardiac output (L/h); C_{inh} is inhaled vapor concentration (mg/L); C_{art} is concentration of vapor in the arterial blood; C_{ven} is concentration of vapor in the mixed venous blood. The equilibrium relationship between the chemical in the alveolar air (C_{alv}) and the chemical in the arterial blood (C_{art}) is determined by the blood/air partition coefficient P_b, e.g., $C_{alv} = C_{art}/P_{b/a}$.

The lung is viewed here as a portal of entry and not as a target organ, and the concentration of a xenobiotic delivered to other organs by the blood, or the arterial concentration of that xenobiotic, is of primary interest. The assumptions of continuous ventilation, rapid equilibration with arterial blood, and no hold-up in lung tissues have proved applicable with many volatile organics. The use of these assumptions simplifies and speeds up model calculations and may be entirely adequate for describing the toxicokinetic behavior of relatively inert vapors with low water solubility.

Liver—The liver is almost always featured as a distinct compartment in physiologic models because biotransformation is an important route of elimination for many toxicants and the liver is considered the major organ for biotransformation of xenobiotics. A simple compartmental structure for the liver is one where uptake into the liver compartment is assumed to be flow-limited. This liver compartment is similar to the general tissue compartment in Figure 7–4, except that the liver compartment contains an additional process for metabolic elimination. Under first-order elimination, the rate of hepatic metabolism (R) by the liver can be presented as:

$$R = Cl_l \cdot C_f$$

where C_f is the free concentration of toxicant in the liver (mg/L), and Cl_l is the clearance of free toxicant within the liver (L/h).

In the case of a single enzyme mediating the biotransformation and Michaelis–Menten kinetics are obeyed, Cl_l is related to the maximum rate of metabolism V_{max} (in mg/h) and the Michaelis constant K_M (in mg/L). As a result, the rate of hepatic metabolism can be expressed in terms of the Michaelis parameters:

$$R = \left[\frac{V_{max}}{K_M + C_f} \right] C_f$$

Under nonsaturating or first-order condition (i.e., $C_f \ll K_M$), Cl_l becomes equal to the ratio of V_{max}/K_M. Because many toxicants at high exposure levels display saturable metabolism, the above equation is often invoked for simulation of toxicant disposition across a wide range of doses.

Other, more complex expressions for metabolism also can be incorporated into physiologic models. Bi-substrate second-order reactions, reactions involving the destruction of enzymes, inhibition of enzymes, or the depletion of cofactors, have been simulated using physiologic models. Metabolism can be also included in other compartments in much the same way as described for the liver.

Blood—In a physiologic model, the tissue compartments are linked together by the circulatory network. The decision to represent blood as an explicit physiologic compartment depends on the role the blood plays in disposition and the type of application. If the toxicokinetics after intravenous injection is to be simulated or if binding to or metabolism by blood components is suspected, a separate compartment for the blood that incorporates these additional processes is required. A blood compartment is obviously needed if the model were developed to explain a set of blood concentration–time data for a toxicant. However, if blood is simply a conduit to the other compartments, as in the case for inhaled volatile organics, an algebraic solution is acceptable.

CONCLUSION

Biological monitoring or biomonitoring is defined as the systematic sampling of body fluids, and at times body tissue, for the purpose of estimating an individual's internal dose from exposure to chemicals in the workplace or assessing the range of internal exposure within a select population to environmental pollutants. The advantages of biomonitoring over traditional environmental monitoring, such as ambient or personal air sampling or dermal dosimetry, include the accounting of other unanticipated routes of exposure, individual differences in toxicant absorption and disposition, and critical personal or lifestyle variables, such as body size and composition, workload that affects pulmonary ventilation, or cigarette smoking that could affect the metabolic status of an individual. Linking environmental exposure or dose to measurements of concentration of the parent chemical or its metabolite(s) in a biological sample is essentially an exercise in toxicokinetics.

Although simpler elements of physiologic models and the important assumptions that underlie model structures are presented, toxicologists are developing increasingly more sophisticated applications. Three-dimensional visualizations of xenobiotic transport, physiologic models of a parent chemical linked in series with one or more active metabolites, models describing biochemical interactions among xenobiotics, and more biologically realistic descriptions of tissues previously viewed as simple lumped compartments are just a few of the more sophisticated applications. Finally, physiologically based toxicokinetic models are now being linked to biologically based toxicodynamic models to simulate the entire exposure → dose → response paradigm that is basic to the science of toxicology.

BIBLIOGRAPHY

Andersen ME: Toxicokinetic modeling and its applications in chemical risk assessment. *Toxicol Lett* 138:9–27, 2003.

Esteban M, Castaño A: Non-invasive matrices in human biomonitoring—a review. *Environ Int* 35:438–449, 2009.

Fowler BA (ed.): *Computational Toxicology: Methods and Applications for Risk Assessment.* New York: Academic Press/Elsevier, 2013.

Lipscomb JC, Ohanian EV: *Toxicokinetics and Risk Assessment.* New York: Informa Healthcare, 2007.

Rowland M, Tozer TN: *Clinical Pharmacokinetics and Pharmacodynamics–Concepts and Applications.* Philadelphia, PA: Wolters Kluwer/Lippincott, Williams & Wilkins, 2011.

QUESTIONS

1. Regarding the two-compartment model of classic toxicokinetics, which of the following is true?
   a. There is rapid equilibration of chemical between central and peripheral compartments.
   b. The logarithm of plasma concentration versus time data yields a linear relationship.
   c. There is more than one dispositional phase.
   d. It is assumed that the concentration of a chemical is the same throughout the body.
   e. It is ineffective in determining effective doses in toxicity studies.

2. When calculating the fraction of a dose remaining in the body over time, which of the following factors need not be taken into consideration?
   a. half-life.
   b. initial concentration.
   c. time.
   d. present concentration.
   e. elimination rate constant.

3. All of the following statements regarding apparent volume of distribution (V_d) are true EXCEPT:
   a. V_d relates the total amount of chemical in the body to the concentration of chemical in the plasma.
   b. V_d is the apparent space into which an amount of chemical is distributed in the body to result in a given plasma concentration.
   c. A chemical that usually remains in the plasma has a low V_d.
   d. V_d will be low for a chemical with high affinity for tissues.
   e. V_d can be used to estimate the amount of chemical in the body if the plasma concentration is known.

4. Chemical clearance:
   a. is independent of V_d.
   b. is unaffected by kidney failure.
   c. is indirectly proportional to V_d.
   d. is performed by multiple organs.
   e. is not appreciable in the GI tract.

5. A chemical with which of the following half-lives ($T_{1/2}$) will remain in the body for the longest period of time when given equal dosage of each?
   a. $T_{1/2} = 30$ min.
   b. $T_{1/2} = 1$ day.
   c. $T_{1/2} = 7$ h.
   d. $T_{1/2} = 120$ s.
   e. $T_{1/2} = 1$ month.

6. With respect to first-order elimination, which of the following statements is FALSE?
   a. The rate of elimination is directly proportional to the amount of the chemical in the body.
   b. A semilogarithmic plot of plasma concentration versus time shows a linear relationship.
   c. Half-life ($T_{1/2}$) differs depending on the dose.
   d. Clearance is dosage-independent.
   e. The plasma concentration and tissue concentration decrease similarly with respect to the elimination rate constant.

7. The toxicity of a chemical is dependent on the amount of chemical reaching the systemic circulation. Which of the following does NOT *greatly* influence systemic availability?
   a. absorption after oral dosing.
   b. intestinal motility.
   c. hepatic first-pass effect.
   d. intestinal first-pass effect.
   e. incorporation into micelles.

8. Which of the following is NOT an advantage of a physiologically based toxicokinetic model?
   a. Complex dosing regimens are easily accommodated.
   b. The time course of distribution of chemicals to any organ is obtainable.
   c. The effects of changing physiologic parameters on tissue concentrations can be estimated.
   d. The rate constants are obtained from gathered data.
   e. The same model can predict toxicokinetics of chemicals across species.

9. Which of the following will not help to increase the flux of a xenobiotic across a biological membrane?
   a. decreased size.
   b. decreased oil:water partition coefficient.
   c. increased concentration gradient.
   d. increased surface area.
   e. decreased membrane thickness.

10. Which of the following statements is true regarding diffusion-limited compartments?
    a. Xenobiotic transport across the cell membrane is limited by the rate at which blood arrives at the tissue.
    b. Diffusion-limited compartments are also referred to as flow-limited compartments.
    c. Increased membrane thickness can cause diffusion-limited xenobiotic uptake.
    d. Equilibrium between the extracellular and intracellular space is maintained by rapid exchange between the two compartments.
    e. Diffusion of gases across the alveolar septa of a healthy lung is diffusion-limited.

C H A P T E R

8

Chemical Carcinogenesis

James E. Klaunig

KEY POINTS

- The term *cancer* describes a subset of neoplastic lesions.
- A *neoplasm* is defined as a heritably altered, relatively autonomous growth of tissue with abnormal regulation of gene expression.
- *Metastases* are secondary growths of cells from the primary neoplasm.
- A *carcinogen* is an agent whose administration to previously untreated animals leads to a statistically significant increased incidence of neoplasms of one or more histogenetic types as compared with the incidence in appropriate untreated animals.

- *Initiation* requires one or more rounds of cell division for the "fixation" of the DNA damage.
- *Promotion* results from the selective functional enhancement of the initiated cell and its progeny by the continuous exposure to the promoting agent.
- *Progression* is the transition from early progeny of initiated cells to the biologically malignant cell population of the neoplasm.

OVERVIEW

Cancer is a disease of cellular mutation, proliferation, and aberrant cell growth. It ranks as one of the leading causes of death in the world. Multiple causes of cancer have been either firmly established or suggested, including infectious agents, radiation, and chemicals. Estimates suggest that 70% to 90% of all human cancers have a linkage to environmental, dietary, and behavioral factors.

Definitions

Table 8–1 lists definitions of terms commonly used in discussing chemical carcinogenesis. For benign neoplasms, the tissue of origin is frequently followed by the suffix "oma"; e.g., a benign fibrous neoplasm would be termed *fibroma*, and a benign glandular epithelium termed an *adenoma*. Malignant neoplasms from epithelial origin are called *carcinomas*, whereas those derived from mesenchymal origin are referred to as *sarcoma*. Thus, a malignant neoplasm of fibrous tissue would be a *fibrosarcoma*, whereas that derived from bone would be an *osteosarcoma*.

Carcinogens may be *genotoxic*, meaning that they interact physically with DNA to damage or change its structure. Other carcinogens may change how DNA expresses information without modifying or directly damaging its structure, or may create a situation in a cell or tissue that makes it more susceptible to DNA damage from other sources. Chemicals belonging to this latter category are referred to as *nongenotoxic* carcinogens. Common features of genotoxic and nongenotoxic carcinogens are shown in Table 8–2.

MULTISTAGE CARCINOGENESIS

The carcinogenesis process involves a series of definable and reproducible stages. Operationally, these stages have been defined as initiation, promotion, and progression (Figure 8–1).

TABLE 8–1   Terminology.

Neoplasia	New growth or autonomous growth of tissue
Neoplasm	The lesion resulting from the neoplasia
Benign	Lesions characterized by expansive growth, frequently exhibiting slow rates of proliferation that do not invade surrounding tissues
Malignant	Lesions demonstrating invasive growth, capable of metastases to other tissues and organs
Metastases	Secondary growths derived from a primary malignant neoplasm
Tumor	Lesion characterized by swelling or increase in size, may or may not be neoplastic
Cancer	Malignant neoplasm
Carcinogen	A physical or chemical agent that causes or induces neoplasia
Genotoxic	Carcinogens that interact with DNA resulting in mutation
Nongenotoxic	Carcinogens that modify gene expression but do not damage DNA

TABLE 8–2   Features of genotoxic and nongenotoxic carcinogens.

Genotoxic carcinogens
- Mutagenic
- Can be complete carcinogens
- Tumorigenicity is dose responsive
- No theoretical threshold

Nongenotoxic carcinogens
- Nonmutagenic
- Threshold, reversible
- Tumorigenicity is dose responsive
- May function at tumor promotion stage
- No direct DNA damage
- Species, strain, tissue specificity

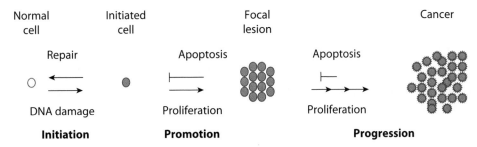

FIGURE 8-1 Multistage model of carcinogenesis.

The defining characteristics of each of these stages are outlined in Table 8–3.

Initiation

The first stage of the cancer process involves *initiation*, a process that is defined as a stable, heritable change. This stage is a rapid, irreversible process that results in a carcinogen-induced mutational event. Chemical and physical agents that interact with cellular components at this stage are referred to as initiators or initiating agents. Initiating agents lead to genetic changes including mutations and deletions. Chemical carcinogens that covalently bind to DNA and form adducts that result in mutations are initiating agents. The initiating event becomes "fixed" when the DNA damage is not correctly or completely repaired prior to DNA synthesis and cell division.

TABLE 8-3 Characteristics of the stages of carcinogenesis process.

Initiation
DNA modification
Mutation
Genotoxic
One cell division necessary to lock-in mutation
Modification is not enough to produce cancer
Nonreversible
Single treatment can induce mutation

Promotion
No direct DNA modification
Nongenotoxic
No direct mutation
Multiple cell divisions necessary
Clonal expansion of the initiated cell population
Increase in cell proliferation or decrease in cell death (apoptosis)
Reversible
Multiple treatments (prolonged treatment) necessary
Threshold

Progression
DNA modification
Genotoxic event
Mutation, chromosome disarrangement
Changes from preneoplasia to neoplasia benign/malignant
Irreversible
Number of treatments needed with compound unknown (may require only single treatment)

Once initiated cells are formed, their fate has multiple potential outcomes: (1) the initiated cell can remain in a static nondividing state; (2) the initiated cell may possess mutations incompatible with viability or normal function and be deleted through apoptotic mechanisms; or (3) the cell may undergo cell division resulting in the proliferation of the initiated cell. Besides the production of an initiated cell through carcinogen binding and misrepair, additional evidence has come forth showing that induction of continual stress, resulting in continual cell proliferation, can also produce new mutated, initiated cells.

Promotion

The second stage of the carcinogenesis process involves the selective clonal expansion of initiated cells to produce a preneoplastic lesion. This is referred to as the *promotion* stage of the carcinogenesis process. Both exogenous and endogenous agents that operate at this stage are referred to as tumor promoters. Tumor promoters are not mutagenic and generally are not able to induce tumors by themselves; rather they act through several mechanisms involving gene expression changes that result in sustained cell proliferation through increases in cell proliferation and/or the inhibition of apoptosis. Promotion is reversible upon removal of the promoting agent, and the focal cells may return to single initiated cell thresholds. In addition, these agents demonstrate a well-documented threshold for their effects—below a certain dose or frequency of application, tumor promoters are unable to induce cell proliferation. Tumor promoters generally show organ-specific effects, e.g., a tumor promoter of the liver, such as phenobarbital, will not function as a tumor promoter in the skin or other tissues.

Progression

Progression involves the conversion of benign preneoplastic lesions into neoplastic cancer. In this stage, due to an increase in DNA synthesis and cell proliferation in the preneoplastic lesions, additional genotoxic events may occur, resulting in further DNA damage including chromosomal aberrations and translocations. The progression stage is irreversible in that neoplasm formation, whether benign or malignant, occurs. With the formation of neoplasia, an autonomous growth and/or lack of growth control is achieved. Spontaneous progression can occur from spontaneous karyotypic changes that occur in mitotically active initiated cells during promotion. An accumulation of nonrandom chromosomal aberrations and karyotypic instability are hallmarks of progression.

MECHANISMS OF ACTION OF CHEMICAL CARCINOGENS

The formation of a neoplasm is a multistage, multistep process that involves the ultimate release of the neoplastic cells from normal growth control processes and creating a tumor microenvironment. The eight properties of carcinogenesis are listed in Table 8–4. An important concept is that tumors are not just a collection of clonal neoplastic cells but a complex tissue with multiple cell populations that interact with one another and function as a unique tissue. This tumor microenvironment involves the recruitment of normal stromal and inflammatory cells that contribute to the growth the development of the neoplasm.

Genotoxic/DNA-Reactive Carcinogens

Genotoxic compounds directly interact with the nuclear DNA of a target cell. If this damage is unrepairable, DNA damage is inherited in subsequent daughter cells. DNA reactive carcinogens can be further subdivided according to whether they are active in their parent form (i.e., direct-acting carcinogens—agents that can directly bind to DNA without being metabolized) and those that require metabolic activation (i.e., indirect-acting carcinogens—compounds that require metabolism in order to react with DNA).

Direct-acting (Activation-independent) Carcinogens—
Direct-acting carcinogens are highly reactive electrophilic molecules that can interact with and bind to nucleophiles, such as cellular macromolecules, including DNA without needing to be biotransformed into a reactive toxicant. Generally, these highly reactive chemicals frequently result in tumor formation at the site of chemical exposure.

The relative carcinogenic strength of direct-acting carcinogens depends in part on the relative rates of interaction between the chemical and genomic DNA, as well as competing reactions with the chemical and other cellular nucleophiles. Chemical stability, transport, and membrane permeability determine the carcinogenic activity of the chemical. Direct-acting carcinogens are typically carcinogenic at multiple sites and in all species examined.

Indirect-acting Genotoxic Carcinogens—
The majority of DNA reactive carcinogens are found as parent compounds, or procarcinogens, chemicals that require subsequent metabolism to be carcinogenic. Terms have been coined to define the parent compound (procarcinogen) and its metabolite form, either intermediate (proximate carcinogen) or final (ultimate carcinogen), that reacts with DNA. The ultimate form of the carcinogen may not be known or may be several forms depending on metabolic pathway, but it is most likely the chemical species that

TABLE 8–4 Proposed modes of action for selected nongenotoxic chemical carcinogens.

Mode of Action	Example
Cytotoxicity	Chloroform Melamine
α_{2u}-Globulin-binding	D-limonene, 1,4-dichlorobenzene
Receptor-mediated CAR	Phenobarbital
PPARα	Trichloroethylene Perchloroethylene Diethylhexylphthalate Fibrates (e.g., clofibrate)
AhR	TCDD Polychlorinated biphenyls (PCBs) Polybrominated biphenyls (PBBs)
Hormonal	Biogenic amines Steroid and peptide hormones DES Phytoestrogens (bisphenol-A) Tamoxifen Phenobarbital
Altered methylation	Phenobarbital Choline deficiency Diethanolamine
Oxidative stress inducers	Ethanol TCDD Lindane Dieldrin Acrylonitrile

results in mutation and neoplastic transformation. It is important to note that besides activation of the procarcinogen to a DNA reactive form, detoxification pathways may also occur resulting in inactivation of the carcinogen.

Indirect-acting genotoxic carcinogens usually produce their neoplastic effects at the target tissue where the metabolic activation of the chemical occurs and not at the site of exposure (as seen with direct-acting genotoxic carcinogens).

Mutagenesis

Effects of mutations depend on when in the cell cycle the adducts are formed, where the adducts are formed, and the type of repair process used in response to the damage. Mutagenesis may result from misread DNA (through transitions or transversions), frame-shifting, or broken DNA strands.

Damage by Alkylating Electrophiles

As noted above, most chemical carcinogens require metabolic activation to exert a carcinogenic effect. The ultimate carcinogenic forms of these chemicals are frequently strong electrophiles (Figure 8–2) that can readily form covalent adducts with nucleophilic targets. In general, the stronger electrophiles

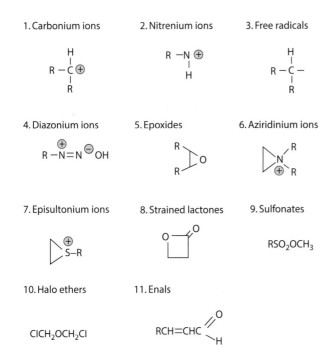

1. Carbonium ions   2. Nitrenium ions   3. Free radicals

4. Diazonium ions   5. Epoxides   6. Aziridinium ions

7. Episultonium ions   8. Strained lactones   9. Sulfonates

RSO_2OCH_3

10. Halo ethers   11. Enals

$ClCH_2OCH_2Cl$

$RCH{=}CHC$

FIGURE 8–2 Structures of reactive electrophiles.

display a greater range of nucleophilic targets, whereas weak electrophiles are only capable of alkylating strong nucleophiles.

An important and abundant source of nucleophiles is contained not only in the DNA bases, but also in the phosphodiester backbone. Different electrophilic carcinogens will often display different preferences for nucleophilic sites in DNA and, thus, a different spectra of damage.

Another common modification to DNA is the hydroxylation of DNA bases. Oxidative DNA adducts have been identified in all four DNA bases. The source of oxidative DNA damage is typically formed from free radical reactions that occur endogenously in the cell or from exogenous sources.

Methylation of DNA results in heritable expression or repression of genes, with hypomethylation associated with active transcription of genes, whereas hypermethylated genes tend to be rarely transcribed. Chemical carcinogens may inhibit DNA methylation by forming covalent adducts, single-strand breaks in the DNA, alteration of methionine pools, and inactivation of the DNA methyltransferase responsible for methylation. Whether a particular DNA adduct will result in mutation depends in part on the process of DNA replication and in part on DNA repair.

DNA Repair

Following the formation of a carcinogen-DNA adduct, the persistence of the adduct is a major determinant of the outcome. This persistence depends on the ability of the cell to repair the altered DNA. However, the presence of a DNA adduct is not sufficient for the carcinogenesis process to proceed. The relative rates or persistence of particular DNA adducts may be an

important determinant of carcinogenicity. Differences in susceptibility to carcinogenesis are likely the result of a number of factors, including DNA replication within a tissue and repair of a DNA adduct. The development of cancer following exposure to chemical carcinogens is a relatively rare event because of a cell's ability to recognize and repair damaged DNA. The DNA region containing the adduct is removed and a new patch of DNA is synthesized, using the opposite intact strand as a template. The new DNA segment is then spliced into the DNA molecule in place of the defective one. To be effective in restoring a cell to normal, repair of DNA must occur prior to cell division.

DNA Repair Mechanisms

Although cells possess mechanisms to repair many types of DNA damage, these are not always completely effective, and residual DNA damage can lead to the synthesis of altered protein. Mutations in an oncogene, tumor-suppressor gene, or gene that controls the cell cycle can result in a clonal cell population with a survival advantage. The development of a tumor requires many such events, occurring over a long period of time, and for this reason human cancer induction often takes place within the context of chronic exposure to chemical carcinogens.

Cells have several mechanisms for repairing DNA damage. Repair of DNA damage does not always occur prior to cell replication, and repair of DNA damage by some chemicals is relatively inefficient.

Mismatch Repair of Single-base Mispairs—Many spontaneous mutations are point mutations, a change in a single-base pair in the DNA sequence. Depurination is a fairly common occurrence and a spontaneous event in mammals, and results in the formation of apurinic sites. All mammalian cells possess apurinic endonucleases that function to cut DNA near apurinic sites. The cut is then extended by exonucleases, and the resulting gap repaired by DNA polymerases and ligases.

Excision Repair—DNA regions containing chemically modified bases, or DNA chemical adducts, are typically repaired by excision repair processes. Proteins that slide along the surface of a double-stranded DNA molecule recognize irregularities in the shape of the double helix, and induce repair of the lesion.

End-joining Repair of Nonhomologous DNA—A cell that has double-strand breaks can be repaired by joining the free DNA ends. The joining of broken ends from different chromosomes, however, will lead to the translocation of DNA pieces from one chromosome to another, translocations that have the potential to enable abnormal cell growth. Homologous recombination is one of two mechanisms responsible for the repair of double-strand breaks. In this process, the double-strand break on one chromosome is repaired using the information on the homologous, intact chromosome.

The predominant mechanism for double-stranded DNA repair in multicellular organisms is nonhomologous repair, which involves the rejoining of the ends of the two DNA molecules. Although this process yields a continuous double-stranded molecule, several base pairs are lost at the joining point. This type of deletion may produce a potentially mutagenic coding change.

Classes of Genotoxic Carcinogens

Polyaromatic Hydrocarbons—Polyaromatic hydrocarbons such as benzo(*a*)pyrene are found at high levels in charcoal broiled foods, cigarette smoke, and in diesel exhaust.

Alkylating Agents—Whereas some alkylating chemicals are direct-acting genotoxic agents, many require metabolic activation to produce electrophilic metabolites that can react with DNA. Alkylating agents readily react with DNA at more than 12 sites. The N^7 position of guanine and the N^3 position of adenine are the most reactive sites in DNA for alkylating chemicals.

Aromatic Amines and Amides—Aromatic amines and amides encompass a class of chemicals with varied structures. Classically, exposure to these chemicals was through the dye industry, although exposure still occurs through cigarette smoke and other environmental sources. The aromatic amines undergo phase-I (hydrolysis, reduction, and oxidation) and phase-II (conjugation) metabolism. Phase-I reactions occur mainly by cytochrome P450–mediated reactions, yielding hydroxylated metabolites that are often associated with adduct formation in proteins and DNA, and produce liver and bladder carcinogenicity.

Inorganic Carcinogens

Several metals exhibit carcinogenicity in experimental animals and/or humans, including arsenic, beryllium, cadmium, chromium, nickel, and lead. The carcinogenic manifestations are varied as well and include increased risk for skin, lung, and liver tumors. Additional discussion of selected metals is in Chapter 23.

Nongenotoxic (Epigenetic) Carcinogens

The targets induced by nongenotoxic carcinogens are often in tissues where a significant incidence of background, spontaneous tumors is seen in the animal model. Prolonged exposure to relatively high levels of chemicals is usually necessary for the production of tumors. Examples of the diverse modes of action for non-DNA-reactive carcinogens are listed in Table 8–4.

Cytotoxicity—Chemicals that function through this mechanism produce sustained cell death that is accompanied by persistent regenerative growth. This results in the potential for the acquisition of "spontaneous" DNA mutations and allowing mutated cells to accumulate and proliferate. This process then gives rise to preneoplastic focal lesions that, upon expansion, can lead to tumor formation. The induction of cytotoxicity may be observed with many carcinogens both genotoxic and nongenotoxic when high toxic exposures occur. Thus, the

induction of cytotoxicity with compensatory hyperplasia may contribute to the observed tumorigenicity of many carcinogenic chemicals at high doses.

Receptor Mediated

P450 Inducers: Phenobarbital-like Carcinogens—Phenobarbital is a commonly studied non-DNA reactive compound that is known to cause tumors by a nongenotoxic mechanism involving liver hyperplasia. The induction of CYP2B by phenobarbital is mediated by activation of the constitutive androstane receptor (CAR), a member of the nuclear receptor family. Other CAR-dependent phenobarbital responses that are critical for tumor formation include increased cell proliferation, inhibition of apoptosis, inhibition of gap junctional communication, hypertrophy, and development of preneoplastic focal lesions in the liver.

Peroxisome Proliferator–activated Receptor-α (PPARα)—Various chemicals are capable of increasing the number and volume of peroxisomes in the cytoplasm of cells. These so-called peroxisome proliferators include chemicals such as herbicides, chlorinated solvents (e.g., trichloroethylene and perchloroethylene), plasticizers (e.g., diethylhexylphthalate and other phthalates), lipid-lowering fibrate drugs (e.g., ciprofibrate and clofibrate), and natural products. The currently accepted mode of action for this class of chemicals involves agonist binding to the nuclear hormone receptor, PPARα. PPARα is highly expressed in cells that have active fatty acid oxidation capacity. PPARα plays a central role in lipid metabolism and acts as a transcription factor to modulate gene expression following ligand activation.

Hormonal Mode of Action—Hormonally active chemicals include biogenic amines, steroids, and peptide hormones that cause tissue-specific changes through interaction with a receptor. A number of non-DNA-reactive chemicals induce neoplasia through receptor-mediated mechanisms, and/or perturbation of hormonal balance. Trophic hormones are known to induce cell proliferation at their target organs. This action may lead to the development of tumors when the mechanisms of hormonal control are disrupted and some hormone shows persistently increased levels.

Estrogenic agents can induce tumors in estrogen-dependent tissue. Individuals with higher circulating estrogen levels and those with exposure to the potent estrogenic agent diethylstilbestrol (DES) are at increased risk of cancer development. DES has been causally linked to the higher incidence of adenocarcinomas of the vagina and cervix in daughters of women treated with the hormone during pregnancy. The effects of steroidal chemicals on the cell cycle and on microtubule assembly may be important in the aneuploidy inducing effects of some hormonal agents.

A number of chemicals that reduce thyroid hormone concentrations (T4 and/or T3) and increase thyroid-stimulating hormone (TSH) have been shown to induce neoplasia in the rodent thyroid. TSH demonstrates proliferative activity in the thyroid, with chronic drug-induced TSH increases leading to progression of follicular cell hypertrophy, hyperplasia, and eventually neoplasia.

DNA Methylation and Carcinogenesis—Post-DNA synthetic methylation of the five position on cytosine is a naturally occurring modification to DNA in higher eukaryotes that influences gene expression. Under normal conditions, DNA is methylated symmetrically on both strands. Immediately following DNA replication, the newly synthesized double-stranded DNA contains hemimethylated sites that signal for DNA maintenance methylases to transfer methyl groups from S-adenosylmethionine to cytosine residues on the new DNA strand. The degree of methylation within a gene inversely correlates with the expression of that gene. Several chemical carcinogens are known to modify DNA methylation, methyltransferase activity, and chromosomal structure. During carcinogenesis, both hypomethylation and hypermethylation of the genome have been observed. Tumor-suppressor genes have been reported to be hypermethylated in tumors. Hypomethylation has been associated with increased mutation rates because many oncogenes are hypomethylated and their expression is amplified.

Reactive oxygen species have also been shown to modify DNA methylation by interfering with the ability of methyltransferases to interact with DNA; the resulting hypomethylation allows for the expression of normally quiescent genes. Also, the abnormal methylation pattern observed in cells transformed by chemical oxidants may contribute to an overall aberrant gene expression and promote tumorigenesis.

Oxidative Stress and Chemical Carcinogenesis—Oxygen radicals can be produced by both endogenous and exogenous sources and are typically counterbalanced by antioxidants. Antioxidant defenses are both enzymatic (e.g., superoxide dismutase, glutathione peroxidase, and catalase) and nonenzymatic (e.g., vitamin E, vitamin C, β-carotene, and glutathione). Endogenous sources of reactive oxygen species include oxidative phosphorylation, P450 metabolism, peroxisomes, and inflammatory cell activation. Through these or other currently unknown mechanisms, a number of chemicals that induce cancer (e.g., chlorinated compounds, radiation, metal ions, barbiturates, and some PPARα agonists) induce reactive oxygen species formation and/or oxidative stress.

Oxidative DNA Damage and Carcinogenesis—Reactive oxygen species left unbalanced by antioxidants can result in damage to cellular macromolecules. In DNA, reactive oxygen species can produce single- or double-stranded DNA breaks, purine, pyrimidine, or deoxyribose modifications, and DNA crosslinks. Although many pathways exist that enable the formation of oxidative DNA damage, mammalian cells also possess specific repair pathways for the remediation of oxidative DNA damage.

Mutations and oxidative damage to mitochondrial DNA have been identified in a number of cancers. Compared to nuclear DNA, the mitochondrial genome is relatively susceptible to oxidative base damage due to (1) close proximity to the electron transport system, a major source of reactive oxygen species; (2) mitochondrial DNA is not protected by histones; and (3) DNA repair capacity is limited in the mitochondria.

Aside from oxidized nucleic acids, oxygen radicals can damage cellular biomembranes resulting in lipid peroxidation. Peroxidation of biomembranes generates a variety of products including reactive electrophiles such as epoxides and aldehydes, including malondialdehyde.

Oxidative Stress and Cell Growth Regulation—Reactive oxygen species production and oxidative stress can affect both cell proliferation and apoptosis. It has been demonstrated that low levels of reactive oxygen species influence signal transduction pathways and alter gene expression. Many xenobiotics, by increasing cellular levels of oxidants, alter gene expression through activation of signaling pathways including cAMP-mediated cascades, calcium-calmodulin pathways, transcription factors such as AP-1 and NF-κB, as well as signaling through mitogen-activated protein (MAP) kinases. Activation of these signaling cascades ultimately leads to altered gene expression for a number of genes including those affecting proliferation, differentiation, and apoptosis.

Gap Junctional Intercellular Communication and Carcinogenesis

Cells within an organism communicate in a variety of ways including through gap junctions, which are aggregates of connexin proteins that form a conduit between two adjacent cells. Gap junctional intercellular communication appears to play an important role in the regulation of cell growth and cell death, in part through the ability to exchange small molecules (<1 kDa) between cells. If cell communication is blocked between tumor and normal cells, the exchange of growth inhibitory signals from normal cells to initiated cells is prevented, thus allowing the potential for unregulated growth and clonal expansion of initiated cell populations.

Modifiers of Chemical Carcinogenic Effects

Genetic and environmental factors have a significant impact on the way in which individuals and/or organisms respond to carcinogen exposure. As with most genes, enzymes that metabolize carcinogens are expressed in a tissue-specific manner. Within tissues, the enzymatic profile can vary with cell type or display differential localization within cells. Further, carcinogen metabolizing enzymes are differentially expressed among species. These differences may represent an underlying factor explaining the differential responses to chemical carcinogens across species.

Polymorphisms in Carcinogen Metabolism and DNA Repair

Genetic polymorphisms arise from human genetic variability. A genetic polymorphism is when a gene has more than one allele. In assessing variability in the human genome project it was found that base variations occurred at approximately once in every 1 000 base pairs. Therefore, there may be over one million genetic variations between any two individuals. A single nucleotide polymorphism (SNP) is a variant in DNA sequence found in greater than 1% of the population. Thus, by definition, changes in DNA sequence go from mutation to polymorphism when a unique genotype is seen in over 1% of the population. Over three million candidate SNPs have been identified to date with up to 10 million being estimated to be present within the human genome. In carcinogenesis, genetic polymorphisms may account for the susceptibility of some individuals to certain cancers. In carcinogenesis, genetic polymorphisms may account for the susceptibility of some individuals to certain cancers. A number of polymorphisms have been described in carcinogen-metabolizing enzymes, with certain alleles linked to altered risk of selective cancers. Glutathione *S*-transferases (GSTs) are highly polymorphic in humans. The GSTM1 isoform is particularly important in carcinogenesis, because of its high reactivity toward epoxides.

Carcinogenic risk depends on both exposure (dose and duration) as well as genetic susceptibility. For example, if the genetic susceptibility is high, then exposure to a chemical carcinogen will result in a higher risk for cancer development.

Proto-oncogenes and Tumor-suppressor Genes

Proto-oncogenes and tumor-suppressor genes encode a wide array of proteins that function to control cell growth and proliferation. Common characteristics of oncogenes and tumor-suppressor genes are shown in Table 8–5. Mutations in both oncogenes and tumor-suppressor genes contribute to the progressive development of human cancers. Accumulated damage to multiple oncogenes and/or tumor-suppressor genes can result in altered cell proliferation, differentiation, and/or survival of cancer cells.

Retroviruses—The *Rous sarcoma virus* (RSV) is capable of transforming a normal cell and producing sarcomas. The genome of RSV and other retroviruses consists of two identical copies of mRNA, which is then reverse transcribed into DNA and incorporated into the host-cell genome. Oncogenic transforming viruses like RSV contain the v-*src* gene, a gene required for cancer induction. Normal cells contain a gene closely related to v-*src* in RSV. This discovery showed that cancer may be induced by the action of normal, or nearly normal, genes.

DNA Viruses—Unlike retroviral oncogenes, which are derived from normal cellular genes and have no function for the virus, the known oncogenes of DNA viruses are integral parts of the viral genome required for viral replication. Infection by small DNA viruses is lethal to most non-host animal cells; however, a small proportion integrates the viral DNA into the host-cell genome. The cells that survive infection become permanently transformed due to the presence of one or more oncogenes in the viral DNA. Papilloma viruses can infect and cause tumors in humans. Some examples of oncogenic DNA viruses include human papilloma viruses, Epstein–Barr virus, hepatitis B virus, and herpes viruses.

Proto-oncogenes—An oncogene encodes a protein that is capable of transforming cells in culture or inducing cancer in animals. Of the known oncogenes, the majority appear to have been derived from normal genes (i.e., proto-oncogenes), and are involved in cell signaling cascades. Because most proto-oncogenes are essential for maintaining viability, they are highly conserved. Activation of proto-oncogenes to oncogenes arises through mutational events occurring within proto-oncogenes. It has been recognized that a number of chemical carcinogens are capable of inducing mutations in proto-oncogenes. Oncogene products can operate at multiple levels of signaling cascades, including ligand, receptor, second messengers, and transcription factor stages of transduction.

TABLE 8–5 Characteristics of proto-oncogenes, cellular oncogenes, and tumor-suppressor genes.

Proto-oncogenes	Oncogenes	Tumor-suppressor Genes
Dominant	Dominant	Recessive
Broad tissue specificity for cancer development	Broad tissue specificity for cancer development	Considerable tissue specificity for cancer development
Germ line inheritance rarely involved in cancer development	Germ line inheritance frequently involved in cancer development	Germ line inheritance frequently involved in cancer development
Analogous to certain viral oncogenes	No known analogs in oncogenic viruses	No known analogs in oncogenic viruses
Somatic mutations activated during all stages of carcinogenesis	Somatic mutations activated during all stages of carcinogenesis	Germ line mutations may initiate, but mutation to neoplasia occurs only during progression stage

the mismatch, stabilization of the binding by the addition of one or more proteins, cutting the DNA at a distance from the mismatch, excision past the mismatch, resynthesis, and ligation.

O⁶-Methylguanine-DNA Methyltransferase Repair—The enzyme O⁶-methylguanine-DNA methyltransferase (MGMT) protects cells against the toxic effects of simple alkylating agents by transferring the methyl group from O⁶-methylguanine in DNA to a cysteine residue in MGMT. The adducted base is reverted to a normal one by the enzyme, which is itself inactivated by the reaction.

Formation of Gene Mutations

Somatic Cells—Gene mutations, considered to be small DNA-sequence changes confined to a single gene, are substitutions, small additions, and small deletions. Base substitutions are the replacement of the correct nucleotide by an incorrect one; they can be further subdivided as transitions, where the change is purine for purine or pyrimidine for pyrimidine, and transversions where the change is purine for pyrimidine or vice versa. Frameshift mutations are the addition or deletion of one or a few base pairs (not in multiples of 3) in protein-coding regions.

The great majority of so-called spontaneous (background) mutations arise from *replication* of an altered template. These DNA alterations are either the result of oxidative damage or produced from the deamination of 5-methyl cytosine to thymine at CpG sites resulting in G:C $\rightarrow$ A:T transitions. Mutations induced by ionizing radiations tend to be deletions ranging in size from a few bases to multilocus events.

Gene mutations produced by a majority of chemicals and nonionizing radiations are base substitutions, frameshifts, and small deletions. Of these mutations, most are produced by errors of DNA *replication* on a damaged template. The relative mutation frequency will be the outcome of the race between repair and replication, that is, the more repair that takes place prior to replication, the lower the mutation frequency for a given amount of induced DNA damage. Significant regulators of the race are cell-cycle checkpoint genes (e.g., *P53*) because if the cell is checked from entering the S phase at a G_1/S checkpoint, then more repair can take place prior to the cell starting to replicate its DNA.

Germ Cells—The mechanism of production of gene mutations in germ cells is basically the same as in somatic cells. Ionizing radiations produce mainly deletions via errors of DNA repair; the majority of chemicals induce base substitutions, frameshifts, and small deletions by errors of DNA replication.

An important consideration for assessing gene mutations induced by chemicals in germ cells is the relationship between exposure and the timing of DNA replication (i.e., if there is damage, is it able to be repaired before replication?). The spermatogonial stem cell is the major contributor to genetic risk assessment because it is present generally throughout the reproductive lifetime of an individual. Each time a spermatogonial stem cell divides, it produces a differentiating spermatogonium and a stem cell. This stem cell can accumulate genetic damage from chronic exposures.

In oogenesis, the primary oocyte arrests prior to birth, and there is no further S phase until the zygote. For this reason, the oocyte is resistant to the induction of gene mutations by most chemicals.

Formation of Chromosomal Alterations
Somatic Cells

Structural Chromosome Aberrations—There are common components between the formation of chromosome aberrations, sister chromatid exchanges (SCEs; the apparently reciprocal exchange between the sister chromatids of a single chromosome), and gene mutations. In particular, damaged DNA serves as the substrate leading to chromosomal aberrations. However, chromosome aberrations induced by ionizing radiations are generally formed by errors of DNA repair, whereas those produced by nonradiomimetic chemicals are generally formed by errors of DNA replication on a damaged DNA template.

The DNA repair errors that lead to the formation of chromosome aberrations following ionizing radiation exposure arise from misligation of double-strand breaks or interaction of coincidentally repairing regions during nucleotide excision repair of damaged bases. Incorrect rejoining of chromosomal pieces during repair leads to chromosomal exchanges within and between chromosomes. Failure to rejoin double-strand breaks or to complete repair of other types of DNA damage leads to terminal deletions.

The failure to incorporate an acentric fragment into a daughter nucleus at anaphase/telophase, or the failure of a whole chromosome to segregate to the cellular poles at anaphase, can result in the formation of a micronucleus that resides in the cytoplasm. Errors of DNA replication on a damaged template can lead to a variety of chromosomal alterations. The majority of these involve deletion or exchanges of individual chromatids but some can involve both chromatids.

Numerical Chromosome Changes—Numerical changes (e.g., monosomies, trisomies, and ploidy changes) can arise from errors in chromosomal segregation due to any of the numerous possible impairments of mitotic control processes. Alteration of various cellular components can result in failure to segregate the sister chromatids to separate daughter cells or in failure to segregate a chromosome to either pole.

Sister Chromatid Exchange—SCEs are produced during S phase and are presumed to be a consequence of errors in the replication process.

Germ Cells—The formation of chromosomal alterations in germ cells is basically the same as that for somatic cells, namely, via misrepair for ionizing radiations and radiomimetic chemicals for treatments in G_1 and G_2, and by errors of replication for all radiations and chemicals for DNA damage present during the S phase.

The types of aberrations formed in germ cells are the same as those formed in somatic cells. The specific segregation of chromosomes during meiosis influences the probability of recovery of an aberration, particularly a reciprocal translocation, in the offspring of a treated parent.

ASSAYS FOR DETECTING GENETIC ALTERATIONS

Introduction to Assay Design

Genetic toxicology assays serve two interrelated but distinct purposes in the toxicologic evaluation of chemicals: (1) identifying mutagens for purposes of hazard identification and (2) characterizing dose–response relationships and mutagenic mechanisms.

Table 9–1 lists many of the assays employed in genetic toxicology. Some assays for gene mutations detect forward mutations, whereas others detect reversion. Forward mutations are genetic alterations in a wild-type gene and are detected by a change in phenotype caused by the alteration or loss of gene function. In contrast, a back mutation or reversion is a mutation that restores gene function in a mutant and thereby brings about a return to the wild-type phenotype. The simplest gene mutation assays rely on selection techniques to detect mutations. By imposing experimental conditions under which only cells or organisms that have undergone mutation can grow, selection techniques greatly facilitate the identification of rare cells that have experienced mutation among the many cells that have not.

Studying mutagenesis in intact animals requires more complex assays, which range from inexpensive short-term tests that can be performed in a few days to complicated assays for mutations in mammalian germ cells. Typically, there remains a gradation in which an increase in relevance for human risk entails more elaborate and costly tests.

Many compounds that are not themselves mutagenic or carcinogenic can be activated into mutagens and carcinogens by mammalian metabolism. Such compounds are called promutagens and procarcinogens. The most widely used metabolic activation system in microbial and cell culture assays is a postmitochondrial supernatant from a rat liver homogenate, along with appropriate buffers and cofactors. Most of the short-term assays in Table 9–1 require exogenous metabolic activation to detect promutagens. Exceptions are those in intact mammals.

Despite their usefulness, in vitro metabolic activation systems cannot mimic mammalian metabolism perfectly. There are differences among tissues in reactions that activate or inactivate foreign compounds, and organisms of the normal flora of the gut can contribute to metabolism in intact mammals. Agents that induce enzyme systems or otherwise alter the physiological state can also modify the metabolism of toxicants, and the balance between activation and detoxication reactions in vitro may differ from that in vivo.

Structural Alerts and In Silico Assays

The first indication that a chemical is a mutagen often lies in chemical structure. Potential electrophilic sites in a molecule serve as an alert to possible mutagenicity and carcinogenicity because such sites confer reactivity with nucleophilic sites in DNA. Developmental work to formalize the structural prediction through automated computer programs has not yet led to an ability to predict mutagenicity and carcinogenicity of new chemicals with great accuracy. These computer-based systems for predicting genotoxicity based on chemical properties are sometimes called in silico assays. These assays include computational and structural programs and the modeling of quantitative structure–activity relationships. Although there is much skepticism that such approaches can replace biological testing, they hold promise of improving the efficiency of testing strategies and reducing current levels of animal use.

DNA Damage and Repair Assays

Some assays measure DNA damage itself rather than mutational consequences of DNA damage. They may do so directly, through such indicators as chemical adducts or strand breaks in DNA, or indirectly, through measurement of biological repair processes. Adducts in DNA can be detected by ^{32}P-postlabeling, high-performance liquid chromatography (HPLC), fluorescence-based methods, mass spectrometry, immunological methods using antibodies against specific adducts, isotope-labeled DNA binding, and electrochemical detection.

A rapid method of measuring DNA damage is the comet assay. In this assay, cells are incorporated into agarose on slides, lysed so as to liberate their DNA, and subjected to electrophoresis. The DNA is stained with a fluorescent dye for observation and image analysis. Because broken DNA fragments migrate more quickly than larger pieces of DNA, a blur of fragments (a "comet") is observed when the DNA is extensively damaged. The extent of DNA damage can be estimated from the length and other attributes of the comet tail. The comet assay appears to be a sensitive indicator of DNA damage with broad applicability among diverse species, including plants, worms, mollusks, fish, and amphibians.

The occurrence of DNA repair can serve as a readily measured indicator of DNA damage. A common excision repair assay in mammalian cells measures unscheduled DNA synthesis (UDS). The occurrence of UDS indicates that the DNA had been damaged. The absence of UDS, however, does not provide evidence that DNA has not been damaged because some classes of damage are not readily excised, and some excisable damage may not be detected as a consequence of assay insensitivity.

Gene Mutations in Prokaryotes

The most common means of detecting mutations in microorganisms is selecting for reversion in strains that have a specific nutritional requirement differing from wild-type members of

TABLE 9–1 Overview of genetic toxicology assays.

Assays

I. Prediction of genotoxicity
   A. Interpretation of chemical structure
       Structural alerts to genotoxicity
   B. In silico predictive models
       Computational and structural programs: MCASE,
         TOPKAT, DEREK
       Quantitative structure–activity relationship (QSAR) modeling

II. DNA damage and repair assays
   A. Direct detection of DNA damage
       Alkaline elution assays for DNA strand breakage
         in hepatocytes
       Comet assay (single-cell gel electrophoresis) for DNA strand
         breakage
       Comet-FISH assay for region-specific DNA damage and repair
       Nonmammalian comets in ecotoxicology
       Assays for chemical adducts in DNA
   B. DNA repair, recombination, and genotoxic stress responses as
      indicators of damage
       Differential killing of repair-deficient and wild-type bacteria
       Induction of the bacterial SOS system
       "Green Screen" for GADD45a gene induction in
         TK6 human cells
       Unscheduled DNA synthesis (UDS) in isolated rat hepatocytes
         or rodents in vivo
       Induction of mitotic recombination

III. Prokaryote gene mutation assays
   A. Bacterial reverse mutation assays
       Salmonella/mammalian microsome assay (Ames test)
       E. coli WP2 tryptophan reversion assay
       Salmonella-specific base-pair substitution assay
         (Ames II assay)
       E. coli lacZ-specific reversion assay
   B. Bacterial forward mutation assays
       E. coli lacI assay
       Resistance to toxic metabolites or analogs in *Salmonella*

IV. Assays in nonmammalian eukaryotes
   A. Fungal assays
       Forward mutations, reversion, and small deletions
       Mitotic crossing over, gene conversion, and homology-
         mediated deletions in yeast
       Genetic detection of mitotic and meiotic aneuploidy in yeast
   B. Plant assays
       Gene mutations affecting chlorophyll in seedlings, the waxy
         locus in pollen, or *Tradescantia stamen* hair color
       Chromosome aberrations and micronuclei in mitotic and
         meiotic cells of corn, *Tradescantia*, and other plants
   C. *Drosophila* assays
       Sex-linked recessive lethal test in germ cells
       Heritable translocation assays
       Mitotic recombination and LOH in eyes or wings

V. Mammalian gene mutation assays
   A. In vitro assays for forward mutations
       tk mutations in mouse lymphoma or human cells
       hprt or *xprt* mutations in Chinese hamster or human cells
       CD59 mutations in CHO-human hybrid AL cells
   B. In vivo assays for gene mutations in somatic cells
       Mouse spot test (somatic cell specific-locus test)
       hprt mutations (6-thioguanine-resistance) in rodent
         lymphocytes
       Pig-a mutations (immunological detection of mutations
         blocking glycosylphosphatidylinositol synthesis)

C. Transgenic assays
       Mutations in the bacterial *lacI* gene in "Big Blue" mice and rats
       Mutations in the bacterial *lacZ* gene in the "Muta Mouse"
       Mutations in the phage *cII* gene in lacI or lacZ transgenic mice
       Point mutations and deletions in the lacZ plasmid mouse
       Point mutations and deletions in delta gpt mice and rats
       Forward mutations and reversions in ΦX174 transgenic mice
       Inversions and deletions arising in pKZ1 mice by
         intrachromosomal recombination

VI. Mammalian cytogenetic assays
   A. Chromosome aberrations
       Metaphase analysis in cultured Chinese hamster or
         human cells
       Metaphase analysis of rodent bone marrow or lymphocytes
         in vivo
       Chromosome painting and other FISH applications in vitro
         and in vivo
   B. Micronuclei
       Cytokinesis-block micronucleus assay in human lymphocytes
       Micronucleus assay in mammalian cell lines
       In vivo micronucleus assay in rodent bone marrow or blood
       In vivo micronucleus assay in tissues other than marrow
         or blood
   C. Sister chromatid exchange
       SCE in human cells or Chinese hamster cells
       SCE in rodent tissues, especially bone marrow
   D. Aneuploidy in mitotic cells
       Hyperploidy detected by chromosome counting or FISH in
         cell cultures or bone marrow
       Micronucleus assay with centromere/kinetochore labeling in
         cell cultures
       Altered parameters in flow-cytometric detection of
         micronuclei in CHO cells
       Mouse bone marrow micronucleus assay with centromere
         labeling

VII. Germ cell mutagenesis
   A. Measurement of DNA damage
       Molecular dosimetry based on mutagen adducts in
         reproductive cells
       UDS in rodent germ cells
       Alkaline elution assays for DNA strand breaks in rodent testes
       Comet assay in sperm and gonadal tissue
   B. Gene mutations
       Mouse specific-locus test for gene mutations and deletions
       Mouse electrophoretic specific-locus test
       Dominant mutations causing mouse skeletal defects or
         cataracts
       ESTR assay in mice
       Germ cell mutations in transgenic assays
   C. Chromosomal aberrations
       Cytogenetic analysis of oocytes, spermatogonia,
         spermatocytes, or zygotes
       Direct detection in sperm by FISH
       Micronuclei in mouse spermatids
       Mouse heritable translocation test
   D. Dominant lethal mutations
       Mouse or rat dominant lethal assay
   E. Aneuploidy
       Cytogenetic analysis for aneuploidy arising by nondisjunction
       Sex chromosome loss test for nondisjunction or breakage
       Micronucleus assay in spermatids with centromere labeling
       FISH with probes for specific chromosomes in sperm

the species; such strains are called auxotrophs. In the Ames assay, one measures the frequency of histidine-independent bacteria that arise in a histidine-requiring strain in the presence or absence of the chemical being tested. Auxotrophic (nutrient-deficient) bacteria are treated with the chemical of interest and plated on medium that is deficient in histidine; if the colony survives, it must have a reversion mutation that allows it to survive without exogenous histidine.

The development of specific reversion assays of histidine mutations in *Salmonella* strains and of *lacZ* mutations in *Escherichia coli* has made the identification of specific base-pair substitutions more straightforward. Bacterial forward mutation assays, such as selections for resistance to arabinose or to purine or pyrimidine analogs in *Salmonella*, are also used in research and testing, although less extensively than reversion assays.

Genetic Alterations in Nonmammalian Eukaryotes

Gene Mutations and Chromosome Aberrations—The fruit fly, *Drosophila*, has long occupied a prominent place in genetic research because of the sex-linked recessive lethal (SLRL) test. The SLRL test permits the detection of recessive lethal mutations at 600 to 800 different loci on the X chromosome by screening for the presence or absence of wild-type males in the offspring of specifically designed crosses. A significant increase over the frequency of spontaneous SLRLs in the lineages derived from treated males indicates mutagenesis. The SLRL test yields information about mutagenesis in germ cells, which is lacking in microbial and cell culture systems.

Genetic and cytogenetic assays in plants continue to find use in special applications, such as in situ monitoring for mutagens and exploration of the metabolism of promutagens by agricultural plants. In situ monitoring entails looking for evidence of mutagenesis in organisms that are grown in the environment of interest.

Mitotic Recombination—Assays in nonmammalian eukaryotes are important for the study of induced recombination. Recombinogenic effects in yeast have long been used as a general indicator of genetic damage. The best characterized assays for recombinogens are those that detect mitotic crossing over and mitotic gene conversion in the yeast *Saccharomyces cerevisiae*.

Gene Mutations in Mammals

Gene Mutations In Vitro—Mutagenicity assays in cultured mammalian cells have some of the same advantages as microbial assays with respect to speed and cost, and they follow quite similar approaches. The most widely used assays for gene mutations in mammalian cells detect forward mutations that confer resistance to a toxic chemical.

Gene Mutations In Vivo—In vivo assays involve treating intact animals and analyzing genetic effects in appropriate tissues. Mutations may be detected either in somatic cells or in germ cells.

The mouse spot test is a traditional genetic assay for gene mutations in somatic cells. Visible spots of altered phenotype in mice heterozygous for coat color genes indicate mutations in the progenitor cells of the altered regions.

Besides determining whether agents are mutagenic, mutation assays also provide information on mechanisms of mutagenesis. Base-pair substitutions and large deletions can be differentiated through the use of probes for the target gene and Southern blotting, in that base substitutions are too subtle to be detectable on the blots. Gene mutations have been characterized at the molecular level by DNA-sequence analysis both in transgenic rodents and in endogenous mammalian genes.

Transgenic Assays—Transgenic animals are products of DNA technology in which the animal contains foreign DNA sequences that have been added to the genome and are transmitted through the germ line. The foreign DNA is therefore represented in all the somatic cells of the animal.

Mice that carry *lac* genes from *E. coli* use either *lacI* or *lacZ* as a target for mutagenesis. After mutagenic treatment of the transgenic animals, the *lac* genes are recovered from the animal, packaged into phage λ, and transferred to *E. coli* for mutational analysis. Mutant plaques are identified on the basis of phenotype, and mutant frequencies can be calculated for different tissues of the treated animals.

Mammalian Cytogenetic Assays

Chromosome Aberrations—Genetic assays without DNA sequencing are indirect, in that one observes a phenotype and reaches conclusions about genes. In contrast, cytogenetic assays use microscopy for direct observation of the effect of interest. In conventional cytogenetics, metaphase analysis is used to detect chromosomal anomalies. Cells should be treated during a sensitive period of the cell cycle (typically S), and aberrations should be analyzed at the first mitotic division after treatment. Examples of chromosome aberrations are shown in Figure 9–3.

It is essential that sufficient cells be analyzed because a negative result in a small sample is equivocal and inconclusive. Results should be recorded for specific classes of aberrations, not just as an overall index of aberrations per cell.

In interpreting results on the induction of chromosome aberrations in cell cultures, questionable positive results have been found at highly cytotoxic doses, high osmolality, and pH extremes. Although excessively high doses may lead to artifactual positive responses, the failure to test sufficiently high doses also undermines the utility of a test; therefore, testing should be conducted at an intermediate dose and extended to a dose at which some cytotoxicity is observed.

In vivo assays for chromosome aberrations involve treating intact animals and later collecting cells for cytogenetic analysis. The main advantage of in vivo assays is that they

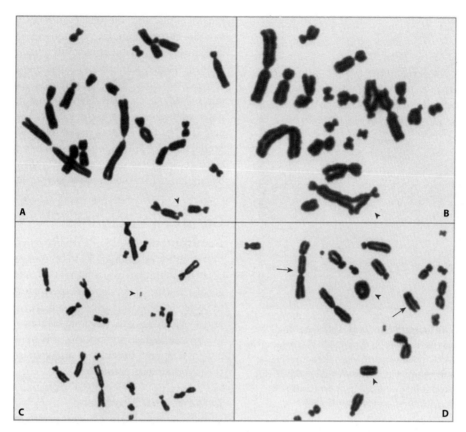

FIGURE 9–3 **Chromosome aberrations induced by x-rays in Chinese hamster ovary (CHO) cells.** *A.* A chromatid deletion (▶). *B.* A chromatid exchange called a triradial (▶). *C.* A small interstitial deletion (▶) that resulted from chromosome breakage. *D.* A metaphase with more than one aberration: a centric ring plus an acentric fragment (▶) and a dicentric chromosome plus an acentric fragment (→).

include mammalian metabolism, DNA repair, and pharmacodynamics. The target is a tissue from which large numbers of dividing cells are easily prepared for analysis such as bone marrow.

In interphase cell analysis by fluorescence in situ hybridization (FISH; Figure 9–4), a nucleic acid probe is hybridized to complementary sequences in chromosomal DNA. The probe is labeled with a fluorescent dye so that the chromosomal location to which it binds is visible by fluorescence microscopy; often, probes are used that cover the whole chromosome, called "chromosome painting."

Chromosome painting facilitates cytogenetic analysis, because aberrations are easily detected by the number of fluorescent regions in a painted metaphase. FISH permits the scoring of stable aberrations, such as translocations and insertions, which are not readily detected in traditional metaphase analysis of unbanded chromosomes.

Micronuclei—Micronuclei are membrane-bounded structures that contain chromosomal fragments, or sometimes whole chromosomes, that were not incorporated into a daughter nucleus at mitosis. Micronuclei usually represent acentric chromosomal fragments, and they are commonly used as simple indicators of chromosomal damage. Micronuclei in a binucleate human lymphocyte are shown in Figure 9–5.

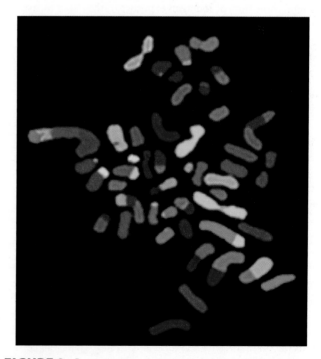

FIGURE 9–4 **Chromosome aberrations identified by FISH.** Human breast cancer cell with aneuploidy for some chromosomes and with reciprocal translocations identified by color switches along a chromosome.

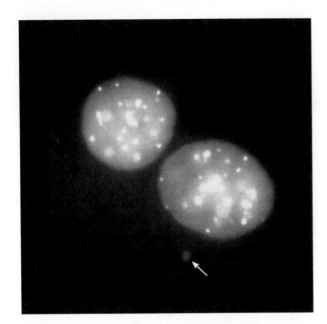

FIGURE 9–5 Micronucleus in a human lymphocyte. The cytochalasin B method was used to inhibit cytokinesis that resulted in a binucleate nucleus. The micronucleus (arrow) resulted from failure of an acentric chromosome fragment or a whole chromosome being included in a daughter nucleus following cell division. (Used with permission of James Allen, Jill Barnes, and Barbara Collins.)

Sister Chromatid Exchange—SCE, in which apparently reciprocal segments have been exchanged between the two chromatids of a chromosome, is visible cytologically through differential staining of chromatids (Figure 9–6). SCE assays are general indicators of mutagen exposure, rather than measures of a mutagenic effect.

Aneuploidy—Assays for aneuploidy include chromosome counting, the detection of micronuclei that contain kinetochores, and the observation of abnormal spindles or spindle–chromosome associations in cells in which spindles and chromosomes have been differentially stained.

The presence of the spindle attachment region of a chromosome (kinetochore) in a micronucleus can indicate that it contains a whole chromosome. Aneuploidy may therefore be detected by means of antikinetochore antibodies with a fluorescent label or FISH with a probe for centromere-specific DNA. Frequencies of micronuclei ascribable to aneuploidy and to clastogenic effects may therefore be determined concurrently by tabulating micronuclei with and without kinetochores.

Germ Cell Mutagenesis

Gene Mutations—Mammalian germ cell assays provide the best basis for assessing risks to human germ cells. Mammalian assays permit the measurement of mutagenesis at different germ cell stages. Late stages of spermatogenesis are often found to be sensitive to mutagenesis, but spermatocytes, spermatids, and spermatozoa are transitory. Mutagenesis in stem cell spermatogonia and resting oocytes is of special interest in genetic risk assessment because of the persistence of these stages throughout reproductive life.

Chromosomal Alterations—Knowledge of the induction of chromosome aberrations in germ cells is important for assessing risks to future generations. A germ cell micronucleus assay has been developed, in which chromosomal damage induced in meiosis is measured by observation of rodent spermatids. Aneuploidy originating in mammalian germ cells may be detected cytologically through chromosome counting for hyperploidy or genetically in the mouse sex-chromosome loss test.

Besides cytological observation, indirect evidence for chromosome aberrations is obtained in the mouse heritable translocation assay, which measures reduced fertility in the offspring of

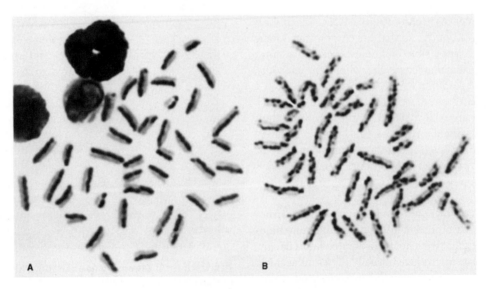

FIGURE 9–6 Sister chromatid exchanges (SCEs) in human lymphocytes. A. SCEs in untreated cell. B. SCEs in cell exposed to ethyl carbamate. The treatment results in a very large increase in the number of SCEs. (Used with permission of James Allen and Barbara Collins.)

treated males. This presumptive evidence of chromosomal rearrangements can be confirmed through cytogenetic analysis.

Dominant Lethal Mutations—The mouse or rat dominant lethal assay offers an extensive database on the induction of genetic damage in mammalian germ cells. Commonly, males are treated on an acute or subchronic basis with the agent of interest and then mated with virgin females. The females are killed and necropsied during pregnancy so that embryonic mortality, assumed to be due to chromosomal anomalies, may be characterized and quantified.

Development of Testing Strategies

Concern about adverse effects of mutation on human health, principally carcinogenesis and the induction of transmissible damage in germ cells, has provided the impetus to identify environmental mutagens. Genetic toxicology assays may be used to screen chemicals to detect mutagens and to obtain information on mutagenic mechanisms and dose–responses that contribute to an evaluation of hazards. Besides testing pure chemicals, environmental samples are tested because many mutagens exist in complex mixtures. The analysis of complex mixtures often requires a combination of mutagenicity assays and refined analytical methods.

Assessment of a chemical's genotoxicity requires data from well-characterized genetic assays. Sensitivity refers to the proportion of carcinogens that are positive in the assay, whereas specificity is the proportion of noncarcinogens that are negative. Sensitivity and specificity both contribute to the predictive reliability of an assay. Assays are said to be validated when they have been shown to perform reproducibly and reliably with many compounds from diverse chemical classes in several laboratories.

Rather than trying to assemble batteries of complementary assays, it is prudent to emphasize mechanistic considerations in choosing assays. Such an approach makes a sensitive assay for gene mutations (e.g., the Ames assay) and an assay for clastogenic effects in mammals pivotal in the evaluation of genotoxicity. Beyond gene mutations, one should evaluate damage at the chromosomal level with a mammalian in vitro or in vivo cytogenetic assay. Other assays offer an extensive database on chemical mutagenesis (*Drosophila* SLRL), a unique genetic end point (i.e., aneuploidy; mitotic recombination), applicability to diverse organisms and tissues (i.e., DNA damage assays, such as the comet assay), or special importance in the assessment of genetic risk (i.e., germ cell assays).

HUMAN POPULATION MONITORING

For cancer risk assessment considerations, the human data utilized most frequently, in the absence of epidemiologic data, are those collected from genotoxicity/mutagenicity assessments in human populations. The studies conducted most frequently are for chromosome aberrations, micronuclei, and SCEs in peripheral lymphocytes.

The size of each study group should be sufficiently large to avoid any confounder having undue influence. Certain characteristics should be matched among exposed and unexposed groups. These include age, sex, smoking status, and general dietary features. Study groups of 20 or more individuals can be used as a reasonable substitute for exact matching because confounders will be less influential on chromosome alteration or mutation frequency in larger groups. In some instances, it might be informative to compare exposed groups with a historical control, as well as to a concurrent control.

Reciprocal translocations are transmissible from cell generation to generation, and frequency can be representative of an accumulation over time of exposure. The importance of this is that stable chromosome aberrations observed in peripheral lymphocytes exposed in vivo, but assessed following in vitro culture, are produced in vivo in hematopoietic stem cells or other precursor cells of the peripheral lymphocyte pool.

NEW APPROACHES FOR GENETIC TOXICOLOGY

The ability to manipulate and characterize DNA, RNA, and proteins has been at the root of the advance in our understanding of basic cellular processes and how they can be perturbed. However, the development of sophisticated molecular biology does not in itself imply a corresponding advance in the utility of genetic toxicology and its application to risk assessment. Knowing the types of studies to conduct and knowing how to interpret the data remain as fundamental as always. There is a need for genetic toxicology to avoid the temptation to use more and more sophisticated techniques to address the same questions and in the end make the same mistakes as have been made previously.

Advances in Cytogenetics

Conventional chromosome staining with DNA stains such as Giemsa or the process of chromosome banding requires considerable expenditure of time and a rather high level of expertise. Chromosome banding does allow for the assessment of transmissible aberrations such as reciprocal translocations and inversions with a fairly high degree of accuracy. Stable aberrations are transmissible from parent to daughter cell, and they represent effects of chronic exposures. The more readily analyzed but cell-lethal, nontransmissible aberrations such as dicentrics and deletions reflect only recent exposures and then only when analyzed at the first division after exposure.

Specific chromosomes, specific genes, and chromosome alterations can be detected readily since the development of FISH. In principle, the technique relies on amplification of DNA from particular genomic regions such as whole chromosomes or gene regions and the hybridization of these amplified DNAs to metaphase chromosome preparations or interphase nuclei. Regions of hybridization can be determined by the use of fluorescent antibodies that detect modified DNA bases incorporated during amplification or by incorporating fluorescent bases during amplification. The fluorescently labeled, hybridized regions are detected by fluorescence micros-copy. Alterations in tumors can also be detected on a whole-genome basis. Comparative genomic hybridization (CGH) has allowed an accurate and sensitive assessment of chromosomal alterations present in tumors. CGH is adapted for automated screening approaches using biochips.

The types of data collected will affect our understanding of how tumors develop. Data on the dose–response characteris-tics for a specific chromosomal alteration as a proximate marker of cancer can enhance the cancer risk assessment pro-cess by describing effects of low exposures that are below those for which tumor incidence can be reliably assessed. Cytogenetic data can also improve extrapolation of data generated with lab-oratory animals to humans.

Molecular Analysis of Mutations and Gene Expression

With technological advances, the exact basis of a mutation at the level of the DNA sequence can be established. With hybrid-ization of test DNAs to oligonucleotide arrays, specific genetic alterations or their cellular consequences can be determined rapidly and automatically. cDNA microarray technologies allow the measurement of changes in expression of hundreds or even thousands of genes at one time. The level of expression at the mRNA level is measured by amount of hybridization of iso-lated cDNAs to oligonucleotide fragments from known genes or expressed sequence tags (EST) on a specifically laid out grid. This technique holds great promise for establishing a cell's response to exposure to chemical or physical agents in the con-text of normal cellular patterns of gene expression.

These microarray-based techniques are now being replaced by massively parallel sequencing or ultrahigh throughput sequencing approaches that can quantitatively assess gene expression changes in response to exposures. Such sequencing-based techniques have the great advantage that they are based on molecule counting approaches rather than on hybridiza-tion, thereby making them more quantitative and able to detect very low level transcripts. There are parallel efforts in the area of proteomics and metabolomics whereby changes in a broad range of cellular proteins can be assessed in response to endog-enous or exogenous factors, potentially leading to the develop-ment of biomarkers of effect.

The move in the field of genetic toxicology is away from the "yes/no" approach to hazard identification and much more toward a mechanistic understanding of how a chemical or physical agent can produce adverse cellular and tissue responses. In turn such knowledge can be used for the develop-ment of informative bioindicators representing the key events along the pathway from initial interactions with cells to adverse outcome. The move is clearly toward analysis at the whole genome level and away from single gene responses.

CONCLUSION

Genetic toxicology demonstrated that ionizing radiations and chemicals could induce mutations and chromosome alterations in plant, insect, and mammalian cells. Various short-term assays for genetic toxicology identified many mutagens and address the relationship between mutagens and carcinogens. Failure of the assays to be completely predictive resulted in the identification of nongenotoxic carcinogens. Key cellular pro-cesses related to mutagenesis have been identified, including multiple pathways of DNA repair, cell-cycle controls, and the role of checkpoints in ensuring that the cell cycle does not pro-ceed until the DNA and specific cellular structures are checked for fidelity. Recent developments in genetic toxicology have improved our understanding of basic cellular processes and alterations that can affect the integrity of the genetic material and its functions. The ability to detect and analyze mutations in mammalian germ cells continues to improve and contribute to a better appreciation for the long-term consequences of muta-genesis in human populations.

BIBLIOGRAPHY

Bansbach CE, Cortez D: Defining genome maintenance pathways using functional genomic approaches. *Crit Rev Biochem Mol Biol* 49:327–341, 2011

Barile FA: *Principles of Toxicology Testing*. Boca Raton, FL: CRC Press, 2013.

Mahadevan B, Snyder RD, Waters MD, et al.: Genetic toxicity in the 21st century: reflections and future directions. *Environ Mol Mutagen* 52:339–364, 2011.

Semizarov D, Blomme E: *Genomics in Drug Discovery and Development*. Hoboken, NJ: John Wiley & Sons, 2009.

QUESTIONS

1. Oncogenes:
   a. maintain normal cellular growth and development.
   b. exert their action in a genetically recessive fashion.
   c. are often formed via translocation to a location with a more active promoter.
   d. can be mutated to form proto-oncogenes.
   e. include growth factors and GTPases, but not transcription factors.

2. Which of the following is NOT one of the more common sources of DNA damage?
   a. ionizing radiation.
   b. UV light.
   c. electrophilic chemicals.
   d. DNA polymerase error.
   e. x-rays.

3. Which of the following pairs of DNA repair mechanisms is most likely to introduce mutations into the genetic composition of an organism?
   a. nonhomologous end-joining (NHEJ) and base excision repair.
   b. nonhomologous end-joining and homologous recombination.
   c. homologous recombination and nucleotide excision repair.
   d. nucleotide excision repair and base excision repair.
   e. homologous recombination and mismatch repair.

4. Which of the following DNA mutations would NOT be considered a frameshift mutation?
   a. insertion of 5 nucleotides.
   b. insertion of 7 nucleotides.
   c. deletion of 18 nucleotides.
   d. deletion of 13 nucleotides.
   e. deletion of 1 nucleotide.

5. Which of the following base-pair mutations is properly characterized as a transversion mutation?
   a. $T \rightarrow C$.
   b. $A \rightarrow G$.
   c. $G \rightarrow A$.
   d. $T \rightarrow U$.
   e. $A \rightarrow C$.

6. All of the following statements regarding nondisjunction during meiosis are true EXCEPT:
   a. Nondisjunction events can happen during meiosis I or meiosis II.
   b. All gametes from nondisjunction events have an abnormal chromosome number.
   c. Trisomy 21 (Down syndrome) is a common example of nondisjunction.
   d. In a nondisjunction event in meiosis I, homologous chromosomes fail to separate.
   e. The incorrect formation of spindle fibers is a common cause of nondisjunction during meiosis.

7. Which of the following diseases does NOT have a recessive inheritance pattern?
   a. phenylketonuria.
   b. cystic fibrosis.
   c. Tay–Sachs disease.
   d. sickle cell anemia.
   e. Huntington's disease.

8. What is the purpose of the Ames assay?
   a. to determine the threshold of UV light that bacteria can receive before having mutations in their DNA.
   b. to measure the frequency of aneuploidy in bacterial colonies treated with various chemicals.
   c. to determine the frequency of a reversion mutation that allows bacterial colonies to grow in the absence of vital nutrients.
   d. to measure rate of induced recombination in mutagen-treated fungi.
   e. to measure induction of phenotypic changes in *Drosophila*.

9. In mammalian cytogenic assays, chromosomal aberrations are measured after treatment of the cells at which sensitive phase of the cell cycle?
   a. interphase.
   b. M phase.
   c. S phase.
   d. G1.
   e. G2.

10. Which of the following molecules is used to gauge the amount of a specific gene being transcribed to mRNA?
    a. protein.
    b. mRNA.
    c. DNA.
    d. cDNA.
    e. CGH.

Developmental Toxicology

John M. Rogers

KEY POINTS

- Developmental toxicology encompasses the study of pharmacokinetics, mechanisms, pathogenesis, and outcomes following exposure to agents or conditions leading to abnormal development.

- Developmental toxicology includes teratology, or the study of structural birth defects.

- *Gametogenesis* is the process of forming the haploid germ cells: the egg and the sperm.

- *Organogenesis* is the period during which most bodily structures are established. This period of heightened susceptibility to malformations extends from the third to the eighth week of gestation in humans.

SCOPE OF PROBLEM—THE HUMAN EXPERIENCE

Successful pregnancy outcome in the general population occurs at a surprisingly low frequency. Estimates of adverse outcomes include postimplantation pregnancy loss, 31%; major birth defects, 2% to 3% at birth and increasing to 6% to 7% at 1 year as more manifestations are diagnosed; minor birth defects, 14%; low birth weight, 7%; infant mortality (prior to 1 year of age), 1.4%; and abnormal neurologic function, 16% to 17%. Thus, less than half of all human conceptions result in the birth of a completely normal, healthy infant. Many hundreds of chemicals are teratogens; most of them produce birth defects by an unknown mechanism. However, Table 10–1 lists chemicals, chemical classes, or conditions known to alter prenatal development in humans.

Thalidomide

In 1960, a large increase in newborns with rare limb malformations of amelia (absence of the limbs) or various degrees of phocomelia (reduction of the long bones of the limbs) was recorded in West Germany. Congenital heart disease; ocular, intestinal, and renal anomalies; and malformations of the external and inner ears were also involved. Thalidomide, identified as the causative agent, was used throughout much of the world as a sleep aid and to ameliorate nausea and vomiting in pregnancy. It had no apparent toxicity or addictive properties in adult humans or rodents at therapeutic exposure levels.

As a result of this catastrophe, regulatory agencies developed requirements for evaluating the effects of drugs on pregnancy outcomes.

Diethylstilbestrol

Diethylstilbestrol (DES) is a synthetic nonsteroidal estrogen widely used from the 1940s to the 1970s in the United States to prevent threatened miscarriage. It was soon linked to clear cell adenocarcinoma of the vagina. Maternal use of DES prior to the 18th week of gestation appeared to be necessary for induction of the genital tract anomalies in offspring; the overall incidence of noncancerous alterations in the vagina and cervix was estimated to be as high as 75%. In male offspring of exposed pregnancies, a high incidence of reproductive tract anomalies along with low ejaculated semen volume and poor semen quality were observed. The realization of the latent and devastating manifestations of prenatal DES exposure has broadened the magnitude and scope of potential adverse outcomes of intrauterine exposures. A recent study in mice suggests that the increased susceptibility to abnormalities conferred by DES exposure may be passed on to future generations of exposed mothers.

Ethanol

Although the developmental toxicity of ethanol can be traced to biblical times (e.g., Judges 13:3–4), only since the description of the Fetal Alcohol Syndrome (FAS) in 1971 has a clear acceptance

TABLE 10–1 Human developmental toxicants.

Radiation
- Atomic fallout
- Radioiodine
- Therapeutic

Infections
- Cytomegalovirus
- Herpes simplex virus 1 and 2
- Parvovirus B-19 (erythema infectiosum)
- Rubella virus
- Syphilis
- Toxoplasmosis
- Varicella virus
- Venezuelan equine encephalitis virus

Maternal trauma and metabolic imbalances
- Alcoholism
- Amniocentesis, early
- Chorionic villus sampling (before day 60)
- Cretinism
- Diabetes
- Folic acid deficiency
- Hyperthermia
- Phenylketonuria
- Rheumatic disease and congenital heart block
- Sjögren's syndrome
- Virilizing tumors

Drugs and chemicals
- Aminoglycosides
- Androgenic hormones
- Angiotensin converting enzyme inhibitors: captopril, enalapril
- Angiotensin receptor antagonists: sartans
- Anticonvulsants: diphenylhydantoin, trimethadione, valproic acid, carbamazepine
- Busulfan
- Carbon monoxide
- Chlorambucil
- Cocaine
- Coumarins
- Cyclophosphamide
- Cytarabine
- Diethylstilbestrol
- Danazol
- Ergotamine
- Ethanol
- Ethylene oxide
- Fluconazole
- Folate antagonists: aminopterin, methotrexate
- Iodides
- Lead
- Lithium
- Mercury, organic
- Methimazole
- Methylene blue
- Misoprostal
- Penicillamine
- Polychlorobiphenyls
- Quinine (high dose)
- Retinoids: accutane, isotretinoin, etretinate, acitretin
- Tetracyclines
- Thalidomide
- Tobacco smoke
- Toluene
- Vitamin A (high dose)

of alcohol's developmental toxicity occurred. FAS comprises craniofacial dysmorphism, intrauterine and postnatal growth retardation, retarded psychomotor and intellectual development, and other nonspecific major and minor abnormalities.

In utero exposure to lower levels of ethanol than those that produce full-blown FAS has been associated with a wide range of effects, including isolated components of FAS and milder forms of neurologic and behavioral disorders that have been termed *fetal alcohol spectrum disorder (FASD)*. Alcohol consumption can affect birth weight in a dose-related fashion.

Tobacco Smoke

Prenatal and early postnatal exposure to tobacco smoke or its constituents may well represent the leading cause of environmentally induced developmental disease and morbidity today. Approximately 25% of women in the United States continue to smoke during pregnancy, despite public health programs aimed at curbing this behavior. The consequences of developmental tobacco smoke exposure include spontaneous abortions, perinatal deaths, increased risk of sudden infant death syndrome (SIDS), increased risk of learning, behavioral, and attention disorders, and lower birth weight. One component of tobacco smoke, nicotine, is a known neuroteratogen in experimental animals and can by itself produce many of the adverse developmental outcomes associated with tobacco smoke. Perinatal exposure to tobacco smoke can also affect branching morphogenesis and maturation of the lung, leading to altered physiologic function. Environmental (second-hand) tobacco smoke also represents a significant risk to the pregnant nonsmoker and her baby, and exposure to second-hand smoke has been associated with many of the effects caused by active maternal smoking.

Cocaine

Cocaine is a local anesthetic with vasoconstrictor properties. Effects on the fetus are complicated and controversial and demonstrate the difficulty of monitoring the human population for adverse reproductive outcomes. Accurate exposure ascertainment is difficult, as many confounding factors including socioeconomic status and concurrent use of cigarettes, alcohol, and other drugs of abuse may be involved. In addition, reported effects on the fetus and infant (neurologic and behavioral changes) are difficult to identify and quantify. Nevertheless, adverse effects reliably associated with cocaine exposure in humans include abruptio placentae, premature labor and delivery, microcephaly, altered prosencephalic development, decreased birth weight, SIDS, and a neonatal neurologic syndrome of abnormal sleep, tremor, poor feeding, irritability, and occasional seizures.

Retinoids

Vitamin A (retinol) exposure can cause malformations of the face, limbs, heart, central nervous system, and skeleton. Spontaneous abortion, live-born infants having at least one major malformation, and numerous exposed children having full-scale IQ scores below 85 at age 5 years have been documented.

Antiepileptic Drugs

Clinical management of women of childbearing age who have epilepsy is difficult. Although control of seizures during pregnancy is crucial, most current antiepileptic drugs (AEDs) have been shown to carry risk of developmental toxicity including birth defects, cognitive impairment, and fetal death. As a class, including phenytoin, carbamazepine, and valproic acid, AEDs are considered human teratogens. Studies to date suggest that newer AEDs such as gabapentin, lamotrigine, oxcarbazone, topiramate, and zonizamide may be safer than the older AEDs.

Angiotensin Converting Enzyme (ACE) Inhibitors and Angiotensin Receptor Antagonists

The renin–angiotensin system is a key controller of blood pressure. The active signaling messenger of this system is angiotensin II, which binds to angiotensin II (AT1) receptors to cause vasoconstriction and fluid retention, resulting in elevation of blood pressure. ACE inhibitors and angiotensin receptor blockers are widely prescribed and, when used in the second half of pregnancy, are known to cause oligohydramnios (low amniotic fluid volume), fetal growth retardation, pulmonary hypoplasia, joint contractures, hypocalvaria, neonatal renal failure, hypotension, and death. Some studies suggest that exposure in the first trimester should be avoided.

PRINCIPLES OF DEVELOPMENTAL TOXICOLOGY

Some basic principles of teratology put forth by Jim Wilson in 1959 are listed in Table 10–2; they are still valid today.

TABLE 10–2 Wilson's general principles of teratology.

I. Susceptibility to teratogenesis depends on the genotype of the conceptus and the manner in which this interacts with adverse environmental factors
II. Susceptibility to teratogenesis varies with the developmental stage at the time of exposure to an adverse influence
III. Teratogenic agents act in specific ways (mechanisms) on developing cells and tissues to initiate sequences of abnormal developmental events (pathogenesis)
IV. The access of adverse influences to developing tissues depends on the nature of the influence (agent)
V. The four manifestations of deviant development are death, malformation, growth retardation, and functional deficit
VI. Manifestations of deviant development increase in frequency and degree as dosage increases, from the no effect to the totally lethal level

Data from Wilson JG: *Environment and Birth Defects*. New York, NY: Academic Press/Elsevier; 1973.

Critical Periods of Susceptibility and End Points of Toxicity

Development is characterized by various changes that are orchestrated by a cascade of factors regulating gene transcription throughout development. Intercellular and intracellular signaling pathways essential for normal development rely on transcriptional, translational, and posttranslational controls. The rapid changes occurring during development alter the nature of the embryo/fetus as a target for toxicity. Timing of some key developmental events in humans and experimental animal species is presented in Table 10–3.

Gametogenesis is the process of forming the haploid germ cells: the egg and the sperm. These gametes fuse in the process of *fertilization* to form the diploid *zygote,* or one-celled embryo. Gametogenesis and fertilization are vulnerable to toxicants. It is now known that the maternal and paternal genomes are not equivalent in their contributions to the zygotic genome. The process of *imprinting* (which involves cytosine methylation and changes in chromatin conformation) occurs during gametogenesis, conferring to certain allelic genes a differential expressivity depending on whether they are of maternal or paternal origin.

Epigenetics refers to the biochemical changes in chromatin that lead to changes in conformation and gene expression. Epigenetic changes include DNA methylation, histone modifications, and expression of microRNAs. There are specific stages of the life cycle during which epigenetic marks may be erased and reestablished, including two periods of development during which large-scale demethylations of the genome are known to occur. One is during migration and proliferation of the primordial gem cells in which imprinted genes are demethylated, with remethylation occurring in a gender-specific manner during gametogenesis in the offspring. The other period of widespread epigenetic reprogramming occurs shortly after formation of the zygote and in the early embryo, with total genomic methylation reaching a nadir at the blastocyst stage.

Following fertilization, the embryo moves down the fallopian tube (oviduct) and implants in the wall of the uterus. The *preimplantation* period comprises mainly an increase in cell number through a rapid series of cell divisions with little growth in size (*cleavage* of the zygote) and cavitation of the embryo to form a fluid-filled blastocoele. This stage, termed the *blastocyst,* contains cells destined to give rise to the embryo proper and other cells that give rise to extraembryonic membranes and support structures.

Toxicity during preimplantation is generally thought to result in no or slight effect on growth (because of regulative growth) or in death (through overwhelming damage or failure

TABLE 10–3 Timing of key developmental events in some mammalian species.*

	Rat	Rabbit	Monkey	Human
Blastocyst formation	3–5	2.6–6	4–9	4–6
Implantation	5–6	6	9	6–7
Organogenesis	6–17	6–18	20–45	21–56
Primitive streak	9	6.5	18–20	16–18
Neural plate	9.5	—	9–21	18–20
First somite	10	—	—	20–21
First branchial arch	10	—	—	20
First heartbeat	10.2	—	—	22
10 somites	10–11	9	23–24	25–26
Upper limb buds	10.5	10.5	25–26	29–30
Lower limb buds	11.2	11	26–27	31–32
Testes differentiation	14.5	20	—	43
Heart septation	15.5	—	—	46–47
Palate closure	16–17	19–20	45–47	56–58
Urethral groove closed in male	—	—	—	90
Length of gestation	21–22	31–34	166	267

*Developmental ages are days of gestation.
Data from Shepard TH: *Catalog of Teratogenic Agents*, 9th ed. Baltimore, MD: The Johns Hopkins University Press; 1998.

to implant). Because of the rapid mitoses occurring during the preimplantation period, chemicals affecting DNA synthesis/integrity or those affecting microtubule assembly would be expected to be particularly toxic if given access to the embryo.

Following implantation the embryo undergoes *gastrulation,* the process of formation of the three primary germ layers—the *ectoderm, mesoderm,* and *endoderm.* During gastrulation, cells migrate through a midline structure called the *primitive streak,* and their movements set up basic morphogenetic fields in the embryo. As a prelude to organogenesis, the period of gastrulation is quite susceptible to teratogens. A number of toxicants administered during gastrulation produce malformations of the eye, brain, and face. These malformations are indicative of damage to the anterior *neural plate,* one of the regions defined by the cellular movements of gastrulation.

The formation of the neural plate in the ectoderm marks the onset of *organogenesis,* during which the rudiments of most bodily structures are established. This period of heightened susceptibility to malformations extends from approximately the third to the eighth week of gestation in humans. The rapid changes of organogenesis require cell proliferation, cell migration, cell–cell interactions, and morphogenetic tissue remodeling. Within organogenesis, there are periods of peak susceptibility for each forming structure. The peak incidence of each malformation coincides with the timing of key developmental events in the affected structure.

The end of organogenesis marks the beginning of the *fetal period,* which is characterized primarily by tissue differentiation, growth, and physiologic maturation. All organs are present and grossly recognizable, although not yet completely developed.

Exposure during the fetal period is most likely to result in effects on growth and functional maturation. Functional anomalies of the central nervous system and reproductive organs—including behavioral, mental, and motor deficits as well as decreases in fertility—are among the possible adverse outcomes.

Over the past two decades, the concept of "developmental programming" has emerged, in which the developmental environment is thought to influence the metabolic parameters of the offspring that will persist throughout life and may affect lifelong risk of disease. Much of the work on fetal programming has focused on the role of maternal nutrition, and there is a paucity of data concerning the long-term effects of chemical exposure during the fetal and early postnatal periods. Some effects could require years to become apparent (such as those noted above for DES), and others may even result in the premature onset of senescence and/or organ failure late in life.

Dose–Response Patterns and the Threshold Concept

The major effects of prenatal exposure, observed at the time of birth in developmental toxicity studies, are embryo lethality, malformations, and growth retardation. For some agents, these end points may represent a continuum of increasing toxicity, with low dosages producing growth retardation and increasing dosages producing malformations and then lethality.

Another key element of the dose–response relationship is the shape of the dose–response curve at low exposure levels. Because of the high restorative growth potential of the mammalian embryo, cellular homeostatic mechanisms, and maternal metabolic defenses, mammalian developmental toxicity has generally been considered a threshold phenomenon. Assumption of a threshold means that there is a maternal dosage below which an adverse response is not elicited because some repair or defense system is able to combat the exposure.

MECHANISMS AND PATHOGENESIS OF DEVELOPMENTAL TOXICITY

The term *mechanisms* refers to cellular-level events that initiate the process leading to abnormal development. *Pathogenesis* comprises the cell-, tissue-, and organ-level sequelae that ultimately manifest in abnormality. Mechanisms of teratogenesis include mutations, chromosomal breaks, altered mitosis, altered nucleic acid integrity or function, diminished supplies of precursors or substrates, decreased energy supplies, altered membrane characteristics, osmolar imbalance, and enzyme inhibition. Although these cellular insults are not unique to development, they may trigger unique pathogenetic responses in the embryo, such as reduced cell proliferation, cell death, altered cell–cell interactions, reduced biosynthesis, inhibition of morphogenetic movements, or mechanical disruption of developing structures.

Cell death plays a critical role in normal morphogenesis. The term *programmed cell death* refers specifically to *apoptosis,* which is under genetic control in the embryo. Apoptosis is necessary for sculpting the digits from the hand plate and for assuring appropriate functional connectivity between the central nervous system and distal structures. Cell proliferation rates change both spatially and temporally during ontogenesis. There is a delicate balance between cell proliferation, cell differentiation, and apoptosis in the embryo. DNA damage might lead to cell cycle perturbations and cell death.

As discussed in Chapter 9, DNA damage can inhibit cell cycle progression at the G_1–S transition, through the S phase, and at the G_2–M transition. If DNA damage is repaired, the cell cycle can return to normal, but if damage is too extensive or cell cycle arrest too long, apoptosis may be triggered. The relationship between DNA damage and repair, cell cycle progression, and apoptosis is depicted in Figure 10–1. From the multiple checkpoints and factors present to regulate the cell cycle and apoptosis, it is clear that different cell populations may respond differently to a similar stimulus, in part because cellular predisposition to apoptosis can vary.

Besides affecting proliferation and cell viability, molecular and cellular insults can alter cell migration, cell–cell interactions, differentiation, morphogenesis, and energy metabolism. Although the embryo has compensatory mechanisms to offset such effects, production of a normal or malformed offspring will depend on the balance between damage and repair at each step in the pathogenetic pathway.

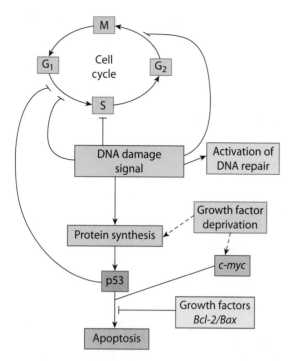

FIGURE 10–1 **Relationships between DNA damage and the induction of cell cycle arrest or apoptosis.** DNA damage can signal inhibition of the cell cycle between G$_1$ and S, in S phase, or between G$_2$ and mitosis. The signal(s) can also activate DNA repair mechanisms and synthesis of proteins, including p53, that can initiate apoptosis. Growth factors and products of the proto-oncogene *c-myc* and the *Bcl-2/Bax* gene family, as well as differentiation state and cell cycle phase, are important determinants of the ultimate outcome of embryonal DNA damage.

Advances in the Molecular Basis of Dysmorphogenesis

Advances in gene targeting and transgenic strategies now allow modification of gene expression at specific points in development and in specific cell types. Conditional knockouts (cKO) or knockins (cKI), inducible gene expression, and other techniques are being used to study the effects of specific gene products on development in great detail. The use of synthetic antisense oligonucleotides allows temporal and spatial restriction of gene ablation by hybridizing to mRNA in the cell, thereby inactivating it. In this way, gene function can be turned off at specific times. RNA interference is a more recent gene knockdown technique, exploiting the discovery of the RNA interference pathway. Small interference (si)RNA, plasmid-, and virus-encoded small RNAs can be used to down-regulate the expression of specific genes posttranscriptionally.

Gain of gene function can also be studied by engineering genetic constructs with an inducible promoter attached to the gene of interest. Ectopic gene expression can be made ubiquitous or site-specific depending on the choice of promoter to drive expression. Transient overexpression of specific genes can be accomplished by adding extra copies using adenoviral transduction.

PHARMACOKINETICS AND METABOLISM IN PREGNANCY

The extent and the form in which chemicals reach the conceptus are important determinants of whether the agent can impact development. The maternal, placental, and embryonic compartments comprise independent, yet interacting, systems that undergo profound changes throughout the course of pregnancy. Alterations in placental physiology can have significant impact on the uptake, distribution, metabolism, and elimination of xenobiotics. For example, decreases in intestinal motility and increases in gastric emptying time result in longer retention of ingested chemicals in the upper gastrointestinal tract in the mother. Cardiac output increases by 50% during the first trimester in humans and remains elevated throughout pregnancy, whereas blood volume increases and plasma proteins and peripheral vascular resistance decrease. The relative increase in blood volume over red cell volume leads to borderline anemia and a generalized edema with a 70% elevation of extracellular space. Thus, the volume of distribution of a chemical and the amount bound by plasma proteins may change considerably during pregnancy. Other changes occur in the renal, hepatic, and pulmonary systems as well. Clearly, maternal handling of a chemical influences the extent of embryotoxicity.

The placenta also influences embryonic exposure by helping to regulate blood flow, offering a transport barrier, and metabolizing chemicals. The placenta acts as a lipid membrane that permits bidirectional transfer of substances between maternal and fetal compartments. It is important to note that virtually any substance present in the maternal plasma will be transported to some extent by the placenta. The passage of most drugs across the placenta seems to occur by simple passive diffusion. Important modifying factors to the rate and extent of transfer include lipid solubility, molecular weight, protein binding, the type of transfer (passive diffusion, and facilitated or active transport), the degree of ionization, and placental metabolism. Blood flow probably constitutes the major rate-limiting step for more lipid-soluble compounds.

Maternal metabolism of xenobiotics is an important and variable determinant of developmental toxicity. As for other health end points, the field of pharmacogenomics offers hope for increasing our ability to predict susceptible subpopulations based on empirical relationships between maternal genotype and fetal phenotype.

RELATIONSHIPS BETWEEN MATERNAL AND DEVELOPMENTAL TOXICITY

Although all developmental toxicity must ultimately result from an insult to the conceptus at the cellular level, the insult may occur through a direct effect on the embryo/fetus, indirectly through toxicity of the agent to the mother and/or the placenta, or a combination of direct and indirect effects. Maternal factors known to affect fetal development include

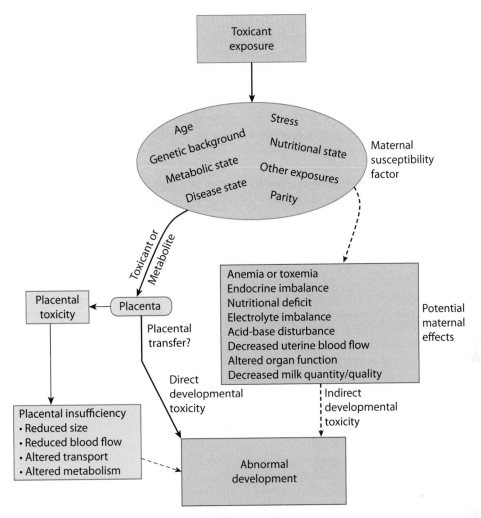

FIGURE 10–2 **Interrelationships between maternal susceptibility factors, metabolism, induction of maternal physiologic or functional alterations, placental transfer and toxicity, and developmental toxicity.** A developmental toxicant can cause abnormal development through any one or a combination of these pathways. Maternal susceptibility factors determine the predisposition of the mother to respond to a toxic insult, and the maternal effects listed can adversely affect the developing conceptus. Most chemicals traverse the placenta in some form, and the placenta can also be a target for toxicity. In most cases, developmental toxicity is probably mediated through a combination of these pathways.

genetics, disease, nutrition, stress, placental toxicity, and maternal toxicity. Some conditions that may adversely affect the fetus are depicted in Figure 10–2.

The distinction between direct and indirect developmental toxicity is important for interpreting safety assessment results in pregnant animals, as the highest dosage level in these experiments is chosen based on its ability to produce some maternal toxicity (e.g., decreased food or water intake, weight loss, and clinical signs). However, maternal toxicity defined only by such crude manifestations gives little insight to the toxic actions of a xenobiotic. When developmental toxicity is observed only in the presence of maternal toxicity, the developmental effects may be indirect (i.e., caused by an inappropriate growing condition because of an altered maternal environment rather than by a direct interaction of the fetus with the toxin). Greater understanding of the physiologic changes underlying the observed

maternal toxicity and elucidation of the association with developmental effects is needed before one can begin to address the relevance of the observations to human safety assessment.

Maternal Factors Affecting Development

Genetics—The genetic makeup of the pregnant female has been well documented as a determinant of developmental outcome in both humans and animals. The incidence of cleft lip and/or palate [CL(P)], which occurs more frequently in whites than in blacks, has been investigated in offspring of interracial couples in the United States. Offspring of white mothers had a higher incidence of CL(P) than offspring of black mothers after correcting for paternal race, whereas offspring of white fathers did not have a higher incidence of CL(P) than offspring of black fathers after correcting for maternal race.

Disease—Chronic hypertension in the mother, uncontrolled maternal diabetes mellitus, and certain infections in the mother (i.e., cytomegalovirus and *Toxoplasma gondii*) are leading causes of several types of defects in the fetus. Exposure to hyperthermia (such as febrile illness in the mother) is also implicated in neural defects in the fetus.

Nutrition—A wide spectrum of dietary insufficiencies ranging from protein-calorie malnutrition to deficiencies of vitamins, trace elements, and/or enzyme cofactors is known to adversely affect pregnancy. In fact, folate supplementation by pregnant women can reduce neural tube defect recurrence by over 70%.

Stress—Diverse forms of maternal toxicity may have in common the induction of a physiologic stress response. Various forms of physical stress have been applied to pregnant animals in attempts to isolate the developmental effects of stress. Noise stress of pregnant rats or mice throughout gestation can produce developmental toxicity. Restraint stress produces increased fetal death in rats, and malformations of cleft palate, fused and supernumerary ribs, and encephaloceles in mice. There is a positive correlation in humans between stress and adverse developmental effects, including low birth weight and congenital malformations.

Placental Toxicity—The placenta is the interface between the mother and the conceptus, providing attachment, nutrition, gas exchange, and waste removal. The placenta also produces hormones critical to the maintenance of pregnancy, and it can metabolize and/or store xenobiotics. Placental toxicity may compromise these functions. Known placental toxicants include cadmium, arsenic or mercury, cigarette smoke, ethanol, cocaine, endotoxin, and sodium salicylate.

Maternal Toxicity—A retrospective analysis of relationships between maternal toxicity and specific types of prenatal effects found species-specific associations between maternal toxicity and specific adverse developmental effects. Various adverse developmental outcomes include increased intrauterine death, decreased fetal weight, supernumerary ribs, and enlarged renal pelvises.

A number of studies directly relate specific forms of maternal toxicity to developmental toxicity, including those in which the test chemical causes maternal effects that exacerbate the agent's developmental toxicity. However, clear delineation of the relative role(s) of indirect maternal and direct embryo/fetal toxicity is difficult.

Diflunisal, an analgesic and anti-inflammatory drug, causes axial skeletal defects in rabbits. Developmentally toxic dosages resulted in severe maternal anemia and depletion of erythrocyte ATP levels. Teratogenicity, anemia, and ATP depletion were unique to the rabbit. The teratogenicity of diflunisal in the rabbit was probably due to hypoxia resulting from maternal anemia.

Phenytoin, an anticonvulsant, can affect maternal folate metabolism in experimental animals, and these alterations may play a role in the teratogenicity of this drug. A mechanism of teratogenesis was proposed relating depressed maternal heart rate and embryonic hypoxia. Supporting studies have demonstrated that hyperoxia reduces the teratogenicity of phenytoin in mice.

DEVELOPMENTAL TOXICITY OF ENDOCRINE-DISRUPTING CHEMICALS

There is the growing concern that exposure to chemicals that can interact with the endocrine system may pose a serious health hazard. An "endocrine disruptor" has been broadly defined as an exogenous agent that interferes with the production, release, transport, metabolism, binding, action, or elimination of natural hormones responsible for the maintenance of homeostasis and the regulation of developmental processes. Due to the critical role of hormones in directing differentiation in many tissues, the developing organism is particularly vulnerable to fluctuations in the timing or intensity of exposure to chemicals with hormonal or antihormonal activity. Various chemical classes induce developmental toxicity via at least three modes of action involving the endocrine system: (1) by serving as ligands of steroid receptors, (2) by modifying steroid hormone metabolizing enzymes, and (3) by perturbing hypothalamic-pituitary release of trophic hormones. Interactions with the functions of estrogens, androgens, and thyroid hormones have been the most studied, but the underlying principles apply to other hormones also.

Laboratory Animal Evidence

Estrogenic or antiestrogenic developmental toxicants include DES, estradiol, antiestrogenic drugs such as tamoxifen and clomiphene citrate, and some pesticides and industrial chemicals. The pattern of outcomes is generally similar across different estrogens. Female offspring are generally more sensitive to these toxicants than males, and altered pubertal development, reduced fertility, and reproductive tract anomalies are common findings.

Antiandrogens represent another major class of endocrine-disrupting chemicals. Principal manifestations of developmental exposure to an antiandrogen are generally restricted to males, and include hypospadias, retained nipples, reduced testes and accessory sex gland weights, and decreased sperm production.

Hypothyroidism during pregnancy and early postnatal development causes growth retardation, cognitive defects, delayed eye-opening, hyperactivity, and auditory defects. Polychlorinated biphenyls (PCBs) may act at several sites to lower thyroid hormone levels during development, and cause these developmental abnormalities.

Human Evidence

Whether human health is being adversely impacted from exposures to endocrine disruptors present in the environment is equivocal. Reports in humans are of two types:

1. Observations of adverse effects on reproductive system development and function following exposure to chemicals with known endocrine activities that are present in medicines, contaminated food, or the workplace. These have tended to involve relatively higher exposure to chemicals with known endocrine effects.

2. Epidemiologic evidence of increasing trends in reproductive and developmental adverse outcomes that have an endocrine basis. For example, secular trends have been reported for cryptorchidism, hypospadias, semen quality, and testicular cancer, but due to the lack of exposure assessment, such studies provide limited evidence of a cause and effect relationship.

Impact on Screening and Testing Programs

The findings of altered reproductive development following early life-stage exposures to endocrine-disrupting chemicals helped prompt revision of traditional safety evaluation tests. These include assessments of female estrous cyclicity, sperm motility, and sperm morphology in both parental and F1 generations, the age at puberty in the F1s, histopathology of target organs, anogenital distance in the F2s, and primordial follicular counts in the parental and F1 generations. For the new prenatal developmental toxicity test guidelines, one important modification aimed at improved detection of endocrine disruptors was the expansion of the period of dosing from the end of organogenesis (i.e., palatal closure) to the end of pregnancy in order to include the developmental period of urogenital differentiation.

MODERN SAFETY ASSESSMENT

Experience with chemicals that have the potential to induce developmental toxicity indicates that both laboratory animal testing and surveillance of the human population (i.e., epidemiologic studies) as well as alert clinical evaluation after potential exposure are all necessary to provide adequate public health protection. Laboratory animal investigations are guided by both regulatory requirements for drug or chemical marketing and the need to understand mechanisms of toxicity.

Regulatory Guidelines for In Vivo Testing

New and internationally accepted testing protocols rely on the investigator to meet the primary goal of detecting and bringing to light any indication of toxicity to reproduction. Key elements of various tests are provided in Table 10–4. The general goal of these studies is to identify the NOAEL, which is the highest dosage level that does not produce a significant increase in adverse effects in the offspring or juvenile animals. These NOAELs are then used in the risk assessment process to assess the likelihood of effects in humans given certain exposure conditions.

Multigeneration Tests

Information pertaining to developmental toxicity can also be obtained from studies in which animals are exposed to the test substance continuously over one or more generations. For additional information on this approach, see Chapter 20.

Children's Health

Infants and children differ both qualitatively and quantitatively from adults in their exposure to pesticide residues in food because of different dietary composition, intake patterns, and different activities, such as crawling on the floor or ground, putting their hands and foreign objects in their mouths, and raising dust and dirt during play. Even the level of their activity (i.e., closer to the ground) can affect their exposure to some toxicants. In addition to exposure differences, children are growing and developing, which makes them more susceptible to some types of insults. Effects of early childhood exposure, including neurobehavioral effects and cancer, may not be apparent until later in life. Debate continues over the approach to be used in risk assessment in consideration of infants and children.

Alternative Testing Strategies

Various alternative test systems have been proposed to refine, reduce, or replace the standard regulatory mammalian tests for assessing prenatal toxicity (Table 10–5). These can be grouped into assays based on cell cultures, cultures of embryos in vitro (including submammalian species), and short-term in vivo tests. It was initially hoped that the alternative approaches would become generally applicable to all chemicals, and help prioritize full-scale testing; this has not yet been accomplished. Indeed, given the complexity of embryogenesis and the multiple mechanisms and target site of potential teratogens, it was perhaps unrealistic to have expected a single test, or even a small battery, to accurately prescreen the activity of chemicals in general.

An exception to the poor acceptance of alternate tests for prescreening for developmental toxicity is the Chernoff/Kavlock in vivo test. In this test, pregnant females are exposed during the period of major organogenesis to a limited number of dosage levels near those inducing maternal toxicity, and offspring are evaluated over a brief neonatal period for external malformations, growth, and viability. It has proven reliable over a large number of chemical agents and classes.

Epidemiology

Reproductive epidemiology studies associations between specific exposures of the father or pregnant woman and her conceptus and the outcome of pregnancy. The likelihood of

TABLE 10–4 Summary of in vivo regulatory protocol guidelines for evaluation of developmental toxicity.

Study	Exposure	End Points Covered	Comments
Segment I: fertility and general reproduction study	Males: 10 weeks prior to mating Females: 2 weeks prior to mating	Gamete development, fertility, pre and postimplantation viability, parturition, lactation	Assesses reproductive capabilities of male and female following exposure over one complete spermatogenic cycle or several estrous cycles
Segment II: teratogenicity test	Implantation (or mating) through end of organogenesis (or term)	Viability, weight, and morphology (external, visceral, and skeletal) of conceptuses just prior to birth	Shorter exposure to prevent maternal metabolic adaptation and to provide high exposure to the embryo during gastrulation and organogenesis. Earlier dosing option for bioaccumulative agents or those impacting maternal nutrition. Later dosing option covers male reproductive tract development and fetal growth and maturation
Segment III: perinatal study	Last trimester of pregnancy through lactation	Postnatal survival, growth, and external morphology	Intended to observe effects on development of major organ functional competence during the perinatal period, and thus may be relatively more sensitive to adverse effects at this time
ICH 4.1.1: fertility protocol	Males: 4 weeks prior to mating Females: 2 weeks prior to mating	Males: Reproductive organ weights and histology, sperm counts, and motility Females: viability of conceptuses at midpregnancy or later	Improved assessment of male reproductive end points; shorter treatment duration than Segment I
ICH 4.1.2: effects on prenatal and postnatal development, including maternal function	Implantation through end of lactation	Relative toxicity to pregnant versus nonpregnant female; postnatal viability, growth, development, and functional deficits (including behavior, maturation, and reproduction)	
ICH 4.1.3: effects on embryo/fetal development	Implantation through end of organogenesis	Viability and morphology (external, visceral, and skeletal) of fetuses just prior to birth	Similar to Segment II study. Usually conducted in two species (rodent and nonrodent)
OECD 414: prenatal developmental	Implantation (or mating) through day prior to cesarean section	Viability and morphology (external, visceral, and skeletal) of fetuses just prior to birth	Similar to Segment II study. Usually conducted in two species (rodent and nonrodent)

linking a particular exposure with a series of case reports increases with the rarity of the defect, the rarity of the exposure in the population, a small source population, a short time span for study, and biological plausibility for the association. In other situations, such as occurred with ethanol and valproic acid, associations are sought through either a case–control or a cohort approach. Both approaches require accurate ascertainment of abnormal outcomes and exposures, and a large enough effect and study population to detect an elevated risk. Another challenge to epidemiologists is the high percentage of human pregnancy failures related to a particular exposure that may go undetected in the general population. With the availability of prenatal diagnostic procedures, additional pregnancies of malformed embryos (particularly neural tube defects) are electively aborted. Thus, the incidence of abnormal outcomes at birth may not reflect the true rate of abnormalities, and the term prevalence, rather than incidence, is preferred when the denominator is the number of live births rather than total pregnancies.

Other issues particularly relevant to reproductive epidemiology include homogeneity, recording proficiency, and confounding. Homogeneity refers to the fact that a particular outcome may be described differently by various recording units and that there can be multiple pathogenetic origins for a given specific outcome. Recording difficulties relate to inconsistencies of definitions and nomenclature, and to difficulties in ascertaining or recalling outcomes as well as exposures. For example, birth weights are usually accurately determined and recalled, but spontaneous abortions and certain malformations may not be. Last, confounding by factors such as maternal age and parity, dietary factors, diseases and drug usage, and social characteristics must be considered in order to control for variables that affect both exposure and outcome.

TABLE 10–5 Brief survey of alternative test methodologies for developmental toxicity.

Assay	Brief Description and End Points Evaluated
Mouse ovarian tumor	Labeled mouse ovarian tumor cells added to culture dishes with concanavalin A-coated disks for 20 min. End Point is inhibition of attachment of cells to disks
Human embryonic palatal mesenchyme	Human embryonic palatal mesenchyme cell line grown in attached culture. Cell number assessed after 3 days
Micromass culture	Midbrain or limb bud cells dissociated from rat embryos and grown in micromass culture for 5 days. Cell proliferation and biochemical markers of differentiation assessed
Mouse embryonic stem cell test (EST)	Mouse embryonic stem cells and 3T3 cells in 96-well plates assessed for viability after 3 and 5 days. Embryonic stem cells grown for 3 days in hanging drops form embryoid bodies which are plated and examined after 10 days for differentiation into cardiocytes
Chick embryo neural retina cell culture	Neural retinas of day 6.5 chick embryos dissociated and grown in rotating suspension culture for 7 days. End points include cellular aggregation, growth, differentiation, and biochemical markers
Drosophila	Fly larvae grown from egg disposition through hatching of adults. Adult flies examined for specific structural defects (bent bristles and notched wing)
Hydra	Hydra attenuata cells are aggregated to form an "artificial embryo" and allowed to regenerate. Dose response compared to that for adult Hydra toxicity
FETAX	Midblastula stage Xenopus embryos exposed for 96 h and evaluated for viability, growth, and morphology
Rodent whole embryo culture	Postimplantation rodent embryos grown in vitro for up to 2 days and evaluated for growth and development
Zebrafish	Zebrafish eggs or blastulae exposed to chemical in water (can be in multiwell plates) for up to 4 days and evaluated for growth, development, and (in some cases) gene expression
Chernoff/Kavlock assay	Pregnant mice or rats exposed during organogenesis and allowed to deliver. Postnatal growth, viability, and gross morphology of litters assessed

Epidemiologic studies of abnormal reproductive outcomes are usually undertaken with three objectives in mind: the first is scientific research into the causes of abnormal birth outcomes and usually involves analysis of case reports or clusters; the second objective is prevention and is targeted at broader surveillance of trends by birth defect registries around the world; and the last objective is informing the public and providing assurance. Cohort studies, with their prospective exposure assessment and ability to monitor both adverse and beneficial outcomes, may be the most methodologically robust approach to identifying human developmental toxicants.

Information on differential genetic susceptibility to birth defects continues to accrue. This new knowledge promises to elucidate links between genetics and disease susceptibility. Understanding the genetic basis of vulnerability to environmentally induced birth defects will allow more inclusive risk assessments and a better appreciation of the mechanisms of action of developmental toxicants.

Concordance of Data

Studies of the similarity of responses of laboratory animals and humans for developmental toxicants support the assumption that results from laboratory tests are predictive of potential human effects. Concordance is strongest when there are positive data from more than one test species. Humans tend to be more sensitive to developmental toxicants than is the most sensitive test species.

Elements of Risk Assessment

Extrapolation of animal test data for developmental toxicity follows two basic directions, one for drugs where exposure is voluntary and usually to high dosages and the other for environmental agents where exposure is generally involuntary and to low levels. For drugs, a use-in-pregnancy rating is utilized, wherein the letters A, B, C, D, and X are used to classify the evidence that a chemical poses a risk to the human conceptus. For example, drugs are placed in category A if adequate, well-controlled studies in pregnant humans have failed to demonstrate a risk, and in category X (contraindicated for pregnancy) if studies in animals or humans, or investigational or postmarketing reports, have shown fetal risk that clearly outweighs any possible benefit to the patient. The default category C (risks cannot be ruled out) is assigned when there is a lack of human studies and animal studies are either lacking or are positive for fetal risk, but the benefits may justify the potential risk. Categories B and D represent areas of relatively lesser or greater concern for risk, respectively.

For environmental agents, the purpose of the risk assessment process for developmental toxicity is generally to define the dose, route, timing, and duration of exposure that induces effects at the lowest level in the most relevant laboratory animal model. The exposure associated with this "critical effect" is then subjected to a variety of safety or uncertainty factors in order to derive an exposure level for humans that is presumed to be relatively safe. In the absence of definitive animal test data, certain default assumptions are generally made:

1. An agent that produces an adverse developmental effect in experimental animals will potentially pose a hazard to humans following sufficient exposure during development.
2. All four manifestations of developmental toxicity (death, structural abnormalities, growth alterations, and functional deficits) are of concern.
3. The specific types of developmental effects seen in animal studies are not necessarily the same as those that may be produced in humans.
4. The most appropriate species is used to estimate human risk when data are available (in the absence of such data, the most sensitive species is appropriate).
5. In general, a threshold is assumed for the dose–response curve for agents that produce developmental toxicity.

Two approaches to aid defining developmental risk include the benchmark-dose approach and biologically based dose–response modeling. The use of uncertainty factors applied to an experimentally derived NOAEL to arrive at a presumed safe level of human exposure assumes that a threshold for developmental toxicity exists. The available USEPA's Benchmark Dose Software is helping to make this approach a method of choice for many risk assessment organizations. The biologically based dose–response model integrates pharmacokinetic data on tissue dosimetry with molecular, cellular and tissue response, and developmental toxicity.

PATHWAYS TO THE FUTURE

There are several mechanisms of normal development that are conserved in diverse animals, including the fruit fly, roundworm, zebrafish, frog, chick, and mouse. Seventeen conserved intercellular signaling pathways are described that are used repeatedly at different times and locations during development

TABLE 10–6 Seventeen intercellular signaling pathways used in development by most metazoans.

Period during Development	Signaling Pathway
Before organogenesis; later for growth and tissue renewal	1. Wingless–Int pathway 2. Transforming growth factor β pathway 3. Hedgehog pathway 4. Receptor tyrosine kinase pathway 5. Notch–Delta pathway 6. Cytokine pathway (STAT pathway)
Organogenesis and cytodifferentiation; later for growth and tissue renewal	7. Interleukin-1-toll nuclear factor-kappa B pathway 8. Nuclear hormone receptor pathway 9. Apoptosis pathway 10. Receptor phosphotyrosine phosphatase pathway
Larval and adult physiology	11. Receptor guanylate cyclase pathway 12. Nitric oxide receptor pathway 13. G-protein-coupled receptor (large G proteins) pathway 14. Integrin pathway 15. Cadherin pathway 16. Gap junction pathway 17. Ligand-gated cation channel pathway

of these and other animal species, as well as in humans (Table 10–6). The conserved nature of these key pathways provides a strong scientific rationale for using these animal models to advantage for developmental toxicology. These organisms have well-known genetics, embryology, and rapid generation times, and they are also amenable to genetic manipulation to enhance the sensitivity of specific developmental pathways or to incorporate human genes to answer questions of interspecies extrapolation.

Increased understanding of human genetic polymorphisms and their contribution to susceptibility to birth defects, use of sensitized animal models for high- to low-dose extrapolation, use of stress/checkpoint pathways as indicators of developmental toxicity, implementation of bioinformatic systems to improve data archival and retrieval, and increased multidisciplinary education and research on the causes of birth defects will aid assessment of the developmental risk of toxicants.

BIBLIOGRAPHY

Harris C, Hansen JM: *Developmental Toxicology: Methods and Protocols.* New York: Humana Press, 2012.

Hood RD: *Developmental and Reproductive Toxicology: A Practical Approach.* New York: Informa Healthcare, 2012.

Robinson JF, Pennings JL, Piersma AH: A review of toxicogenomic approaches in developmental toxicology. *Methods Mol Biol* 889:347–371, 2012.

QUESTIONS

1. Diethylstilbestrol (DES):
   a. was used to treat morning sickness from the 1940s to the 1970s.
   b. was found to affect only female offspring in exposed pregnancies.
   c. greatly affects the development of the fetal brain.
   d. exposure increases the risk of clear cell adenocarcinoma of the vagina.
   e. is now used to treat leprosy patients.

2. Early (prenatal) exposure to which of the following teratogens is most often characterized by craniofacial dysmorphism?
   a. thalidomide.
   b. retinol.
   c. ethanol.
   d. tobacco smoke.
   e. diethylstilbestrol (DES).

3. The nervous system is derived from which of the following germ layers?
   a. ectoderm.
   b. mesoderm.
   c. epidermal placodes.
   d. paraxial mesoderm.
   e. endoderm.

4. Toxin exposure during which of the following periods is likely to have the LEAST toxic effect on the developing fetus?
   a. gastrulation.
   b. organogenesis.
   c. preimplantation.
   d. third trimester.
   e. first trimester.

5. Regarding prenatal teratogen exposure, which of the following statements is FALSE?
   a. Major effects include growth retardation and malformations.
   b. Exposure to teratogens during critical developmental periods will have more severe effects on the fetus.
   c. There is considered to be a toxin level threshold below which the fetus is capable of repairing itself.
   d. The immune system of the fetus is primitive, so the fetus has little to no ability to fight off chemicals and repair itself.
   e. Embryo lethality becomes more likely as the toxic dose is increased.

6. Which of the following stages of the cell cycle are important in monitoring DNA damage and inhibiting progression of the cell cycle?
   a. G_1–S, anaphase, M–G_1.
   b. G_1–S, S, G_2–M.
   c. S, prophase, G_1.
   d. G_2–M, prophase.
   e. M–G_1, anaphase.

7. Which of the following molecules is NOT important in determining the ultimate outcome of embryonal DNA damage?
   a. p53.
   b. Bax.
   c. Bcl-2.
   d. c-Myc.
   e. NF-κB.

8. Which of the following is NOT a physiologic response to pregnancy?
   a. increased cardiac output.
   b. increased blood volume.
   c. increased peripheral vascular resistance.
   d. decreased plasma proteins.
   e. increased extracellular space.

9. All of the following statements are true EXCEPT:
   a. Offspring of white mothers have a higher incidence of cleft lip or palate than do black mothers, after adjusting for paternal race.
   b. Cytomegalovirus (CMV) is a common viral cause of birth defects.
   c. Folate supplementation during pregnancy decreases the risk of neural tube defects.
   d. Cigarette smoke and ethanol are both toxic to the placenta.
   e. In humans, there is a negative correlation between stress and low birth weight.

10. Which of the following is NOT a mechanism involving the endocrine system by which chemicals induce developmental toxicity?
    a. acting as steroid hormone receptor ligands.
    b. disrupting normal function of steroid hormone metabolizing enzymes.
    c. disturbing the release of hormones from the hypothalamus.
    d. disturbing the release of hormones from the pituitary gland.
    e. elimination of natural hormones.

C H A P T E R

11

Toxic Responses of the Blood

John C. Bloom, Andrew E. Schade, and John T. Brandt

BLOOD AS A TARGET ORGAN

Hematotoxicology is the study of adverse effects of exogenous chemicals on blood and blood-forming tissues. The delivery of oxygen to tissues throughout the body, maintaining vascular integrity and providing the many affector and effector immune functions necessary for host defense, requires a prodigious proliferative and regenerative capacity. Each of the various blood cells (erythrocytes, granulocytes, and platelets) is produced at a rate of approximately 1–3 million/s in a healthy adult; this characteristic makes hematopoietic tissue a particularly sensitive target for cytoreductive or antimitotic agents, such as those used to treat cancer, infection, and immune-mediated disorders. This tissue is also susceptible to secondary effects of toxic agents that affect the supply of nutrients, such as iron; the clearance of toxins and metabolites, such as urea; or the production of vital growth factors, such as erythropoietin (EPO) and granulocyte colony-stimulating factor (G-CSF). The consequences of direct or indirect damage to blood cells and their precursors are predictable and potentially life-threatening. They include hypoxia, hemorrhage, and infection.

Hematotoxicity may be regarded as *primary toxicity*, where one or more blood components are directly affected, or *secondary*, where the toxic effect is a consequence of other tissue injury or systemic disturbances. Primary toxicity is regarded as among the serious effects of xenobiotics, particularly drugs. Secondary toxicity is exceedingly common, due to the propensity of blood cells to reflect various local and systemic effects of toxicants on other tissues.

HEMATOPOIESIS

The production of blood cells, or *hematopoiesis*, is a highly regulated sequence of events by which blood cell precursors proliferate and differentiate. The location of hematopoiesis changes throughout one's life. For instance, fetal hematopoiesis is located in the liver, spleen, bone marrow, thymus, and lymph nodes, while the primary location in adults is the bone marrow of the axial skeleton and proximal limbs. Two types of bone marrow exist: (1) red marrow, which is active in hematopoiesis, and (2) yellow marrow, which is called so because it turns fatty as it ceases participation in hematopoiesis.

Whereas the central function of bone marrow is hematopoiesis and lymphopoiesis (production of a subset of white blood cells), bone marrow is also one of the sites of the mononuclear phagocyte system (MPS), contributing monocytes that differentiate into phagocytic cells in other tissues. A complex interplay of developing cells with stromal (connective tissue) cells, extracellular matrix components, and cytokines makes up the *hematopoietic inductive microenvironment.* Each lineage is supported within a specific niche, and an array of cytokines and chemokines directs a particular progenitor cell to the appropriate niche.

TOXICOLOGY OF THE ERYTHRON

The Erythrocyte

Erythrocytes (red blood cells [RBCs]) comprise 40% to 45% of the circulating blood volume and serve as the principal vehicle for transportation of oxygen from the lungs to peripheral tissues and of carbon dioxide from tissues to the lung. Erythrocytes are also involved as a carrier and/or reservoir for drugs and toxins. Xenobiotics may affect the production, function, and survival of erythrocytes. These effects most frequently manifest as a change in the circulating red cell mass, usually resulting in a decrease (anemia). Occasionally, agents that affect the oxygen affinity of hemoglobin lead to an increase in the red cell mass (erythrocytosis), but this is distinctly less common. Shifts in plasma volume can alter the relative concentration of erythrocytes (and, therefore, hemoglobin concentration) and can be confused with true anemia or erythrocytosis.

Two general mechanisms that lead to true anemia are either decreased production or increased destruction of erythrocytes.

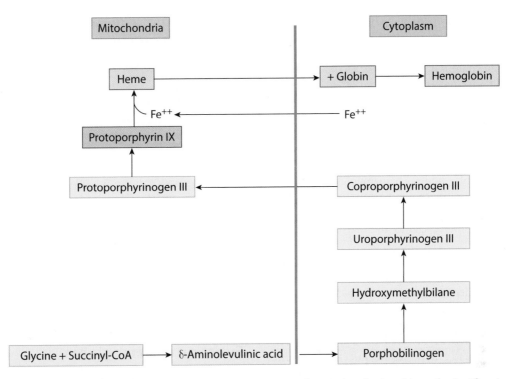

FIGURE 11–1 **Heme and hemoglobin synthesis.** The initial step in heme synthesis is the mitochondria synthesis of δ-aminolevulinic acid, a step that is commonly affected by xenobiotics, including lead. Ferrochelatase catalyzes the incorporation of ferrous iron into the tetrapyrrole protoporphyrin IX. Inhibition of the synthetic pathway leading to protoporphyrin IX, as occurs in the sideroblastic anemias, can cause an imbalance between iron concentration and ferrochelatase activity, resulting in iron deposition within mitochondria. Mitochondrial accumulation of iron is the hallmark lesion of the sideroblastic anemias.

The usual parameters of a complete blood count (CBC), including RBC count, hemoglobin concentration, and hematocrit (also referred to as packed cell volume [PCV]) can establish the presence of anemia. Two additional parameters that are helpful in classifying an anemia are the mean corpuscular volume (MCV) and the reticulocyte count. Increased destruction is usually accompanied by an increase in reticulocytes (young erythrocytes containing residual RNA). Two related processes contribute to the increased number of reticulocytes in humans. First, increased destruction is accompanied by a compensatory increase in bone marrow production, with an increase in the number of cells being released from the marrow into the circulation. Second, during compensatory erythroid hyperplasia, the marrow releases reticulocytes earlier in their life span and thus the reticulocytes persist for a longer period in the peripheral blood.

Alterations in Red Cell Production

Erythrocyte production is a continuous process that is dependent on frequent cell division and a high rate of hemoglobin synthesis. Adult hemoglobin (hemoglobin A) is a tetramer composed of two α-globin chains and two β-globin chains, each with a heme residue.

Abnormalities that lead to decreased hemoglobin synthesis are relatively common (e.g., iron deficiency). An imbalance

between α- and β-chain production is the basis of congenital thalassemia syndromes and results in decreased hemoglobin production and microcytosis. Xenobiotics can affect globin chain synthesis and alter the composition of hemoglobin within erythrocytes.

Synthesis of heme requires incorporation of iron into a porphyrin ring (Figure 11–1). Iron deficiency is usually the result of dietary deficiency or increased blood loss. Any drug that contributes to blood loss may potentiate the risk of developing *iron deficiency anemia.* Defects in the synthesis of porphyrin ring of heme can lead to *sideroblastic anemia,* with its characteristic accumulation of iron in bone marrow erythroblasts. The accumulated iron precipitates within mitochondria causing injury. A number of xenobiotics (Table 11–1) interfere with

TABLE 11–1 **Xenobiotics associated with sideroblastic anemia.**

Chloramphenicol	Isoniazid
Copper chelation/deficiency	Lead intoxication
Cycloserine	Pyrazinamide
Ethanol	Zinc intoxication

one or more steps in erythroblast heme synthesis and result in sideroblastic anemia.

Hematopoiesis requires active DNA synthesis and frequent mitoses. Folate and vitamin B_{12} are necessary to maintain synthesis of thymidine for incorporation into DNA. Deficiency of folate and/or vitamin B_{12} results in *megaloblastic anemia*, a result of improper cell division. Xenobiotics that may contribute to a deficiency of vitamin B_{12} and/or folate are listed in Table 11–2.

Many antiproliferative agents used in the treatment of malignancy predictably inhibit hematopoiesis, including erythropoiesis. The resulting bone marrow toxicity may be dose-limiting. Drugs, such as amifostine, have been developed that may help protect against the marrow toxicity of these agents.

Drug-induced *aplastic anemia* may represent either a predictable or idiosyncratic reaction to a xenobiotic. This life-threatening disorder is characterized by peripheral blood pancytopenia, reticulocytopenia, and bone marrow hypoplasia. Agents associated with the development of aplastic anemia are listed in Table 11–3. *Pure red cell aplasia* is a syndrome that may be due to genetic defects, infection, immune-mediated injury, myelodysplasia, drugs, or other toxicants, in which the decrease in marrow production is limited to the erythroid lineage.

TABLE 11–2 Xenobiotics associated with megaloblastic anemia.

B_{12} Deficiency	Folate Deficiency
Antimetabolites	Neomycin
p-Aminosalicylic acid	Omeprazole
Carbamazepine	Phenobarbital
Cholestyramine	Phenytoin
Colchicine	Primidone
Ethanol	Sulfasalazine
Fish tapeworm	Triamterine
Hemodialysis	Zidovudine
Malabsorption syndromes	

Alterations in the Respiratory Function of Hemoglobin

Hemoglobin transports oxygen and carbon dioxide between the lungs and tissues. The individual globin units show cooperativity in the binding of oxygen, resulting in the

TABLE 11–3 Drugs and chemicals associated with the development of aplastic anemia.

Allopurinol	Diclofenac	Penicillin
Amphotericin B	Dinitrophenol	Phenylbutazone
Azidothymidine	Ethosuximide	Potassium perchlorate
Benzene	Felbamate	Propylthiouracil
Bismuth	Gold	Pyrimethamine
Carbamazepine	Indomethacin	Quinacrine
Carbimazole	Isoniazid	Streptomycin
Carbon tetrachloride	Mefloquine	Sulfamethoxypyridazine
Carbutamide	Mepazine	Sulfisoxazole
Chloramphenicol	Meprobamate	Sulfonamides
Chlordane	Mercury	Tetracycline
Chlordiazepoxide	Methazolamide	Thiocyanate
Chlorphenothane	Methicillin	Ticlopidine
Chlorpropamide	Methylphenylethylhydantoin	Tolbutamide
Chlorpromazine	Methylmercaptoimidazole	Trifluoroperazine
Chlortetracycline	Metolazone	Trimethadione
Cimetidine	Organic arsenicals	Tripelennamine
D-Penicillamine	Parathion	

familiar sigmoid shape to the oxygen dissociation curve (Figure 11–2).

Homotropic Effects—One of the most important homotropic (intrinsic) properties of oxyhemoglobin is the slow but consistent oxidation of heme iron to the ferric state to form methemoglobin, which is not capable of binding and transporting oxygen. The presence of methemoglobin in a hemoglobin tetramer results in a leftward shift of the oxygen dissociation curve (Figure 11–2). The combination of decreased oxygen content and increased affinity may significantly impair delivery of oxygen to tissues, as the oxygen will not be readily released from hemoglobin in the periphery.

The normal erythrocyte has metabolic mechanisms for reducing heme iron back to the ferrous state. Failure of these control mechanisms leads to increased levels of methemoglobin, or *methemoglobinemia*. Various chemicals that cause methemoglobinemia are shown in Table 11–4. Most patients tolerate low levels (< 10%) of methemoglobin without clinical symptoms. Higher levels lead to tissue hypoxemia that is eventually fatal.

Heterotropic Effects—There are three major heterotropic (extrinsic) effectors of hemoglobin function: pH, erythrocyte 2,3-bisphosphoglycerate (2,3-BPG, formerly designated 2,3-diphosphoglycerate [2,3-DPG]) concentration, and temperature. A decrease in pH (e.g., lactic acid and carbon dioxide) lowers the affinity of hemoglobin for oxygen causing a right shift in the oxygen dissociation curve and facilitating the delivery of oxygen to tissues (Figure 11–2). As bicarbonate and carbon dioxide equilibrate in the lung, the hydrogen ion concentration decreases, which results in increased affinity of hemoglobin for oxygen and facilitated oxygen uptake.

Binding of 2,3-BPG to deoxyhemoglobin results in reduced oxygen affinity (a shift to the right of the oxygen dissociation curve), which promotes oxygen delivery to peripheral tissues. The conformational change induced by binding of oxygen to hemoglobin alters the binding site for 2,3-BPG and results in release of 2,3-BPG from hemoglobin. This facilitates uptake of more oxygen in the lungs for delivery to tissues. The concentration of 2,3-BPG increases whenever there is tissue hypoxemia but may decrease in the presence of acidosis or hypophosphatemia.

The oxygen affinity of hemoglobin decreases as the body temperature increases. This facilitates delivery of oxygen to tissues during periods of extreme exercise and febrile illnesses associated with increased temperature. Correspondingly, oxygen affinity increases and delivery decreases during hypothermia.

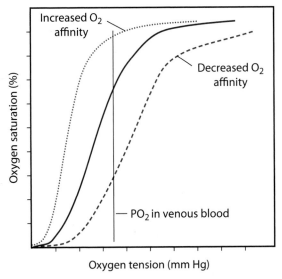

FIGURE 11–2 Hemoglobin-oxygen dissociation curves. The normal oxygen dissociation curve (*solid line*) has a sigmoid shape due to the cooperative interaction between the four globin chains in the hemoglobin molecule. Fully deoxygenated hemoglobin has a relatively low affinity for oxygen. Interaction of oxygen with one heme–iron moiety induces a conformational change in that globin chain. Through surface interactions, that conformational change affects the other globin chains, causing a conformational change in all of the globin chains that increases their affinity for oxygen. Homotropic and heterotropic parameters also affect the affinity of hemoglobin for oxygen. An increase in oxygen affinity results in a shift to the left in the oxygen dissociation curve. Such a shift may decrease oxygen delivery to the tissues. A decrease in oxygen affinity results in a shift to the right in the oxygen dissociation curve, facilitating oxygen delivery to the tissues.

TABLE 11–4 Environmental and therapeutic agents associated with methemoglobinemia.

Aminobenzenes	Nitrobenzenes
Amyl nitrate	Nitroethane
Aniline dyes and aniline derivatives	Nitroglycerin
Benzocaine	Nitrotoluenes
Beta-naphthol disulfonate	*ortho*-Toluidine
Butyl nitrite	*para*-Toluidine
Dapsone	Potassium chlorate
Flutamide	Prilocaine
Gasoline additives	Primaquine
Isobutyl nitrite	Phenacetin
Lidocaine	Phenazopyridine
Methylene blue	Quinones
Nitrates	Silver nitrate
Nitric oxide	Sulfonamide
Nitrites	Trinitrotoluene

The respiratory function of hemoglobin may also be impaired by blocking the ligand binding site with other substances. Carbon monoxide has a relatively low rate of association with deoxyhemoglobin but shows high affinity once bound, and causes a left shift in the oxygen dissociation curve, further compromising oxygen delivery to the tissues. Nitric oxide, an important vasodilator that modulates vascular tone, binds avidly to heme iron. Erythrocytes can influence the availability of nitric oxide in parts of the circulation because the nitric oxide is bound to erythrocyte hemoglobin.

Alterations in Erythrocyte Survival

The normal survival of erythrocytes in the circulation is about 120 days. During this period, erythrocytes are exposed to a various oxidative injuries and must negotiate the tortuous passages of the microcirculation and the spleen. This requires a deformable cell membrane and energy to maintain the sodium–potassium gradients and repair mechanisms. Very little protein synthesis occurs during this time, as erythrocytes are anucleate when they enter the circulation and residual mRNA is rapidly lost over the first 1 to 2 days in the circulation. Consequently, senescence occurs over time until the aged erythrocytes are removed by the spleen, where the iron is recovered for reutilization in heme synthesis. Any insult that increases oxidative injury, decreases metabolism, or alters the membrane may cause a decrease in erythrocyte concentration and a corresponding anemia.

Nonimmune Hemolytic Anemia

Microangiopathic Anemias—Intravascular fragmentation of erythrocytes gives rise to the *microangiopathic hemolytic anemias*. The hallmark of this process is the presence of schistocytes (fragmented RBCs) in peripheral blood. The formation of fibrin strands in the microcirculation is a common mechanism for RBC fragmentation. This may occur in the setting of disseminated intravascular coagulation, sepsis, hemolytic-uremic syndrome (HUS), and thrombotic thrombocytopenic purpura (TTP). The erythrocytes are essentially sliced into fragments by the fibrin strands that extend across the vascular lumen and impede the flow of erythrocytes through the vasculature. Excessive fragmentation can also be seen in the presence of abnormal vasculature. The high shear associated with malignant hypertension may also lead to RBC fragmentation.

Other Mechanical Injuries—RBC destruction can also occur as a result of mechanical stress. For instance, march hemoglobinuria is an episodic anemia resulting from mechanical trauma to the feet from prolonged activity. Major thermal burns are also associated with a hemolytic process. The erythrocyte membrane becomes unstable as temperature increases to the point where small RBC fragments break off and the membrane reseals. Consequently, these abnormal cell fragments are removed by the spleen, leading to anemia.

Infectious Diseases—Infectious diseases may be associated with significant hemolysis, by either direct effect on the erythrocyte or an immune-mediated hemolytic process. Erythrocytes parasitized in malaria and babesiosis may undergo destruction. Clostridial infections are associated with release of hemolytic toxins that enter the circulation and lyse erythrocytes.

Oxidative Hemolysis—Molecular oxygen is a reactive and potentially toxic chemical species; consequently, the normal respiratory function of erythrocytes generates oxidative stress on a continuous basis. There are several mechanisms that protect against oxidative injury in erythrocytes including NADH-diaphorase, superoxide dismutase, catalase, and the glutathione pathway.

Xenobiotics capable of inducing oxidative injury in erythrocytes are listed in Table 11–5. These agents appear to potentiate the normal redox reactions and are capable of overwhelming the usual protective mechanisms. The interaction between these xenobiotics and hemoglobin leads to the formation of free radicals that denature critical proteins, including hemoglobin, thiol-dependent enzymes, and components of the erythrocyte membrane. Significant oxidative injury usually occurs when the concentration of the xenobiotic is high enough to overcome the normal protective mechanisms, or, more commonly, when there is an underlying defect in the protective mechanisms.

The most common enzyme defect associated with oxidative hemolysis is glucose-6-phosphate dehydrogenase (G-6-PD) deficiency, a sex-linked disorder characterized by diminished G-6-PD activity. It is often clinically asymptomatic until the erythrocytes are exposed to oxidative stress from the host response to infection or exposure to xenobiotics.

Nonoxidative Chemical-induced Hemolysis—Exposure to some xenobiotics is associated with hemolysis without

TABLE 11–5 Xenobiotics associated with oxidative injury.

Acetanilide	Phenacetin
Aminosalicylic acid	Phenol
Chlorates	Phenylhydrazine
Dapsone	Primaquine
Furazolidone	Phenazopyridine
Hydroxylamine	Sodium sulfoxone
Methylene blue	Sulfamethoxypyridazine
Nalidixic acid	Sulfanilamide
Naphthalene	Sulfasalazine
Nitrofurantoin	Toluidine blue
Nitrobenzene	

significant oxidative injury. For example, inhalation of gaseous arsenic hydride (arsine) can result in severe hemolysis, with anemia, jaundice, and hemoglobinuria. Several elements are known to cause hemolysis in the absence of oxidative damage, namely, lead, copper, and chromium. Additionally, significant hemolysis may occur with biologic toxins found in insect and snake venoms.

Immune Hemolytic Anemia—Immunologic destruction of erythrocytes is mediated by the interaction of IgG or IgM antibodies with antigens expressed on the surface of the erythrocyte. In the case of autoimmune hemolytic anemia, the antigens are intrinsic components of the patient's own erythrocytes.

A number of mechanisms have been implicated in xenobiotic-mediated antibody binding to erythrocytes. Some drugs, of which penicillin is a prototype, appear to bind to the surface of the cell, with the "foreign" drug acting as a *hapten* and eliciting an immune response. The antibodies that arise in this type of response only bind to drug-coated erythrocytes. Other drugs, of which quinidine is a prototype, bind to components of the erythrocyte surface and induce a conformational change in one or more components of the membrane. A third mechanism, for which α-methyldopa is a prototype, results in production of a *drug-induced autoantibody* that cannot be distinguished from the antibodies arising in idiopathic autoimmune hemolytic anemia.

TOXICOLOGY OF THE LEUKON

Components of Blood Leukocytes

The leukon consists of leukocytes, or white blood cells, including granulocytes, which may be subdivided into neutrophils, eosinophils, and basophils; monocytes; and lymphocytes. Granulocytes and monocytes are nucleated ameboid cells that are phagocytic. They play a central role in the inflammatory response and host defense. Unlike the RBC, which resides exclusively within blood, granulocytes and monocytes merely pass through the blood on their way to extravascular tissues, where they reside in large numbers.

Granulocytes are defined by the characteristics of their cytoplasmic granules as they appear on a blood smear. Neutrophils, the largest component of blood leukocytes, are highly specialized in the mediation of inflammation and the ingestion and destruction of pathogenic microorganisms. Eosinophils and basophils modulate inflammation through the release of various mediators.

Evaluation of Granulocytes

In the blood, neutrophils are distributed between *circulating* and *marginated* pools, which are of equal size in humans and in constant equilibrium. A blood neutrophil count assesses only the circulating pool, which remains remarkably constant (1800 to $7500\ \mu L^{-1}$) in a healthy adult human. During inflammation, an increased number of immature (non-segmented) granulocytes may be seen in peripheral blood. In certain conditions, neutrophils may show morphological changes indicative of toxicity.

Toxic Effects on Granulocytes

Effects on Proliferation—The high rate of proliferation of neutrophils makes their progenitor and precursor granulocyte pool particularly susceptible to inhibitors of mitosis. Such effects by cytotoxic drugs are generally nonspecific as they similarly affect cells of the dermis, gastrointestinal tract, and other rapidly dividing tissues. Agents that affect both neutrophils and monocytes pose a greater risk for toxic sequelae, such as infection. Such effects tend to be dose-related, with mononuclear phagocyte recovery preceding neutrophil recovery.

Myelotoxicity is commonly seen with cytoreductive cancer chemotherapy agents, which often act to inhibit DNA synthesis or directly attack its integrity through the formation of DNA adducts or enzyme-mediated breaks. However, this is changing, as more cancer cell-targeted, normal-tissue-sparing anticancer agents are being developed. The toxicity associated with cytotoxic drugs, however, remains important in that it is often dose-limiting (even with some of the newer drugs) with serious manifestations that include febrile neutropenia associated with life-threatening infections. While these drugs can be toxic to both resting and actively dividing cells, nonproliferating cells such as metamyelocytes, bands, and mature neutrophils are relatively resistant. Because stem cells cycle slowly, they are minimally affected by a single administration of a cytotoxic drug. Sustained exposure to drugs affecting stem cells is believed to cause more prolonged myelosuppression.

Two innovations have had a dramatic impact on cancer chemotherapy and the dose-limiting myelotoxicity associated with these drugs: (1) the development of drugs with cancer cell–specific molecular targets that are relatively bone marrow sparing, such as those that target aberrant growth factor receptor signaling, apoptosis, angiogenesis, and other metabolic, immune, inflammatory, and mutation-promoting pathways that selectively advantage tumor cells, and (2) cotreatment with hematopoietic growth factors mitigates or successfully rescues patients from the effects of myelosuppression. Cytokine-induced differentiation therapy of leukemias is another exciting treatment modality. The prospect of exaggerated pharmacology and off-target effects of these sophisticated interventions should provide the preclinical toxicologist and oncologist with interesting hematotoxicologic challenges.

Effects on Function—While there are a variety of disorders associated with defects in the parameters of neutrophil function discussed above, demonstrable in vivo effects associated with drugs and nontherapeutic chemicals are surprisingly few. Examples include ethanol and glucocorticoids, which impair phagocytosis and microbe ingestion. Iohexol and ioxaglate, components of radiographic contrast media, have also been reported to inhibit phagocytosis. Superoxide production, required for microbial killing and chemotaxis, is reportedly reduced in patients using parenteral heroin as well as in former opiate abusers on long-term methadone maintenance. Chemotaxis is also impaired following treatment with zinc salts in antiacne preparations.

Idiosyncratic Toxic Neutropenia—Of greater concern are agents that unexpectedly damage neutrophils and granulocyte precursors and induce *agranulocytosis,* which is characterized by a profound depletion in blood neutrophils to less than 500 μL^{-1}. Such injury occurs in specifically conditioned individuals, and is therefore termed *idiosyncratic.*

Idiosyncratic xenobiotic-induced agranulocytosis may involve a sudden depletion of circulating neutrophils concomitant with exposure, which may persist as long as the agent or its metabolites persist in the circulation. Hematopoietic function is usually restored when the agent is detoxified or excreted. Toxicants affecting uncommitted stem cells induce total marrow failure, as seen in aplastic anemia. After agents that affect more differentiated precursors, surviving uncommitted stem cells eventually produce recovery, provided that

TABLE 11–6 Examples of toxicants that cause immune and nonimmune idiopathic neutropenia.

Drugs Associated with WBC Antibodies	Drugs Not Associated with WBC Antibodies
Aminopyrine	Allopurinol
Ampicillin	Ethambutol
Aprindine	Flurazepam
Azulfidine	Hydrochlorothiazide
Chlorpropamide	Isoniazide
Clozapine	Phenothiazines
CPZ/phenothiazines	Rifampicin
Dicloxacillin	
Gold	
Levamisole	
Lidocaine	
Methimazole	
Metiamide	
Phenytoin	
Procainamide	
Propylthiouracil	
Quinidine	
Tolbutamide	

the risk of infection is successfully managed during the leukopenic episodes.

Mechanisms of Toxic Neutropenia—In *immune-mediated neutropenia,* antigen–antibody reactions lead to destruction of peripheral neutrophils, granulocyte precursors, or both. As with RBCs, an immunogenic xenobiotic can act as a hapten, where the agent must be physically present to cause cell damage, or alternatively, may induce immunogenic cells to produce antineutrophil antibodies that do not require the drug to be present.

Non-immune-mediated toxic neutropenia often shows a genetic predisposition. Direct damage may cause inhibition of granulopoiesis or neutrophil function. Some studies suggest that a buildup of toxic oxidants generated by leukocytes can result in neutrophil damage.

Examples of agents associated with immune and nonimmune neutropenia/agranulocytosis are listed in Table 11–6.

LEUKEMOGENESIS AS A TOXIC RESPONSE

Human Leukemias

Leukemias are proliferative disorders of hematopoietic tissue that are monoclonal and originate from individual bone marrow cells. Historically they have been classified as myeloid or lymphoid, referring to the major lineages for erythrocytes, granulocytes, thrombocytes, or lymphocytes, respectively. Poorly differentiated phenotypes have been designated as "acute," including acute lymphoblastic leukemia (ALL) and acute myelogenous leukemia (AML), whereas well-differentiated ones are referred to as "chronic" leukemias, which include chronic lymphocytic leukemia (CLL), chronic myelogenous leukemia (CML), and the myelodysplastic syndromes (MDS).

There is considerable evidence supporting the notion that leukemogenesis is a multievent progression, which suggest that factors involved in the regulation of hematopoiesis also influence neoplastic transformation. Such factors include cellular growth factors (cytokines), proto-oncogenes, and other growth-promoting genes, as well as additional genetic and epigenetic factors that govern survival, proliferation, and differentiation.

Secondary leukemia is a term used to describe patients with AML or MDS who have a history of environmental, occupational, or therapeutic exposure to hematotoxins or radiation. It also includes patients with AML evolving from antecedent myelodysplastic or other myeloid stem cell disorders. *Therapy-related AML and MDS* is a term applied to the former group; both are used to distinguish from features of AML that arise de novo. Various cytogenetic findings have been associated with prognosis and response to therapy. It has been suggested that secondary leukemias be redefined as any leukemia with a specific cytogenic or molecular poor prognostic feature due to a presumed predisposing factor.

Mechanisms of Toxic Leukemogenesis

AML is the dominant leukemia associated with drug or chemical exposure, followed by MDS. This represents a continuum of one toxic response that has been linked to cytogenetic abnormalities, particularly the loss of all or part of chromosomes 5 and 7. Remarkably, the frequency of these deletions in patients who develop MDS and/or AML after treatment with alkylating or other antineoplastic agents ranges from 67% to 95%, depending on the study. Some of these same changes have been observed in AML patients occupationally exposed to benzene, who also show aneuploidy with a high frequency of involvement of chromosome 7. The relatively low frequency of deletions in chromosomes 5 and 7 in de novo as compared with secondary AML suggests that these cytogenetic markers can be useful in discriminating between toxic exposures and other etiologies of this leukemia.

Leukemogenic Agents

Most *alkylating agents* used in cancer chemotherapy can cause MDS and/or AML. Of the *aromatic hydrocarbons,* only benzene has been proven to be leukemogenic. Treatment with the *topoisomerase II inhibitors,* etoposide and teniposide, can induce AML.

Exposure to *high-dose γ- or x-ray radiation* has long been associated with ALL, AML, and CML, as demonstrated in survivors of the atom bombings of Nagasaki and Hiroshima. Less clear is the association of these diseases with low-dose radiation secondary to fallout or diagnostic radiographs. Other *controversial agents* include 1,3-butadiene, nonionizing radiation (electromagnetic, microwave, infrared, visible, and the high end of the ultraviolet spectrum), cigarette smoking, and formaldehyde.

TOXICOLOGY OF PLATELETS AND HEMOSTASIS

Hemostasis, the stoppage of bleeding or blood flow through an organ, is a multicomponent system responsible for preventing the loss of blood from sites of vascular injury and maintaining circulating blood in a fluid state. Loss of blood is prevented by formation of stable hemostatic plugs. The major constituents of the hemostatic system include circulating platelets, a variety of plasma proteins, and vascular endothelial cells. Alterations in these components or systemic activation of this system can lead to the clinical manifestations of deranged hemostasis, including excessive bleeding and thrombosis. The hemostatic system is a frequent target of therapeutic intervention as well as inadvertent expression of the toxic effect of a variety of xenobiotics.

Toxic Effects on Platelets

The Thrombocyte—Platelets are essential for formation of a stable hemostatic plug in response to vascular injury. Platelets initially adhere to the damaged blood vessel wall through binding of von Willebrand factor (vWF) with the platelet Ib/IX/V (GP Ib/IX/V) receptor complex. Activation of a pathway of several factors permits fibrinogen and other multivalent adhesive molecules to form cross-links between nearby platelets, resulting in platelet aggregation. Xenobiotics may interfere with the platelet response by causing thrombocytopenia (low platelet levels) or interfering with platelet function.

Thrombocytopenia—Like anemia, thrombocytopenia may be due to decreased production or increased destruction of platelets. Thrombocytopenia is a common side effect of intensive chemotherapy, due to the predictable effect of antiproliferative agents on hematopoietic precursors. Thrombocytopenia is a clinically significant component of idiosyncratic xenobiotic-induced aplastic anemia. Indeed, the initial manifestation of aplastic anemia may be mucocutaneous bleeding secondary to thrombocytopenia.

Exposure to xenobiotics may cause increased immune-mediated platelet destruction through any one of the several mechanisms. Penicillin is an example of a drug that functions as a hapten, which is a small molecule that only produces a specific immune response if bound to a protein carrier. The responding antibody then binds to the hapten on the platelet surface, leading to removal of the antibody-coated platelet from the circulation.

A second mechanism of immune thrombocytopenia is initiated by a change in a platelet membrane glycoprotein caused by the xenobiotic. This elicits an antibody response, with the responding antibody binding to this altered platelet antigen in the presence of drug, resulting in removal of the platelet from the circulation by the mononuclear phagocytic system.

Thrombocytopenia is an uncommon, but serious, complication of drugs that inhibit the platelet glycoprotein IIb/IIIa receptor. Inhibitors like abciximab can change the conformation of this receptor, causing exposure of certain peptides (called neoepitopes because they are newly exposed to the immune system) on the factors that react with endogenous antibodies. This leads to phagocytosis of the platelets associated with these factors. Thus, exposure of epitopes that react with naturally occurring antibodies represents a third mechanism of immune-mediated platelet destruction.

Heparin-induced thrombocytopenia (HIT) represents a fourth mechanism of immune-mediated platelet destruction. When heparin (an anticoagulant) binds to certain clotting factors, a neoepitope is exposed, and an immune response is mounted against the neoepitope. This results in platelet activation and aggregation instead of heparin's normal function of preventing clot formation, which can lead to a risk of thrombosis (pieces of clots falling off and lodging in microvasculature, impairing circulation).

Thrombotic thrombocytopenic purpura (TTP) is a syndrome characterized by the sudden onset of thrombocytopenia, a microangiopathic hemolytic anemia, and multisystem organ failure. The syndrome tends to occur following an infectious disease but may also occur following administration of some drugs. The pathogenesis of TTP appears to be related to the ability of unusually large vWf multimers to activate platelets, even in the absence of significant vascular damage. Acquired TTP is associated with the development of an antibody that inhibits the protease responsible for processing very large vWf multimers into smaller multimers; the large multimers persist in circulation and inappropriately activate the platelets. The organ failure and hemolysis in TTP is due to the formation of platelet-rich microthrombi throughout the circulation. The development of TTP or TTP-like syndromes has been associated with drugs such as ticlopidine, clopidogrel, cocaine, mitomycin, and cyclosporine.

Hemolytic uremic syndrome (HUS) is a disorder with clinical features similar to those of TTP, but with less severe neurologic complications and predominant renal failure. Sporadic HUS cases have been linked to *Escherichia coli* infection, but HUS can also occur during therapy with some drugs, including mitomycin. Unlike TTP, the vWf-cleaving protease is normal and the pathogenesis is thought to be related to endothelial cell damage with subsequent platelet activation and thrombus formation.

Toxic Effects on Platelet Function—Platelet function is dependent on the coordinated interaction of a number of biochemical response pathways. Major drug groups that affect platelet function include nonsteroidal anti-inflammatory drugs (NSAIDs), β-lactam-containing antibiotics, cardiovascular drugs (particularly β-blockers), psychotropic drugs, anesthetics, antihistamines, and some chemotherapeutic agents.

Xenobiotics may interfere with platelet function through a variety of mechanisms. Some drugs inhibit the phospholipase A_2/cyclooxygenase pathway and synthesis of thromboxane A_2 (e.g., NSAIDs). Other agents appear to interfere with the interaction between platelet agonists and their receptors (e.g., antibiotics, ticlopidine, and clopidogrel). As the platelet response is dependent on rapid increase in cytoplasmic calcium, any agent that interferes with translocation of calcium may inhibit platelet function (e.g., calcium channel blockers). Occasionally, drug-induced antibodies will bind to a critical platelet receptor and inhibit its function.

Toxic Effects on Fibrin Clot Formation

Coagulation—Fibrin clot formation results from sequential activation of a series of serine proteases that culminates in the formation of thrombin. Thrombin is a multifunctional enzyme that converts fibrinogen to fibrin; activates factors V, VIII, XI, XIII, protein C, and platelets; and interacts with a variety of cells (e.g., leukocytes and endothelial cells), activating cellular signaling pathways.

Decreased Synthesis of Coagulation Proteins—Most proteins involved in the coagulation cascade are synthesized in the liver. Therefore, any agent that impairs liver function may cause a decrease in production of coagulation factors. The common tests of the coagulation cascade, the prothrombin time (PT) and activated partial thromboplastin time (aPTT),

TABLE 11–7 Conditions associated with abnormal synthesis of vitamin K–dependent coagulation factors.

Warfarin and analogs	Intravenous α-tocopherol
Rodenticides (e.g., brodifacoum)	Dietary deficiency
Broad-spectrum antibiotics	Cholestyramine resin
N-Methyl-thiotetrazole cephalosporins	Malabsorption syndromes

may be used to screen for liver dysfunction and a decrease in clotting factors.

Factors II, VII, IX, and X are dependent on vitamin K for their complete synthesis. Anything that interferes with absorption of vitamin K from the intestine or with the reduction of vitamin K epoxide may lead to a deficiency of these factors and a bleeding tendency (Table 11–7).

Increased Clearance of Coagulation Factors—Idiosyncratic reactions to xenobiotics include the formation of antibodies that react with coagulation proteins, forming an immune complex that is rapidly cleared from the circulation resulting in deficiency of the factor. The factors that are most often affected by xenobiotics are listed in Table 11–8. In addition to causing increased clearance from the circulation, these antibodies often inhibit the function of the coagulation factor. Other antibodies have catalytic activity, resulting in proteolysis of the target coagulation factor.

Lupus anticoagulants are antibodies that are directed against phospholipid binding proteins like prothrombin, can potentiate procoagulant mechanisms and interfere with the protein C system, increasing the risk of thrombosis. The development of lupus anticoagulants has been seen in association with chlorpromazine, procainamide, hydralazine, quinidine, phenytoin, and viral infections.

Toxicology of Agents Used to Modulate Hemostasis

Oral Anticoagulants—Oral anticoagulants (e.g., warfarin) interfere with vitamin K metabolism by preventing the reduction of vitamin K epoxide, resulting in a functional deficiency of reduced vitamin K. These drugs are widely used for prophylaxis and therapy of venous and arterial thrombosis. The therapeutic window for oral anticoagulants is relatively narrow, and there is considerable interindividual variation in the response to a given dose. A number of factors, including concurrent medications and genetics, affect the individual response to oral anticoagulants. For these reasons, therapy with these drugs must be routinely monitored to maximize both safety and efficacy. This is routinely performed with the PT, with results expressed in terms of the international normalized ratio (INR).

A number of xenobiotics, including foods, have been found to affect the response to oral anticoagulants. Mechanisms for interference with oral anticoagulants include induction or

TABLE 11–8 Relationship between xenobiotics and the development of specific coagulation factor inhibitors.

Coagulation Factor	Xenobiotic
Thrombin	Topical bovine thrombin Fibrin glue
Factor V	Streptomycin Penicillin Gentamicin Cephalosporins Topical bovine thrombin
Factor VIII	Penicillin Ampicillin Chloramphenicol Phenytoin Methyldopa Nitrofurazone Phenylbutazone
Factor XIII	Isoniazid Procainamide Penicillin Phenytoin Practolol
von Willebrand factor	Ciprofloxacin Hydroxyethyl starch Valproic acid Griseofulvin Tetracycline Pesticides

inhibition of biotransformation; interference with absorption of warfarin from the gastrointestinal tract; displacement of warfarin from albumin in plasma, which temporarily increases the bioavailability of warfarin until equilibrium is reestablished; diminished vitamin K availability; and inhibition of the reduction of vitamin K epoxide, which potentiates the effect of oral anticoagulants. Additionally, administration of oral anticoagulants may affect the activity or the half-lives of other medications.

Oral anticoagulants have been associated with warfarin-induced skin necrosis, which is due to development of microvascular thrombosis in skin. This uncommon effect occurs most commonly in patients deficient in proteins C or S or in patients administered high doses of warfarin too rapidly.

Vitamin K is also necessary for the synthesis of osteocalcin, a major component of bone. Long-term administration of warfarin has been associated with bone demineralization.

Administration of warfarin, particularly during the first 12 weeks of pregnancy, is associated with congenital anomalies in 25% to 30% of exposed infants. Many of the anomalies are related to abnormal bone formation. It is thought that warfarin may interfere with synthesis of additional proteins critical for normal structural development.

Heparin—Heparin is widely used for both prophylaxis and therapy of acute venous thromboembolism. The major complication associated with heparin therapy is bleeding, which is a direct manifestation of its anticoagulant activity. The aPTT is commonly used to monitor therapy with unfractionated heparin, a naturally occurring polysaccharide. Long-term administration of heparin is associated with an increased risk of clinically significant osteoporosis.

Fibrinolytic Agents—Fibrinolytic agents dissolve pathogenic thrombi by converting plasminogen, an inactive zymogen, to plasmin, an active proteolytic enzyme. Plasmin is normally tightly regulated and is not freely present in the circulation. However, administration of fibrinolytic agents regularly results in the generation of free plasmin leading to systemic fibrin(ogen)olysis, which is characterized by prolongation of the PT, aPTT, and thrombin time. All of these effects increase the risk of bleeding. Platelet inhibitors and heparin are commonly used in conjunction with fibrinolytic therapy to prevent recurrent thrombosis.

Streptokinase is a protein derived from group C β-hemolytic streptococci that is antigenic in humans. Allergic reactions to the protein can result from streptococcal infection or from exposure to streptokinase-containing fibrinolytic drugs. Acute allergic reactions may occur in 1% to 5% of patients exposed to streptokinase. Allergic reactions also occur with other fibrinolytic agents containing streptokinase (e.g., anisoylated plasminogen–streptokinase complex, alteplase) or streptokinase-derived peptides.

Inhibitors of Fibrinolysis—Antifibrinolytics are commonly used to control bleeding in patients with congenital abnormalities of hemostasis, such as von Willebrand disease. Tranexamic acid and ε-aminocaproic acid are small molecules that block the binding of plasminogen and plasmin to fibrin. Although relatively well tolerated, there is some evidence that administration of these chemicals may increase the risk of thrombosis due to the inhibition of the fibrinolytic system.

Aprotinin is a naturally occurring polypeptide inhibitor of serine protease clotting factors that is immunogenic when administered to humans.

RISK ASSESSMENT

Assessing the risk that exposure to new chemical products poses to humans—in terms of significant toxic effects on hematopoiesis and the functional integrity of blood cells and hemostatic mechanisms—is challenging. This is due in part to the complexity of hematopoiesis and the range of important tasks that these components perform. Risk assessment includes preclinical testing of animals and clinical trials in humans. It is hoped that in preclinical trials, the test animals will react similarly to humans on exposure to the xenobiotic, and the animals are examined in detail for signs of toxicity.

TABLE 11–9 Examples of problem-driven tests used to characterize hematologic observations in preclinical toxicology.

Reticulocyte count
Heinz body preparation
Cell-associated antibody assays (erythrocyte, platelet, neutrophil)
Erythrocyte osmotic fragility test
Erythrokinetic/ferrokinetic analyses
Cytochemical/histochemical staining
Electron microscopy
In vitro hematopoietic clonogenic assays
Platelet aggregation
Plasma fibrinogen concentration
Clotting factor assays
Thrombin time
Bleeding time

Subsequent clinical trials are conducted in humans and measure myriad parameters of potential toxicity to determine the relative safety or toxicity of the test substance.

Tests used to assess blood and bone marrow in preclinical toxicology studies should provide information on the effects of single- and multiple-dose exposure on erythrocyte parameters (RBC, hemoglobin, PCV, MCV, and MCHC), leukocyte parameters (WBC and absolute differential counts), thrombocyte counts, coagulation tests (PT and aPTT), peripheral blood cell morphology, and bone marrow cytologic and histologic examinations. Additional tests should be employed in a problem-driven fashion as required to better characterize hematotoxicologic potential. Examples of these tests are listed in Table 11–9.

Patient- or population-related risk factors include pharmacogenetic variations in drug metabolism and detoxification that lead to reduced clearance of the agent or production of novel intermediate metabolites, histocompatibility antigens, interaction with drugs or other agents, increased sensitivity of hematopoietic precursors to damage, preexisting disease of the bone marrow, and metabolic defects that predispose to oxidative or other stresses associated with the agent.

A central issue in drug and nontherapeutic chemical development is the *predictive value* of preclinical toxicology data and the expansive but inevitably limited clinical database for the occurrence of significant hematotoxicity on broad exposure to human populations.

BIBLIOGRAPHY

Evans GO: *Animal Hematotoxicology: A Practical Guide for Toxicologists and Biomedical Researchers.* Boca Raton, FL: CRC Press, 2008.

Hillman R, Ault KA, Rinder HM: *Hematology in Clinical Practice: A Guide to Diagnosis and Management,* 4th ed. New York: McGraw-Hill, 2005.

Kaushansky K, Lichtman MA, Beutler E, Kipps TJ, Seligsohn U, Prchal JT (eds.): *Williams Hematology,* 8th ed. New York: McGraw-Hill, 2010.

QUESTIONS

1. Which of the following statements is FALSE regarding true anemia?
    a. Alterations of the mean corpuscular volume are characteristic of anemia.
    b. Increased destruction of erythrocytes can lead to anemia.
    c. Decreased production of erythrocytes is not a common cause of anemia because the bone marrow is continuously renewing the red blood cell pool.
    d. Reticulocytes will live for a longer period of time in the peripheral blood when a person is anemic.
    e. The main parameters in diagnosing anemia are RBC count, hemoglobin concentration, and hematocrit.

2. Which of the following types of anemia is properly paired with its cause?
    a. iron deficiency anemia—blood loss.
    b. sideroblastic anemia—vitamin B_{12} deficiency.
    c. megaloblastic anemia—folate supplementation.
    d. aplastic anemia—ethanol.
    e. megaloblastic anemia—lead poisoning.

3. The inability to synthesize the porphyrin ring of hemoglobin will most likely result in which of the following?
    a. iron deficiency anemia.
    b. improper RBC mitosis.
    c. inability to synthesize thymidine.
    d. accumulation of iron within erythroblasts.
    e. bone marrow hypoplasia.

4. Which of the following will cause a right shift in the oxygen dissociation curve?
    a. increased pH.
    b. decreased carbon dioxide concentration.
    c. decreased body temperature.
    d. increased 2,3-BPG concentration.
    e. fetal hemoglobin.

5. All of the following statements regarding erythrocytes are true EXCEPT:
    a. Aged erythrocytes are removed by the liver, where the iron is recycled.
    b. Erythrocytes have a life span of approximately 120 days.
    c. Red blood cells generally lose their nuclei before entering the circulation.
    d. Reticulocytes are immature RBCs that still have a little RNA.
    e. Persons with anemia have a higher than normal reticulocyte:erythrocyte ratio.

6. All of the following statements regarding oxidative hemolysis are true EXCEPT:
    a. Reactive oxygen species are commonly generated by RBC metabolism.
    b. Superoxide dismutase and catalase are enzymes that protect against oxidative damage.
    c. Reduced glutathione (GSH) increases the likelihood of oxidative injuries to RBCs.
    d. Glucose-6-phosphate dehydrogenase deficiency is commonly associated with oxidative hemolysis.
    e. Xenobiotics can cause oxidative injury to RBCs by overcoming the protective mechanisms of the cell.

7. Which of the following sets of leukocytes is properly characterized as granulocytes because of the appearance of cytoplasmic granules on a blood smear?
    a. neutrophils, basophils, and monocytes.
    b. basophils, eosinophils, and lymphocytes.
    c. eosinophils, neutrophils, and lymphocytes.
    d. basophils, eosinophils, and neutrophils.
    e. lymphocytes, neutrophils, and basophils.

8. All of the following statements are true EXCEPT:
    a. Xenobiotics can greatly slow down the proliferation of neutrophils and monocytes, increasing the risk of infection.
    b. Ethanol and cortisol decrease phagocytosis and microbe ingestion by the immune system.
    c. Agranulocytosis is predictable and can be caused by exposure to a number of environmental toxins.
    d. Heroin and methadone abusers have reduced ability to kill microorganisms due to drug-induced reduction in superoxide production.
    e. Toxic neutropenia may be mediated by the immune system.

9. Leukemias:
    a. are often due to cytogenic abnormalities, particularly damage to or loss of chromosomes 8 and 11.
    b. are rarely caused by agents used in cancer chemotherapy.
    c. originate in circulating blood cells.
    d. are characterized as "acute" if their effects are short-lived and severe.
    e. have long been associated with exposure to x-ray radiation.

10. Regarding platelets and thrombocytopenia, which of the following statements is FALSE?
    a. Platelets can be removed from the circulation through a hapten-mediated pathway that is induced by drugs or chemicals.
    b. Cortisol decreases platelet activity by inhibiting thromboxane prostaglandin synthesis.
    c. Toxins can induce a change in a platelet membrane glycoprotein, leading to recognition and removal of the platelet by phagocytes.
    d. Heparin administration can result in platelet aggregation and cause thrombocytopenia.
    e. Thrombotic thrombocytopenic purpura is most commonly caused by infectious disease, but can also be associated with administration of pharmacologic agents.

Toxic Responses of the Immune System

Barbara L.F. Kaplan, Courtney E.W. Sulentic,
Michael P. Holsapple, and Norbert E. Kaminski

- Immunity is a series of delicately balanced, complex, multicellular, and physiologic mechanisms that allow an individual to distinguish foreign material from "self" and to neutralize and/or eliminate that foreign matter.
- Innate immunity, which eliminates most potential pathogens before significant infection occurs, includes physical and biochemical barriers both inside and outside of the body as well as immune cells designed for specific responses.
- Acquired immunity involves producing a specific immune response to each infectious agent (*specificity*) and remembering that agent so as to mount a faster response to a future infection by the same agent (*memory*).
- Autoimmunity occurs when the reactions of the immune system are directed against the body's own tissues, resulting in tissue damage and disease.
- Hypersensitivity reactions require prior exposure leading to sensitization in order to elicit a reaction on subsequent challenge.
- Xenobiotics that alter the immune system can upset the balance between immune recognition and destruction of foreign invaders and the proliferation of these microbes and/or cancer cells.

Immunity is a homeostatic process, a series of delicately balanced, complex, multicellular, and physiologic mechanisms that allow an individual to distinguish foreign material from "self" and to neutralize and/or eliminate the foreign matter. Decreased immunocompetence (immunosuppression) may result in repeated, more severe, or prolonged infections as well as the development of cancer. Immunoenhancement may lead to immune-mediated diseases such as hypersensitivity responses, and if some integral bodily tissue is not identified as self, an autoimmune disease may be the end result.

THE IMMUNE SYSTEM

The immune system comprises numerous lymphoid organs and different cellular populations with a variety of functions. The bone marrow and the thymus support the production of mature T and B lymphocytes and myeloid cells, such as macrophages and polymorphonuclear cells (PMN), and are referred to as primary lymphoid organs.

Within the bone marrow, the cells of the immune system developmentally "commit" to either the lymphoid or myeloid lineages. Cells of the lymphoid lineage make a further commitment to become either T cells or B cells. T-cell precursors are programmed to leave the bone marrow and migrate to the thymus, where they differentiate further.

Mature naive or virgin lymphocytes (those T and B cells that have never undergone antigenic stimulation) are first brought into contact with exogenously derived antigens within the spleen and lymph nodes, otherwise known as the secondary lymphoid organs.

Lymphoid tissues associated with the skin and the mucosal lamina propria of the gut, respiratory tract, and genitourinary tract can be classified as tertiary lymphoid tissues. Tertiary lymphoid tissues are primarily effector sites where memory and effector cells exert immunologic and immunoregulatory functions.

Antigen Recognition

Immunity—Mammalian immunity can be classified into two functional divisions: innate immunity and acquired (adaptive) immunity. Innate immunity is a nonspecific, first-line defense response with no associated immunologic memory. The innate immune response to a foreign organism is the same for a secondary or tertiary exposure as it is for the primary exposure. Acquired immunity is characterized by both specificity and memory, resulting in a much greater immune response on secondary challenge.

Antigen—The primary determinant in either type of immune response is the ability of the immune system components to recognize self versus non-self. A broad definition of non-self is anything other than that encoded in one's own germline genome, which includes foreign DNA, RNA, protein, carbohydrates, and even mutated self-proteins. A non-self substance that can be recognized by the immune system is called an antigen, immunogen, or allergen. Antigens are usually (but not absolutely) biological molecules that can be cleaved and rearranged for presentation to other immune cells. Generally, antigens are at least 10 kDa in size. Smaller antigens are termed "haptens" and must be conjugated with carrier molecules (larger antigens) in order to elicit a specific response.

Antibody—Antibodies are produced by B cells and are functionally defined both by the antigen with which they react and their subtype, termed "isotypes" (e.g., IgM, IgG, IgE, IgD, and IgA). Antibodies of a known specificity are labeled as such, e.g., an IgM antibody against sheep red blood cells (sRBCs) is called an anti-sRBC IgM. Antibodies of unknown specificity are referred to as immunoglobulin (Ig) until they can be defined by their specific antigen.

The basic components of an Ig are the same regardless of isotype, namely, heavy chains, light chains, constant regions (Fc),

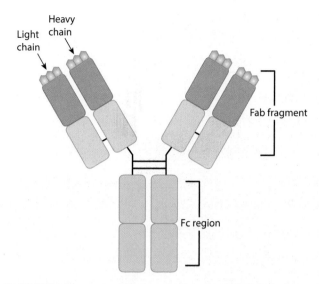

FIGURE 12-1 Ig structure. Igs are composed of two heavy chains and two light chains, which are connected by disulfide bonds. Orange areas are variable regions and green areas at top are antigen recognition regions.

and variable regions (Fab). The general structure of antibodies are also conserved across isotypes (Figure 12–1). There are two genes coding for light chains (V and J) and three genes coding for heavy chains (V, D, and J). Isotype is determined by which Fc of the heavy chain is transcribed and translated (heavy chain genes μ, γ, ε, δ, or α encode for the IgM, IgG, IgE, IgD, or IgA heavy chain proteins, respectively).

The immune system generates antibodies to thousands of antigens with which the host may or may not ever contact. During this process called somatic recombination, V and J segments for light chains as well as V, D, and J segments for heavy chains are combined, within the B cell, to form an Ig. The Fab regions of both the heavy and light chains determine antibody specificity and interact directly with antigen. In addition to isotype determination, the Fc region is also responsible for the various effector functions, such as complement activation (e.g., IgM and some subclasses of IgG) and phagocyte binding (via Fc receptors).

Antibodies possess several functions: (1) opsonization, which is coating of a pathogen with antibody to enhance Fc receptor-mediated endocytosis by phagocytic cells; (2) initiation of the classic pathway of complement-mediated lysis; (3) neutralization of viral infection by binding to viral particles and preventing further infection; and (4) enhancement of the specificity of effectors of cell-mediated immunity (CMI) by binding to specific antigens on target cells, which are then recognized and eliminated by effector cells such as natural killer (NK) cells or cytotoxic T lymphocytes (CTLs).

Complement—The complement system is a series of about 30 serum proteins whose primary functions are the destruction of membranes of infectious agents, opsonization to facilitate phagocytosis, and the promotion of an inflammatory response (see the "Inflammation" section). Complement activation occurs with each component sequentially acting on others, in

a manner similar to the blood-clotting cascade (Figure 12–2). The final components that can enter the membrane and disrupt its integrity are termed the membrane attack complex (MAC). Three pathways have been identified in the activation of the complement cascade, the classical pathway (antibody:antigen-dependent), the alternative pathway (spontaneous activation of C3), and the mannin-binding lectin pathway (a hepatogenic molecule that binds to pathogens).

Antigen Processing—To elicit an acquired immune response to a particular antigen, that antigen must be taken up and processed by accessory cells for presentation to lymphocytes. Accessory cells that perform this function are termed antigen-presenting cells (APCs) and include macrophages, B cells, and dendritic cells (DCs). Of these, the most proficient APC is the DC. There are several subtypes of DC, including plasmacytoid DCs (pDCs), conventional DCs (cDCs), specialized DCs in the skin called Langerhans cells, and follicular DCs in germinal centers within secondary lymphoid organs.

In most tissues, DCs are in an immature state in which they capture antigens through phagocytosis, pinocytosis, or receptor-mediated endocytosis. DCs then process the antigen (intracellular denaturation and catabolism) and display fragments of it on the extracellular side of their cell membrane through direct association with special cell surface molecules (major histocompatibility complex [MHC] classes MHCI and MHCII).

Antigen presentation of the kind discussed here primarily occurs via MHCII (Figure 12–3), although certain types of antigens are processed and presented via MHCI. The pathway of presentation between these two classes have similarities, but the major differences between the MHCI and MHCII pathways are (1) antigens processed and presented via MHCI are not limited to professional APC; (2) all nucleated cells express MHCI; (3) the mechanisms by which the antigen is processed and loaded onto MHCI are slightly different than MHCII; (4) the MHCI antigenic peptides are usually smaller, often 8 to 10 amino acids in length; (5) the MHCI antigens to be processed are usually aberrantly expressed proteins, such as viral-associated proteins or mutated proteins; (6) MHCI facilitates antigen presentation to CD8+ T cells, whereas MHCII facilitates antigen presentation to CD4+ T cells. MHCI antigen processing and presentation is the major pathway by which virally infected cells are detected and killed by the acquired immune system.

Regardless of the MHC utilized to present antigens to lymphocytes, T cells are able to recognize antigen in the context of MHC with their T-cell receptor (TCR). Similar to Ig, the ability of T cells to specifically recognize thousands of antigens is due to somatic recombination. All TCRs are composed of two different subunits, each encoded from a distinct gene (most abundant T-cell population expresses αβ, but γδ also exist). All TCR subunits are made up of constant and variable regions. For α subunits, two separate gene segments (V and J) are combined to form the variable region, which is then joined to one constant region. For β subunits, three separate gene segments (V, D, and J) are combined to form the variable region, which

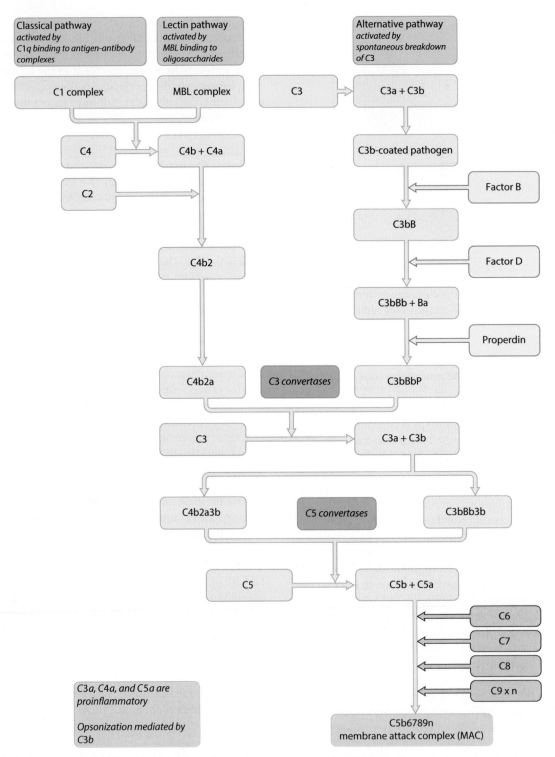

FIGURE 12–2 **The complement cascade.** The complement cascade can be activated in three different ways. Cytolysis occurs via generation of the MAC. Various complement proteins generated along the pathway are either pro-inflammatory mediators (C3a, C5a) or result in opsonization (C3b).

is then joined to one of the two constant regions. Similar to the Ig genes, there are several light chain V and J genes, and several heavy chain V, D, and J genes.

With regard to T and B cells, key events that occur following antigen encounter are (1) specific antigen recognition either in the context of MHCI or MHCII for T cells or through the Ig receptor for B cells, (2) cellular activation and initiation of intracellular signaling cascades that contribute to production and release of cytokines and other cellular mediators, (3) clonal expansion (proliferation) of antigen-specific cells, and (4) differentiation of antigen-stimulated lymphocytes into effector and memory cells.

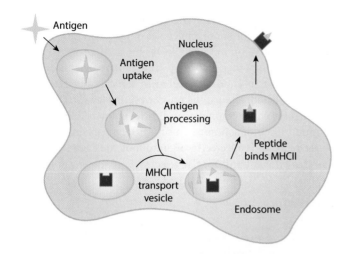

FIGURE 12–3 **Antigen processing by the MHCII pathway.** Antigen is engulfed by an APC (DC, macrophage, or B cell), degraded, and loaded onto MHCII. The MHCII–peptide complex is then expressed on the surface of the APC for presentation to CD4+ Th cells.

Innate Immunity

Innate immunity acts as a first line of defense against infectious agents, eliminating most potential pathogens before significant infection occurs. It includes physical and biochemical barriers both inside and outside of the body as well as immune cells designed for specific responses. There is no immunologic memory associated with innate immunity.

Externally, the skin provides an effective barrier, as most organisms cannot penetrate intact skin. Most infectious agents enter the body through the respiratory system, gut, or genitourinary tract. Innate defenses present to combat infection from pathogens entering through the respiratory system include mucus secreted along the nasopharynx, the presence of lysozyme in most secretions, and cilia lining the trachea and main bronchi. In addition, reflexes such as coughing, sneezing, and elevation in body temperature are also a part of innate immunity. Pathogens that enter the body via the digestive tract are met with severe changes in pH (acidic) within the stomach and a host of microorganisms living in the intestines.

Cellular Components: Neutrophils, Macrophages, Natural Killer Cells, NKT, and γδ T Cells—Neutrophils (also known as polymorphonuclear cells [PMNs]) are phagocytic cells that develop from the myeloid lineage of HSCs. They enter the bloodstream where they circulate for about 10 h, after which they enter tissues and perform effector functions for one or two days. Neutrophils are a primary line of defense because of their ability to pass between the endothelial cells of blood vessels (termed extravasation) and access peripheral tissues. They are excellent phagocytic cells and can eliminate most microorganisms through the release of various reactive oxygen species (ROS), such as superoxide, singlet oxygen, ozone, hydrogen peroxide, and hydroxyl radicals. Their phagocytic activity is greatly enhanced by the presence of complement and antibody

deposited on the surface of the foreign target. They are also important in the induction of an inflammatory response.

Macrophages are terminally differentiated monocytes that are developed from the myeloid lineage of HSCs. Upon exiting the bone marrow, monocytes circulate within the bloodstream for about one day. At that time, they begin to distribute to the various tissues where they can then differentiate into macrophage subsets. Tissue-specific macrophages include Kupffer cells (liver), alveolar macrophages (lung), microglial cells (CNS), and peritoneal and splenic macrophages. Macrophages can be classified as classically activated macrophages (M1), which are pro-inflammatory and participate in antigen presentation, or alternatively activated macrophages (M2), which do not present antigen well, but are efficient in apoptotic cell removal. Based on this classification, M1 macrophages are also APCs.

Like other immune cells, natural killer (NK) cells are derived from a HSC. The two major functions of NK cells are cytokine (soluble protein messenger) production and cytolysis. NK cells are the predominant producer of the cytokine, IFN-γ, which promotes DC maturation. In this way, NK cells serve as a bridge between innate and adaptive immunity. NK cells also mediate both antibody-independent and antibody-dependent cellular cytotoxicity (ADCC) using a variety of mechanisms, including perforin and granzyme, Fas L, TRAIL, and TNF-α. Antigen-dependent cell-mediated cytotoxicity occurs via the FcγRIIIA, which is present on most NK cell subsets. NKT cells are one such subset of NK cells that express both NK- and T-cell markers, which allows the NKT cell to present self and exogenous antigenic glycolipids.

Another cell type that has recently been shown to facilitate the innate-adaptive immunity bridge is the γδ T cell. These cells migrate predominantly to "exposed" tissues, including skin, lung, gut, and reproductive organs, and are also expressed highly in the liver. In part through the expression of TLRs, γδ T cells can acquire effector functions similar to those of NK cells. There is also a subpopulation of B cells that also bridge innate and adaptive immunity. Unlike the conventional B-2 cells, B-1 cells predominate in embryonic life and are later found mostly in the peritoneal and pleural cavities. B-1 cells are self-renewing and spontaneously produce polyspecific IgM antibodies (i.e., natural antibodies) independent of T-cell help.

Historically, innate immunity was defined as nonspecific. It is now clear that innate cells express receptors that respond to soluble components (e.g., Fc or complement receptors) or to certain antigenic motifs. Pattern recognition receptors are a family of receptors that recognize pathogen-derived molecules or cell-derived molecules produced in response to cellular stress ("danger" molecules). Receptors that recognize pathogen-associated molecular patterns (PAMPs) are toll-like receptors (TLRs); receptors that recognize danger-associated molecular patterns (DAMPs) include NOD-like receptors (NLR) and RIG-like receptors (RLR). TLRs are expressed both extracellularly and intracellularly in endosomes, which confers the ability to respond to a variety of pathogenic components, such as bacterial cell wall lipids, single- and double-stranded nucleic acids, or fungal and parasitic products. Functional consequences of TLR engagement on cells include expression of adhesion molecules, chemokines, or cytokines to stimulate T- or B-cell differentiation, enhance phagocytosis, or facilitate maturation of DCs.

Soluble Factors—A common effector mechanism for many immune cells, is cytokine, chemokine, or interferon (IFN) production. The primary function of cytokines, chemokines, and IFNs include cellular activation, initiation or termination of intracellular signaling events, proliferation, differentiation, migration, trafficking, or effector functions (Table 12–1). Although some of these molecules might be constitutively expressed, most are inducible in response to antigens, cellular stressors, or other cytokines. Thus, many cytokines, chemokines, and IFNs are not stored in the cell, but rather are tightly regulated, often at the transcriptional level, so that they are quickly generated on demand. Also, many cytokines share common receptor subunits. This means if a particular subunit of one receptor is affected by an immunotoxic agent, all others that share this subunit are also affected.

TABLE 12–1 Cytokines: sources and functions in immune regulation.

Cytokine	Source	Physiologic Actions
IL-1	Macrophages Epithelial cells	Activation and proliferation of T cells Pro-inflammatory Induces fever and acute-phase proteins Induces synthesis of pro-inflammatory cytokines
IL-2	T cells	Primary T-cell growth factor Growth factor for B and NK cells
IL-4	Th2 cells Mast cells	Proliferation of activated T cells and B cells B-cell differentiation and IgE isotype switching functions Antagonizes IFN-γ Inhibits Th1 responses
IL-5	Th2 cells Mast cells	Proliferation and differentiation of eosinophils
IL-6	Macrophages Th2 cells B cells Endothelial cells	Enhances B-cell differentiation and immunoglobulin secretion Induction of acute-phase proteins by liver Pro-inflammatory Proliferation of T cells and increased IL-2 receptor expression Synergizes with IL-4 to induce secretion of IgE
IL-10	Tregs Bregs	Inhibits T-cell and macrophage responses
IL-12	DCs Macrophages	Activates BK cells Induces TH1 responses
IL-13	Th2 cells	Stimulates B-cell growth Inhibits Th1 responses
IL-17	Th17 cells NK cells $\gamma\delta$ T cells Neutrophils	Pro-inflammatory Inhibits Tregs
Interferon-α/β (IFN-α/β) (type 1 IFN)	Leukocytes DCs Fibroblasts	Induction of MHC class I expression Antiviral activity Stimulation of NK cells
Interferon-γ (IFN-γ)	T cells NK cells	Induction of MHCI and MHCII Activates macrophages
Transforming growth factor-β (TGF-β)	Macrophages Megakaryocytes T cells	Enhances monocyte/macrophage chemotaxis Enhances wound healing: angiogenesis, fibroblast proliferation, deposition of extracellular matrix Inhibits T- and B-cell proliferation Inhibits antibody secretion Primary inducer of isotype switch to IgA
GM-CSF	T cells Macrophages Endothelial cells Fibroblasts	Stimulates growth and differentiation of monocytes and granulocytes

Other soluble components of innate immunity include the complement cascade (discussed earlier), acute-phase proteins, granzyme and perforin, and various cytokines, chemokines and IFNs. Complement is important in innate immunity because of its activation through the mannin-binding lectin pathway. Furthermore, C3a and C5a, which are chemokines generated during the cascade, recruit phagocytic cells to the site of complement activation. Acute-phase proteins, such as serum amyloid A, serum amyloid P, and C-reactive protein, participate in an acute-phase response to infection by binding bacteria and facilitating complement activation. Granzyme and perforin work in conjunction, with perforin disrupting the target cell membrane, allowing granzyme to enter and mediate cell lysis by several mechanisms.

Acquired (Adaptive) Immunity

If the primary defenses against infection (innate immunity) are breached, the acquired arm of the immune system is activated and produces a specific immune response to each infectious agent. This branch of immunity can protect the host from future infection by the same agent. Two key features that distinguish acquired immunity are specificity and memory. Acquired immunity may be further subdivided into humoral and cell-mediated immunity (CMI). Humoral immunity is directly dependent on the production of antigen-specific antibody by B cells and involves the coordinated interaction of APCs, T cells, and B cells. CMI is that part of the acquired immune system in which effector cells, such as phagocytic cells, helper T cells (Th cells), T-regulatory cells (Tregs), APCs, CTLs, or T memory cells, play the critical role(s) without antibody involvement.

Cellular Components: APCs, B Cells, and T Cells—
APCs, which have been discussed previously in the "Antigen Processing" section, include professional APCs such as B cells, macrophages, and DCs. Although all cells may act as APCs with internal antigen processing through the MHCI pathway, what distinguishes a professional APC from the others is the ability to internalize external antigens and process them through the MHCII pathway for presentation to T cells.

Besides serving as APCs, B lymphocytes are also the effector cells of humoral immunity, producing a number of Ig isotypes with varying specificities and affinities. Upon antigen binding to surface Ig (part of the B-cell receptor [BCR]), the mature B cell becomes activated and, after proliferation, undergoes differentiation into either a memory B cell or an antibody-forming cell ([AFC]; also known as a plaque-forming cell [PFC]) that actively secretes antigen-specific antibody.

T-cell precursors migrate from the bone marrow to the thymus where, in a manner analogous to B cells, they begin to rearrange their TCRs. These immature cells then undergo positive and negative selection to (1) eliminate cells that do not produce a functional TCR or produce TCRs with no affinity for self-MHC (positive selection) or (2) eliminate cells that strongly bind MHC plus self-peptide (negative selection).

This rigorous selection process produces T cells that can recognize MHC plus foreign peptides and eliminates autoreactive T cells.

Additionally, expression of CD4 or CD8 will determine to which MHC class the αβ TCR will bind. CD4 will facilitate binding to MHCII expressed on APCs; T cells expressing CD4 (helper T cells, Th) help activate other cells of the adaptive immune response. CD8 will facilitate binding to MHCI, which is expressed on all nucleated cells; generally, T cells expressing CD8 mediate cell killing (CTL). The γδ T cells do not express CD4 or CD8 and therefore do not interact with MHC and do not undergo positive or negative selection. Since γδ T cells are not negatively selected for autoreactivity, these cells may be associated with the development of hypersensitivity and autoimmunity (see subsequent sections).

Mature T cells are found in the lymph nodes, spleen, and peripheral blood. Upon binding of the TCR to MHC plus antigen, the mature T cell becomes activated and, after proliferation, undergoes differentiation into either an effector cell or a memory T cell. There are many subsets of effector Th cells and two subsets, Th1 and Th2, dictate whether CMI or humoral immunity will predominate, respectively. Th1 cells predominantly express IL-2, IFN-γ, and lymphotoxin, which promote CMI and humoral defense against intracellular invaders. Th2 cells predominantly express IL-3, IL-4, IL-5, IL-6, IL-10, and IL-13, which promote humoral defense against extracellular invaders. Although the two populations are not mutually exclusive, they do negatively regulate each other, such that a strong Th1 response suppresses a Th2 response and vice versa.

The ability of APCs, B cells, and T cells to communicate with each other is dependent on a variety of receptor–ligand interactions between cell types. These interactions also help dictate the type of immune response (i.e., humoral versus CMI) and the magnitude of the immune response. The duration and extent of an acquired immune response is also controlled by specialized regulatory cells found in both the T-cell and B-cell lineages.

For the T-cell lineage, there is a small population of CD4+ cells that develop into T-regulatory cells (Tregs), which help to control various immune responses, including those directed against self. The mechanisms by which Tregs suppress immune responses involve direct Treg-cell contact. Several subsets of regulatory B cells have already been identified, but more are being discovered recently. These cells generally play a suppressive role in hypersensitivity and autoimmune diseases. The regulatory T- and B-cell subsets also appear to reciprocally activate or suppress each other and may cooperatively control immune responses.

Humoral and Cell-mediated Immunity—
Humoral immunity is that part of the acquired immune system in which antibody is involved, and CMI is that part of the immune system in which various effector cells perform a wide variety of functions to eliminate invaders. These two branches are often coordinated, as depicted in Figure 12–4.

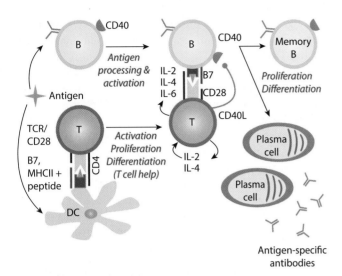

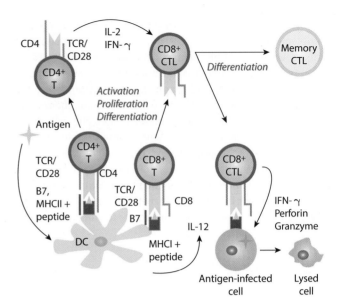

FIGURE 12–4 Cellular interactions in the humoral immune response. Antigen is engulfed by an APC (usually DC) and the antigenic peptide is presented to CD4⁺ T cells in the context of MHCII. CD4⁺ T cells then become activated, proliferate, and differentiate into Th cells, which release cytokines to help B cells that had also encountered the same antigen. B cells then become activated, proliferate, and differentiate into memory B cells or antigen-producing plasma cells.

FIGURE 12–5 Cellular interactions in the CTL response. Antigen is engulfed by an APC (usually DC) and the antigenic peptide is presented to CD4⁺ and CD8⁺ T cells in the context of MHCII and I, respectively. CD4⁺ T cells then become activated, proliferate, and differentiate into Th cells, which release cytokines to help CD8⁺ T cells that had also encountered the same antigen. Especially in the presence of IL-12 produced by the DC, CD8⁺ T cells become activated, proliferate, and differentiate into CTL that can kill other antigen-infected cells.

In general, B cells produce antibodies specific to an antigen, which may act to opsonize or neutralize the invader, or the antibodies act to recruit other factors, such as the complement cascade. The production of antigen-specific IgM requires 3 to 5 days after the primary (initial) exposure to antigen. Upon secondary antigenic challenge, the B cells undergo isotype switching, producing primarily IgG antibody, which is of higher affinity for the activating antigen. In addition, there is a higher serum antibody titer associated with a secondary antibody response.

CMI functions include delayed-type hypersensitivity (DTH) and cell-mediated cytotoxicity. Cell-mediated cytotoxicity responses may occur in numerous ways: (1) MHC-dependent recognition of specific antigens (such as viral particles or tumor proteins) by CTL (Figure 12–5); (2) indirect antigen-specific recognition by the binding of Fc receptors on NK cells to antibodies coating target cells; and (3) receptor-mediated recognition of complement-coated foreign targets by macrophages.

In cell-mediated cytotoxicity, the CTL or NK effector cell binds in a specific manner to the target cell. The majority of CTLs express CD8 and recognize either foreign MHCI on the surface of allogeneic cells or antigen in association with self-MHCI (e.g., viral particles). Once the CTL or NK cells interact with the target cell, the effector cell releases granules containing perforin and other enzymes. This degranulation damages the target cell, after which the effector cell can release and attack other target cells In addition, CTLs induce the target to undergo apoptosis through activation of the Fas and cytotoxic cytokine (i.e., TNF and lymphotoxin) pathways.

Inflammation

Inflammation refers to a complex reaction to injury, irritation, or foreign invaders characterized by pain, swelling, redness, and heat. Inflammation involves various stages, including release of chemotactic factors following the insult, increased blood flow, increased capillary permeability allowing for cellular infiltration, followed by either an acute resolution of tissue damage or persistence of the response that might contribute to fibrosis or subsequent organ failure. It is important to emphasize that while inflammation is a natural reaction to repair tissue damage or attack foreign invaders, the process often results in destruction of adjacent cells and/or tissues. Thus, there is overwhelming evidence that inflammation plays a critical role in many diseases, including asthma, multiple sclerosis, cardiovascular disease, Alzheimer's disease, bowel disorders, and cancer. In addition, inflammation exacerbates idiosyncratic reactions to drugs and other chemicals.

Cellular Components: Macrophages, Neutrophils, and T Cells—Many of the cellular components described in the sections above are critical to initiation and maintenance of an inflammatory response. Major cellular contributors to an inflammatory response are macrophages, neutrophils, and T cells. Neutrophils are often the first, and most numerous, responders to sites of insult. In response to either host- or pathogen-derived signals, neutrophils secrete chemotactic factors to recruit other pro-inflammatory cells, such as macrophages, to the area.

Macrophages can be activated by a variety of mechanisms at the site of insult, such as activation via toll-like receptor, pro-inflammatory cytokines, or recognition of opsonized particles by Fc receptors or complement receptors. Macrophages and neutrophils also induce apoptosis of cells in the insult area through the release of nitric oxide and other ROS, resulting in disruption of extracellular structures that compromise tissue structure and function. Both neutrophils and macrophages are phagocytic cells and can contribute to clearing of apoptotic cells.

Later in the inflammatory response, T cells are critical for generating an adaptive immune response. T cells are attracted to the insult area by adhesion molecules and integrins, and are activated in response to antigen presented in the context of MHC, often by a DC. Depending on the signals that the T cell receives from the cytokine milieu, distinct subpopulations of T cells are induced.

Immune-mediated Disease

While the primary purpose of the immune system is to preserve the integrity of the individual from disease states, situations arise in which the individual's immune system responds in a matter producing tissue damage, resulting in self-induced disease. These disease states fall into two categories: (1) hypersensitivity, or allergy, and (2) autoimmunity.

Hypersensitivity

Classification of Hypersensitivity Reactions—There are four types of hypersensitivity reactions as classified by Coombs and Gell. One characteristic common to all four types of hypersensitivity reactions is the necessity of prior exposure leading to sensitization in order to elicit a reaction upon subsequent challenge. In the case of types I, II, and III, prior exposure to antigen leads to the production of allergen-specific antibodies (IgE, IgM, or IgG) and, in the case of type IV, the generation of allergen-specific memory T cells. Figure 12–6 illustrates the mechanisms of hypersensitivity reactions.

Type I (Immediate or IgE-mediated Hypersensitivity): Using penicillin as an example, Figure 12–7 depicts the major events involved in a type I hypersensitivity reaction (what most people think of as "allergy" and is clinically referred to as "atopy"). Sensitization occurs as the result of dermal exposure to antigens or by exposure to antigens through the respiratory or gastrointestinal tract. Most people would mount an IgM, IgG, or IgA immune response to these antigens and clear them without causing any allergic symptoms. It is unclear why these antigens become allergens in certain individuals who respond by mounting an IgE immune response instead, but appears to involve genetic and/or environmental determinants and likely some type of triggering event (e.g., acute pathogen exposure and emotional stress).

Once produced, soluble IgE not only binds to local tissue mast cells, but also enters the circulation, where it binds to circulating mast cells, basophils, and tissue mast cells at distant sites. Once an individual is sensitized, reexposure to the antigen

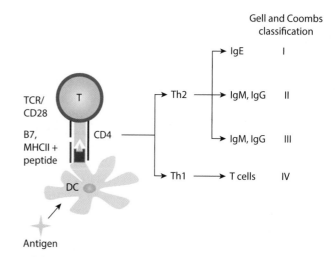

FIGURE 12–6 Overview of classification of hypersensitivity reactions. Hypersensitivity reactions are mediated via T cells and antibody production.

results in binding to IgE on local mast cells and degranulation with the release of preformed mediators and cytokines which recruit and activate circulating eosinophils, basophils, macrophages, and neutrophils leading to the synthesis and release of more cytokines and of leukotrienes and thromboxanes. These mediators promote vasodilation, bronchial constriction, and inflammation. Clinical manifestations can vary from urticarial skin reactions (wheals and flares) to signs of hay fever, including rhinitis and conjunctivitis, to more serious diseases, such as asthma and potentially life-threatening anaphylaxis.

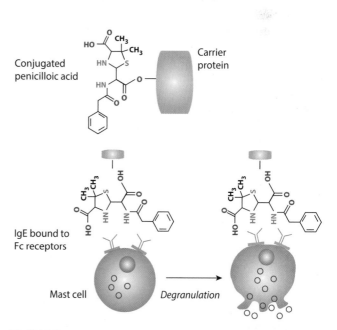

FIGURE 12–7 Type I hypersensitivity reaction. Metabolized penicillin is a hapten that conjugates with a protein. The conjugated hapten cross-links IgE antibodies on mast cells. IgE cross-linking causes mast-cell degranulation and releasing histamine and other pro-inflammatory mediators.

These responses may begin within minutes of reexposure to the offending antigen; therefore, type I hypersensitivity is often referred to as immediate hypersensitivity.

Type II (Antibody-dependent Cytotoxic Hypersensitivity): Type II hypersensitivity is IgG- or IgM-mediated. The antibody response may be mediated by a foreign antigen attached to the surface of a cell or tissue. Conversely, an antibody response could be mediated by an autoantibody due to a breakdown in tolerance and the resulting response would be part of an autoimmune disease (e.g., autoimmune hemolytic anemias and Goodpasture's syndrome). Figure 12–8 shows the mechanisms of action for complement-independent and complement-dependent cytotoxic reactions. Tissue damage may result from the direct action of cytotoxic cells, such as macrophages, neutrophils, or eosinophils, linked through the Fc receptor to antibody-coated target cells (complement-independent) or by antibody-induced activation of the classic complement pathway.

Type III (Immune Complex-mediated Hypersensitivity): Type III hypersensitivity reactions also involve IgG or IgM. The distinguishing feature of type III is that, unlike type II, in which Ig production is against specific cellular or tissue-associated antigen, Ig production is against soluble antigen in the serum (Figure 12–9). This allows for the formation of circulating immune complexes composed of a lattice of antigen and Ig, which may result in widely distributed tissue damage in areas where immune complexes are deposited. The most common location is the vascular endothelium in the lung, joints, and kidneys. The skin and circulatory systems may also be involved. Pathology results from the inflammatory response initiated by the activation of complement. Macrophages, neutrophils, and platelets attracted to the deposition site contribute to the tissue damage. As with type II hypersensitivity, responses similar to type III hypersensitivity can be induced in autoimmune diseases due to autoantibodies directed against soluble antigens such as double-stranded DNA or small nuclear proteins as seen with systemic lupus erythematosus (SLE).

Autoimmunity—Autoimmune disease occurs when the reactions of the immune system are directed against the body's own tissues and is characterized by a genetic susceptibility. These diseases can be either tissue-specific or nonspecific, and the targets from the perspective of the primary sites of tissue damage in autoimmune disease are many and varied. Both humoral immunity and CMI can be involved as effector mechanisms in causing the damage in autoimmune conditions.

Although the resulting pathology may be the same for autoimmune reactions and hypersensitivity, mechanisms of true autoimmune disease are distinguished from hypersensitivity. In cases of autoimmunity, self-antigens are the target, and in the case of chemical-induced autoimmunity, the disease state is induced by a modification of host tissues or immune cells by the chemical and not the chemical acting as an antigen/hapten as in hypersensitivity reactions.

Mechanisms of Autoimmunity—The rearrangement and recombination of the genes that comprise Ig and TCR result

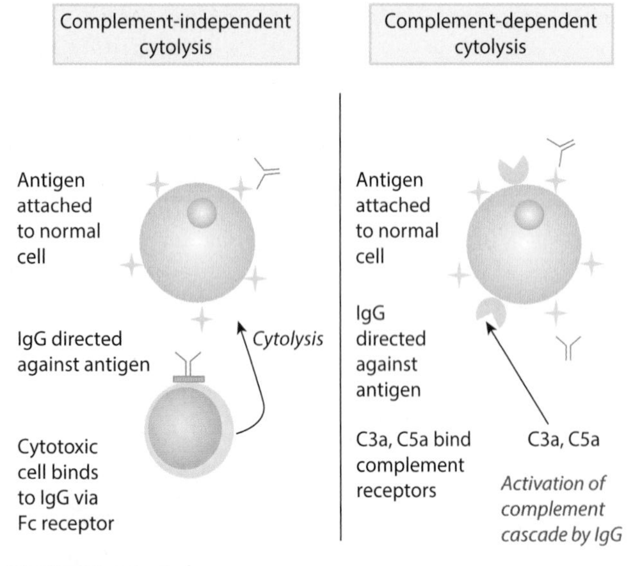

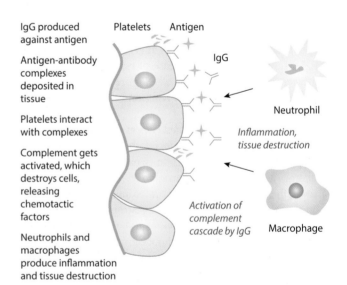

FIGURE 12–8 **Type II hypersensitivity reactions.** In complement-independent cytolysis, antigen becomes attached to a normal cell, which can be recognized by IgG. A cell capable of cytolysis (CTL, NK cell) binds to IgG via its Fc receptor and kills the antigen-coated cell. In complement-dependent cytolysis, antigen becomes attached to a normal cell, which can be recognized by IgG. Complement gets activated by the classical pathway (antigen–antibody complexes) and C3a and C5a bind complement receptors.

FIGURE 12–9 **Type III hypersensitivity reactions.** IgG is produced against an antigen and antigen–antibody complexes form, which can become deposited in tissue. Complement gets activated by the classical pathway (antigen–antibody complexes), and platelets also interact with complexes. Following complement-mediated cytolysis, released chemotactic factors attract neutrophils and macrophages, causing additional inflammation and tissue damage.

in tremendous diversity in the potential antigen recognition of B cells and T cells, respectively. Ideally, during development those lymphocytes recognizing self-antigens will largely be deleted by negative selection as central tolerance is established. Autoreactive clones that escape central tolerance and migrate to the periphery are normally controlled by peripheral tolerance mediated by various mechanisms that ultimately induce anergy or clonal deletion. For autoimmune disease to occur, an autoreactive clone must escape central tolerance, pass into the periphery, and bind with specificity to its self-antigen, then mechanisms of peripheral tolerance must fail and the autoreactive clone must induce a detrimental immunological response.

Autoimmunity is multifaceted and has been associated with several mechanisms primarily related to insufficient peripheral tolerance, while defects in central tolerance are rarely encountered. Several mechanisms have been associated with the breakdown of peripheral tolerance and prime events for the onset of autoimmune disease. These mechanisms include inflammation; molecular mimicry by pathogen antigens; inherent defects in T or B cells including regulatory subsets, APCs, cytokines, or complement; and epitope spreading.

Effector mechanisms in autoimmune disease can be the same as those described earlier for types II and III hypersensitivity or, in the case of pathology associated with solid tissues, they may involve CD8$^+$ cytotoxic T lymphocytes. Tissue damage associated with CTL may be the result of direct cell membrane damage and lysis, or the result of cytokines produced and released by the T cell. TNF-β has the ability to kill susceptible cells, and IFN-γ may increase the expression of MHCI on cell surfaces, making them more susceptible to CD8$^+$ cells. Cytokines may also be chemotactic for macrophages, which can cause tissue damage directly or indirectly through the release of pro-inflammatory cytokines. As is the case with hypersensitivity reactions, autoimmune disease is often the result of more than one mechanism working simultaneously.

Developmental Immunology

A sequential series of carefully timed and coordinated developmental events, beginning early in embryonic/fetal life and continuing through the early postnatal period, is required to establish a functional immune system in all mammals. The immune system develops initially from a population of pluripotent HSCs that gives rise to all circulating blood cell lineages, including cells of the immune system. The bone marrow and thymus are the primary sites of lymphopoiesis and appear to be unique in providing the microenvironment factors necessary for the development of functionally competent immune cells.

Immune system development does not cease at birth, but continues to develop until 5 to 12 years of age in humans. After birth, immunocompetent cells continue to be produced from proliferating progenitor cells in the bone marrow and thymus. These cells subsequently migrate via the blood to the secondary immune organs: spleen, lymph nodes, and mucosal lymphoid tissues. The onset of functional immune competence

depends on the specific parameter being measured, and varies across species with striking differences noted between rodents and humans.

Exposure to specific antigens during the perinatal period results in a rapidly expanding accumulation of lymphocyte specificities in the pool of memory cells in secondary lymphoid tissues. As thymic function wanes and thymocytes are no longer produced in that tissue, it is this pool of memory B and T cells that maintains immune competence for the life of the individual. Senescence of immunity is associated with reductions in both innate and acquired immune responses to antigens during the last quartile of life. This failure of the immune response is due, in part, to a continual reduction in the production of newly formed cells, and to the decreased survival of long-lived memory cells in lymphoid tissues.

One feature of the developing immune system that clearly distinguishes it from the mature immune system, especially during gestation, is the role played by organogenesis. Defects in the development of the immune system due to heritable changes in the lymphoid elements have provided clinical and experimental examples of the devastating consequences of impaired immune development. Therefore, the effects of chemicals on the genesis of critical immune organs in the developing fetus may be more important than effects on these tissues after having been populated by hematopoietic and lymphoid cells. Interestingly, immune organs, such as the thymus, spleen, and/ or bone marrow, are not typically assessed in routine developmental and reproductive toxicology studies.

Neuroendocrine Immunology

Cytokines, neuropeptides, neurotransmitters, and hormones (as well as their receptors) are an integral and interregulated part of the central nervous system, the endocrine system, and the immune system. Because receptors for neuropeptides, neurotransmitters, and hormones are present on lymphoid cells, some chemicals may exert their immunomodulatory effects indirectly on the immune system by modulating the activity of the nervous or endocrine systems. In addition, immune cells are capable of secreting peptide hormones and neurotransmitters, which can have autocrine (immune system) and paracrine (endocrine and nervous systems) effects.

ASSESSMENT OF IMMUNOLOGIC INTEGRITY

Xenobiotics can have significant effects on the immune system. Among the unique features of immune cells is their ability to be removed from the body and to function in vitro. This unique quality offers the toxicologist an opportunity to comprehensively evaluate the actions of xenobiotics on the immune system.

Many medical devices may have intimate and prolonged contact with the body. Possible immunologic consequences of this contact could be envisioned to include immunosuppression, immune stimulation, inflammation, and sensitization.

Methods to Assess Immunocompetence

General Assessment—All studies of immunocompetence should include toxicologic studies (such as organ weights, serum characteristics, hematologic parameters, and bone marrow function) to investigate the effects of immune modulation on other body organs. Histopathology of lymphoid organs also may provide insight into potential immunotoxicants. Moreover, use of fluorescently labeled monoclonal antibodies to cell surface markers in conjunction with a flow cytometer enables accurate enumeration of lymphocyte subsets and whether the xenobiotic may affect maturation.

Functional Assessment

Innate Immunity—Innate immunity encompasses all those immunologic responses that do not require prior exposure to an antigen and that are nonspecific in nature. These responses include recognition of tumor cells by NK cells, phagocytosis of pathogens by macrophages, and the lytic activity of the complement system.

To evaluate phagocytic activity, macrophages are placed in culture plates and incubated with radiolabeled red blood cells. Those cells that are not bound by the macrophages are removed, as are the cells that are bound but not phagocytized. The macrophages are then lysed to determine the amount of cells that were phagocytized. This test provides information about both the binding and phagocytizing activity of the macrophages and can also be performed in vivo by measuring the uptake of the radiolabeled red blood cells by certain tissue macrophages.

Another method to evaluate phagocytosis in vitro is to evaluate the uptake of latex spheres by macrophages. Evaluation of the ability of NK cells to lyse tumor cells is achieved by incubating radiolabeled target cells with NK cells and measuring the amount of radioactivity released into solution from the target cells.

Acquired Immunity: Humoral—The plaque (antibody)-forming cell (PFC or AFC) assay tests the ability of the host to mount an antibody response to a specific antigen, which requires the coordinated interaction of several different immune cells: macrophages, T cells, and B cells. Therefore, an effect on any of these cells (e.g., antigen processing and presentation, cytokine production, proliferation, or differentiation) can have a profound impact on the ability of B cells to produce antigen-specific antibody.

A standard PFC assay involves immunizing mice with sRBC. The antigen is taken up in the spleen and an antibody response occurs. Four days after immunization, spleens are removed and splenocytes are mixed with RBCs, complement, and agar, the mixture plated, and incubated until the B cells secrete anti-sRBC IgM antibody. This antibody then coats the surrounding sRBCs, and areas of hemolysis (plaques) can be seen.

The PFC assay can be evaluated in vivo using serum from peripheral blood of immunized mice and an enzyme-linked immunosorbent assay (ELISA). Serum from mice immunized with sRBCs is incubated in microtiter plates that have been coated with sRBC membranes to serve as the antigen

for sRBC-specific IgM or IgG to bind. After incubation, an enzyme-conjugated monoclonal antibody (the secondary antibody) against IgM (or IgG) is added. This antibody recognizes the IgM (or IgG) and binds specifically to that antibody. Then, the enzyme substrate (chromogen) is added. When the substrate comes into contact with the enzyme on the secondary antibody, a color change occurs that can be detected by measuring absorbance with a plate reader.

Acquired Immunity: Cell-mediated—Of numerous assays of CMI, three routinely performed tests are the cytotoxic T lymphocyte (CTL) assay, the delayed hypersensitivity response (DHR), and the T-cell proliferative responses to antigens.

The CTL assay measures the in vitro ability of splenic T cells to recognize allogeneic or antigenically distinct target cells by evaluating the ability of the CTLs to proliferate and then lyse the target cells. CTLs are incubated with target cells that have been treated so that they cannot themselves proliferate. CTLs recognize the target cells and proliferate until they are harvested. Then, they are incubated with radiolabeled target cells. CTLs that have acquired memory recognize the foreign MHC class I on target cells and lyse them.

The DHR evaluates the ability of memory T cells to recognize foreign antigen, proliferate and migrate to the site of the antigen, and secrete cytokines in vivo. Mice are sensitized by a subcutaneous injection of the chemical. Radiolabeled iodine is allowed to be incorporated into the mouse's mononuclear cells by injecting it into the mouse's bloodstream. Then, some of the sensitizing chemical is injected into the ear, and, after euthanizing the mouse, the ear is evaluated for the presence of radiolabeled mononuclear cells.

Several mechanisms exist to evaluate proliferative capacity of T cells in CMI. The mixed lymphocyte response (MLR) measures the ability of T cells to recognize foreign MHC class I and undergo proliferation.

Flow Cytometric Analysis—Flow cytometry employs light scatter, fluorescence, and absorbance measurements to analyze large numbers of cells on an individual basis. Usually, fluorochrome-conjugated monoclonal antibodies raised against a specific protein are employed for detection. This approach can be used to provide insight into which specific T-cell subsets are targeted after exposure to a xenobiotic, and to identify putative effects on T-cell maturation.

Molecular Biology Approaches to Immunotoxicology—Proteomics (the study of all expressed proteins in a particular cell, and thus the functional expression of the genome) and genomics (the study of all genes encoded by an organism's DNA), combined with bioinformatics, facilitate the evaluation of xenobiotic-induced alterations in the pathways and signaling networks of the immune system.

Mechanistic Approaches to Immunotoxicology—Once an agent has been identified as being an immunotoxicant, it may be necessary to further characterize its mechanism.

A general strategy involves the following steps: (1) identifying the cell type(s) targeted by the agent, (2) determining whether the effects are mediated by the parent compound or by a metabolite of the parent, (3) determining whether the effects are mediated directly or indirectly by the xenobiotic, and (4) elucidating the molecular events responsible for altered leukocyte function.

Regulatory Approaches to the Assessment of Immunotoxicity

The NTP Tier Approach—The National Toxicology Program screens for potential immunotoxic agents using a tier approach. Tier I provides assessment of general toxicity (immunopathology, hematology, and body and organ weights) as well as end-line functional assays (proliferative responses, PFC assay, and NK assay). Tier II was designed to further define an immunotoxic effect and includes tests for CMI (CTL and DHR), secondary antibody responses, enumeration of lymphocyte populations, and host resistance models.

Health Effects Test Guidelines—Guidelines for functional immunotoxicity assessments in regulatory studies recommend conduct of three tests. Assessment of immunotoxicity begins by exposure for a minimum of 28 days to the chemical followed by assessment of humoral immunity (PFC assay or anti-sRBC ELISA). If the chemical produces significant suppression of the humoral response, surface marker assessment by flow cytometry may be performed. If the chemical produces no suppression of the humoral response, an assessment of innate immunity (NK assay) may be performed.

Animal Models in Immunotoxicology

Rats and mice have been the animals of choice for studying the actions of xenobiotics on the immune system because (1) there is a vast database available on the immune system, (2) rodents are less expensive to maintain than larger animals, and (3) a wide variety of reagents (cytokines, antibodies, etc.) are available. Many reagents that are available for studying the human immune system can also be used in rhesus and cynomolgus monkeys. Chicken and fish are being used to evaluate the immunotoxicity of xenobiotics as alternative animal models with heightened environmental consciousness.

The manipulation of the embryonic genome, creating transgenic and knockout mice, may allow complex immune responses to be dissected into their components. In this way, the mechanisms by which immunotoxicants act can be better understood. Severe combined immunodeficient (SCID) mice have been used to study immune regulation, hematopoiesis, hypersensitivity, and autoimmunity.

Evaluation of Mechanisms of Action

Direct effects on the immune system may include chemical effects on immune function, structural alterations in lymphoid organs or on immune cell surfaces, or compositional changes in lymphoid organs or in serum. Xenobiotics may exert an indirect action on the immune system as well. They may be metabolically activated to their toxic metabolites, and may also have effects on other organ systems (e.g., liver damage) that then impact the immune system.

IMMUNE MODULATION BY XENOBIOTICS

The expansive and versatile nature of the immune system renders it susceptible to modulation by a wide variety of xenobiotics (Table 12–2). Many xenobiotics exhibit immunosuppressive actions, whereas some are immunomodulatory, meaning they might produce immune suppression and immune enhancement. Regardless of the end effect (immune suppression, immune enhancement, hypersensitivity, or autoimmunity) of a particular xenobiotic on the immune system, several common themes exist regarding the mechanisms by which these chemicals act. First, the mechanisms by which a xenobiotic affects immune function are likely to be multifaceted, involving several proteins, signaling cascades, or receptors. In fact, there is evidence to suggest that immune system effects for some xenobiotics are both xenobiotic-specific receptor-dependent and independent. Second, whether a xenobiotic produces a particular immune effect might depend on the concentration or dose of the xenobiotic, the mode and/or magnitude of cellular stimulation, and the kinetic relationship between exposure to the xenobiotic and exposure to the immune stimulant (i.e., antigen, mitogen, and pharmacological agent). Third, xenobiotic exposures rarely occur in one chemical at a time; thus, the effects and/or mechanisms observed might be attributable to several chemicals or classes of chemicals. Finally, determination of immune system effects and/or mechanisms by xenobiotics in humans might be further confounded by the physiological or immunological state of the individual.

Halogenated Aromatic Hydrocarbons

Few classes of xenobiotics have been as extensively studied for immunotoxicity as the halogenated aromatic hydrocarbons (HAHs). The majority of the biochemical and toxic effects produced by the HAHs are mediated via HAH binding to the cytosolic aromatic hydrocarbon receptor (AHR). Binding of HAH to AHR ultimately results in upregulation of certain proteins with a net immunosuppressive effect. Interestingly, the degree of immunosuppression is positively correlated with the binding affinity of the HAH for the AHR.

Pesticides

Pesticides include all xenobiotics whose specific purpose is to kill another form of life, including insects (insecticides), small rodents (rodenticides), or even vegetation (herbicides). Exposure to pesticides occurs most often in occupational settings, in which manufacturers, those applying the pesticides, or those harvesting treated agricultural products, are exposed.

TABLE 12–2 Xenobiotics capable of immunosuppression.

Halogenated aromatic hydrocarbons	**Aromatic hydrocarbons**
Polychlorinated biphenyls Polybrominated biphenyls Polychlorinated dibenzodioxins Polychlorinated dibenzofurans	Carbon tetrachloride Ethylene glycol monomethyl ether 2-Methoxyethanol
Polycyclic aromatic hydrocarbons	**Mycotoxins**
Nitrosamines	Aflatoxin Ochratoxin Tricothecenes Vomitoxin
Pesticides	**Natural and synthetic hormones**
Organophosphate pesticides Organochlorine pesticides Organotin pesticides Carbamate pesticides Pyrethroids	Estrogens Androgens Glucocorticoids
Metals	**Therapeutics**
Arsenic Beryllium Cadmium Chromium Cobalt Gold Lead Mercury Nickel Platinum	AIDS therapeutics Biologics Anti-inflammatory agents
	Immunosuppressive drugs
	Azathioprine Cyclophosphamide Cyclosporin A Leflunomide Rapamycin Stavudine (2′,3′-didehydro-2′,3′-dideoxythymidine) Videx (2′,3′-dideoxyinosine; ddl) Zalcitabine (2′,3′-dideoxycytidine; ddC) Zidovudine (3′-azido-3′-deoxythymidine; AZT)
Inhaled substances	
Asbestos Ethylenediamine Formaldehyde Silica Tobacco smoke Urethane	**Drugs of abuse**
	Cannabinoids Cocaine Ethanol Opioids: heroin and morphine
Oxidant gases	
Ozone (O_3) Nitrogen dioxide (NO_2) Sulfur dioxide (SO_2) Phosgene	

Pesticides act through a variety of mechanisms and can be both immunosuppressive and immunoenhancing (see Chapter 22).

Metals

Generally speaking, metals target multiple organ systems and exert their toxic effects via an interaction of the free metal with targets, such as enzyme systems, membranes, or cellular organelles. In considering their immunotoxicity, metals at high concentrations usually exert immunosuppressive effects; however, at lower concentrations, immune enhancement is often observed. Furthermore, as with most immunotoxicants, exposures to metals are likely not single exposures, although one metal might dominate depending on the exposure conditions (e.g., high levels of mercury in fish or high levels of lead

from paint). Many metals are immunotoxic and the interested reader is referred to Chapter 23.

Solvents and Related Chemicals

There is limited, but substantive, evidence that exposure to organic solvents and their related compounds can produce immune suppression. Chemicals in this category are aromatic hydrocarbons, such as benzene, haloalkanes and haloalkenes, glycols and glycol ethers, and nitrosamines. The interested reader is referred to Chapter 24.

Mycotoxins

Mycotoxins are structurally diverse secondary metabolites of fungi (see Chapter 26). This class of chemicals comprises such

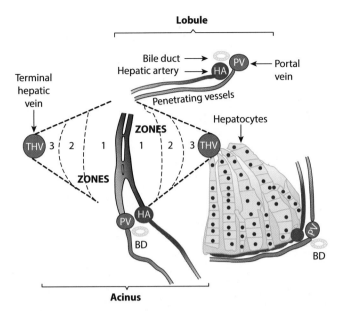

FIGURE 13–1 Schematic of liver operational units, the classic lobule and the acinus. The lobule is centered around the terminal hepatic vein (central vein), where the blood drains out of the lobule. The acinus has as its base the penetrating vessels, where blood supplied by the portal vein and hepatic artery flows down the acinus past the cords of hepatocytes. Zones 1, 2, and 3 of the acinus represent metabolic regions that are increasingly distant from the blood supply.

Well-documented acinar gradients exist for bile salts, bilirubin, and many organic anions as well.

Heterogeneities in protein levels of hepatocytes along the acinus generate gradients of metabolic functions. Hepatocytes in the mitochondria-rich zone 1 are predominant in fatty acid oxidation, gluconeogenesis, and ammonia detoxification to urea. Gradients of enzymes involved in the bioactivation and detoxification of xenobiotics have been observed along the acinus by immunohistochemistry (exploiting the immune system's specificity to stain tissue). Notable gradients for hepatotoxicants are the higher levels of glutathione in zone 1 and the greater amounts of cytochrome P450 proteins in zone 3, particularly the CYP2E1 isozyme inducible by ethanol.

Hepatic sinusoids are the channels between cords of hepatocytes where blood percolates on its way to the terminal hepatic vein. The three major types of cells in the sinusoids are endothelial cells, Kupffer cells, and stellate (Ito) cells. Sinusoids are lined by thin, discontinuous endothelial cells with numerous fenestrae (or pores) that allow molecules smaller than 250 kDa to cross the interstitial space (known as the space of Disse) between the endothelium and hepatocytes. The numerous fenestrae and the lack of basement membrane facilitate exchanges of fluids and molecules, such as albumin, between the sinusoid and hepatocytes, but hinder movement of particles larger than chylomicron remnants.

Kupffer cells, the resident macrophages of the liver, constitute approximately 80% of the fixed macrophages in the body. Kupffer cells are situated within the lumen of the sinusoid. The primary function of Kupffer cells is to ingest and degrade particulate matter. Also, Kupffer cells are a major source of cytokines and eicosanoids and can act as antigen-presenting cells (APCs). Ito cells (also known as *fat-storing cells* and *stellate cells*) are located between endothelial cells and hepatocytes. Ito cells synthesize collagen and are the major storage site for vitamin A in the body.

Bile Formation

Bile contains bile acids, glutathione, phospholipids, cholesterol, bilirubin, and other organic anions, proteins, metals, ions, and xenobiotics. Formation of this fluid is a specialized function of the liver. Adequate bile formation is essential for uptake of lipid nutrients from the small intestine (Table 13–1), protection of the small intestine from oxidative insults, and excretion of endogenous and xenobiotic compounds. Hepatocytes begin the process by transporting bile acids, glutathione, and other solutes including xenobiotics and their metabolites into the canalicular lumen (the space formed by specialized regions of the plasma membrane between adjacent hepatocytes). The canaliculi are separated from the intercellular space between hepatocytes by tight junctions, which form a barrier permeable only to water, electrolytes, and to some degree to small organic cations. These canaliculi form channels between hepatocytes that connect to a series of larger and larger channels or ducts within the liver. The large extrahepatic bile ducts merge into the common bile duct. Bile can be stored and concentrated in the gallbladder before its release into the first segment of the small intestine, the duodenum.

The major driving force of bile formation is the active transport of bile salts and other osmolytes into the canalicular lumen. Most conjugated bile acids (taurine and glycine conjugates) and some unconjugated bile acids are transported into hepatocytes by sodium-dependent transporters. Sodium-independent uptake of conjugated and unconjugated bile acids is performed by members of the organic anion-transporting polypeptides (OATPs). OATPs also transport numerous drugs and hepatotoxicants. Lipophilic cationic drugs, estrogens, and lipids are exported by the canalicular multiple-drug resistance (MDR) P-glycoproteins, one of which is exclusive for phospholipids. Conjugates of glutathione, glucuronide, and sulfate are exported by multidrug resistance–associated protein 2 (MRP2). The many different transporters are shown in Figure 13–2.

Metals are excreted into bile by a series of processes that include (1) uptake across the sinusoidal membrane by facilitated diffusion or receptor-mediated endocytosis; (2) storage in binding proteins or lysosomes; and (3) canalicular secretion via lysosomes, a glutathione-coupled event, or use of a specific canalicular membrane transporter, e.g., MRP2. Biliary excretion is important in the homeostasis of metals, notably copper, manganese, cadmium, selenium, gold, silver, and arsenic. Inability to export Cu into bile is a central problem in Wilson's disease, a rare genetic disorder characterized by accumulation of Cu in the liver and then in other tissues.

Canalicular lumen bile is propelled forward into larger channels by dynamic, ATP-dependent contractions of the

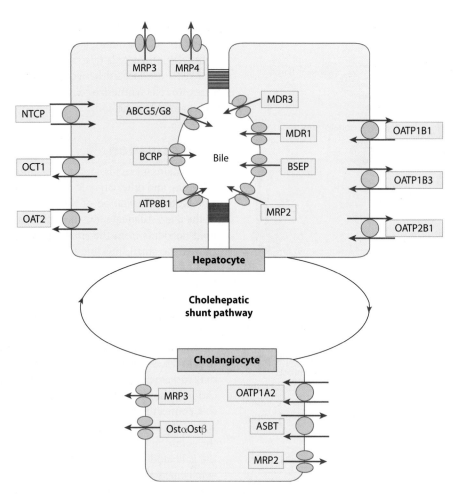

FIGURE 13–2 **Transport proteins in human hepatocytes and cholangiocytes.** Efflux transporters (blue ovals with blue arrows): BSEP, bile salt export pump; MDR, multidrug resistance protein; MRP, multidrug resistance-associated protein; ABCG5/8, heterodimeric ATP binding cassette transporter G5/G8; BCRP, breast cancer resistance protein; Ostα/Ostβ, heterodimeric organic solute transporter alpha and beta. Uptake transporters (green circles with red arrows): ASBT, apical sodium–dependent bile salt transporter; NTCP, sodium taurocholate cotransporting polypeptide; OATP, organic anion-transporting polypeptide; OCT, organic cation transporter; OAT, organic anion transporter. Transporters localized to the sinusoidal membrane extract solutes from the blood. Exporters localized to canalicular membrane move solutes into the lumen of the canaliculus. Exporters of particular relevance to canalicular secretion of toxic chemicals and their metabolites are the canalicular multiple organic anion transporter (MOAT) system and the family of multiple-drug resistant (MDR) P-glycoproteins. MDR3 (ABCB4) flops phosphotidylcholine from the inner to the outer leaflet of the canalicular membrane. ATP8B1 flips phosphatidylserine from the outer to inner membrane to maintain the lipid asymmetry of the canalicular membrane. (Reproduced with permission from Pauli-Magnus C, Meier PJ: Hepatobiliary transporters and drug-induced cholestasis, *Hepatology,* 2006 Oct;44(4):778–787.)

pericanalicular cytoskeleton. Bile ducts modify bile by absorption and secretion of solutes. Biliary epithelial cells also express a variety of phase I and phase II enzymes, which may contribute to the biotransformation of toxicants present in bile.

Secretion into biliary ducts is usually, but not always, a prelude to toxicant clearance by excretion in feces or urine. Exceptions occur when compounds are repeatedly delivered into the intestinal lumen via bile, efficiently absorbed from the intestinal lumen, and then redirected to the liver via portal blood, a process known as *enterohepatic cycling.*

Toxicant-related impairments of bile formation are more likely to have detrimental consequences in populations with other conditions where biliary secretion is marginal. For example,

neonates exhibit delayed development of bile salt synthesis and the expression of sinusoidal and canalicular transporters. Neonates are more prone to develop jaundice when treated with drugs that compete with bilirubin for biliary clearance.

LIVER PATHOPHYSIOLOGY

Mechanisms and Types of Toxicant-induced Liver Injury

Hepatic response to insults by chemicals (Table 13–2) depends on the intensity of the insult, the population of cells affected, and whether the exposure is acute or chronic.

TABLE 13-2 Types of hepatobiliary injury.

Type of Injury or Damage	Representative Toxins
Fatty liver	Amiodarone, CCl₄, ethanol, fialuridine, tamoxifen, valproic acid
Hepatocyte death	Acetaminophen, allyl alcohol, Cu, dimethylformamide, ethanol
Immune-mediated response	Diclofenac, ethanol, halothane, tienilic acid
Canalicular cholestasis	Chlorpromazine, cyclosporin A, 1,1-dichloroethylene, estrogens, Mn, phalloidin
Bile duct damage	Alpha-naphthylisothiocyanate, amoxicillin, methylene dianiline, sporidesmin
Sinusoidal disorders	Anabolic steroids, cyclophosphamide, microcystin, pyrrolizidine alkaloids
Fibrosis and cirrhosis	CCl₄, ethanol, thioacetamide, vitamin A, vinyl chloride
Tumors	Aflatoxin, androgens, arsenic, thorium dioxide, vinyl chloride

Cell Death—Based on morphology, liver cells can die by two different modes, necrosis or apoptosis. Necrosis is characterized by cell swelling, leakage, nuclear disintegration (karyolysis), and an influx of inflammatory cells. When necrosis occurs in hepatocytes, the associated plasma membrane leakage can be detected biochemically by assaying plasma (or serum) for liver cytosol-derived enzymes such as aspartate or alanine aminotransferases (AST or ALT) or γ-glutamyltranspeptidase (GGT). In contrast, apoptosis is characterized by cell shrinkage, nuclear fragmentation, formation of apoptotic bodies, and a lack of inflammation. It is always a single cell event with the main purpose of removing cells no longer needed during development or eliminating aging cells.

Hepatocyte death can occur in a focal, zonal, or panacinar (widespread) pattern. Focal cell death is characterized by the randomly distributed death of single hepatocytes or small clusters of hepatocytes. Zonal necrosis is death to hepatocytes in certain functional regions. Panacinar necrosis is massive death of hepatocytes with only a few or no remaining survivors.

Mechanisms of toxicant-induced injury to liver cells include lipid peroxidation, binding to cell macromolecules, mitochondrial damage, disruption of the cytoskeleton, and massive calcium influx. Independent of the initial insult, the mitochondrial membrane permeability transition pore opens causing collapse of the membrane potential and depletion of cellular ATP, and necrotic cell death. The loss of ATP inhibits the ion pumps in the plasma membrane, which results in the loss of cellular ion homeostasis and causes the characteristic swelling of oncotic necrosis.

Canalicular Cholestasis—Defined physiologically as a decrease in the volume of bile formed or an impaired secretion of specific solutes into bile, cholestasis is characterized biochemically by elevated serum levels of compounds normally concentrated in bile, particularly bile salts and bilirubin. When biliary excretion of the yellowish bilirubin pigment is impaired, this pigment accumulates in the skin and eyes, producing jaundice, and spills into urine, which becomes bright yellow or dark brown. Toxicant-induced cholestasis can be transient or chronic; when substantial, it is associated with cell swelling, cell death, and inflammation. Many different types of chemicals cause cholestasis (Table 13–2).

The molecular mechanisms of cholestasis are related to expression and function of transporter systems in the basolateral and canalicular membranes. An increased hepatic uptake, decreased biliary excretion, and increased biliary reabsorption (cholehepatic shunting) of a drug may contribute to its accumulation in the liver.

Bile formation is vulnerable to toxicant effects on the functional integrity of sinusoidal transporters, canalicular exporters, cytoskeleton-dependent processes for transcytosis, and the contractile closure of the canalicular lumen (Figure 13–3). Changes that weaken the junctions that form the structural barrier between the blood and the canalicular lumen allow solutes to leak out of the canalicular lumen. These paracellular junctions provide a size and charge barrier to the diffusion of solutes between the blood and the canalicular lumen while water and

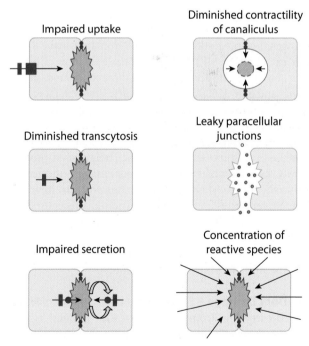

FIGURE 13-3 Schematic of six potential mechanisms for cholestasis. Inhibited uptake, diminished transcytosis, impaired secretion, diminished canalicular contractility, leakiness of the junctions that seal the canalicular lumen from the blood, and detrimental consequences of high concentrations of toxic entities in the pericanalicular area are possible. Note that impaired secretion across the canalicular membrane can result from inhibition of a transporter or retraction of a transporter away from the canalicular membrane.

small ions diffuse across these junctions. One hepatotoxicant that causes tight-junction leakage is α-napthylisothiocyanate.

Compounds that produce cholestasis do not necessarily act by a single mechanism or at just one site. Chlorpromazine impairs bile acid uptake and canalicular contractility. Multiple alterations have been well documented for estrogens, a well-known cause of reversible canalicular cholestasis. Estrogens and progestins decrease bile salt uptake by effects at the sinusoidal membrane including a decrease in the Na^+,K^+-ATPase necessary for Na-dependent transport of bile salts across the plasma membrane and changes in lipid component of this membrane. At the canalicular membrane, estrogens diminish the transport of glutathione conjugates and reduce the number of bile salt transporters.

An additional mechanism for canalicular cholestasis is concentration of reactive forms of chemicals in the pericanalicular area (Figure 13–3). Most chemicals that cause canalicular cholestasis are excreted in bile. Therefore, the proteins and lipids in the canalicular region encounter a high concentration of these chemicals. Observations consistent with this concentration mechanism have been reported for Mn, reactive thioether glutathione conjugates of 1,1-dichloroethylene, and sporidesmin.

Although no case of drug toxicity has been reported in response to modifications of basolateral uptake, OATPs can contribute to the liver injury potential of toxicants. The hepatotoxicity of phalloidin, microcystin, and amanitin is facilitated by the uptake through OATPs. Furthermore, there is a growing list of drugs including rifampicin, bosentan, and troglitazone, which are known to directly inhibit bile salt export pump (BSEP). Estrogens and progestins inhibit BSEP from the canalicular side after excretion by MRP2. A substantial inhibition of bile salt excretion can lead to accumulation of these compounds in hepatocytes and may directly cause cell injury. However, more recent findings indicate that most of the bile acids accumulating in the liver after obstructive cholestasis are nontoxic and instead of cell death cause proinflammatory gene expression in hepatocytes.

While liver injury after obstructive cholestasis is produced mainly by inflammatory cells, compensatory mechanisms within the hepatocyte itself can limit this potential injury. Bile acids are substrates for the nuclear farnesoid X receptor (FXR), down-regulate NTCP and limit bile acid uptake. In addition, FXR activation causes increased expression of transporters on the canalicular and basolateral membranes, which all work to limit the amount of bile acid accumulation.

Bile Duct Damage—Damage to the intrahepatic bile ducts (which carry bile from the liver to the GI tract) is called *cholangiodestructive cholestasis*. A useful biochemical index of bile duct damage is a sharp elevation in serum alkaline phosphatase activity. In addition, serum levels of bile salts and bilirubin are elevated, as observed with canalicular cholestasis. Initial lesions following a single dose of cholangiodestructive agents include swollen biliary epithelium, debris of damaged cells within lumens of the biliary tract, and inflammatory cell infiltration of portal tracts. Chronic administration of chemicals that cause bile duct destruction can lead to

biliary proliferation and fibrosis resembling biliary cirrhosis. A rare response is the loss of bile ducts, a condition known as *vanishing bile duct syndrome.* This persisting problem has been reported in patients receiving antibiotics, anabolic steroids, contraceptive steroids, or the anticonvulsant carbamazepine.

Sinusoidal Damage—The sinusoid is, in effect, a specialized capillary with numerous fenestrae for high permeability. Functional integrity of the sinusoid can be compromised by dilation or blockade of its lumen or by progressive destruction of its endothelial cell wall. Dilation of the sinusoid will occur whenever efflux of hepatic blood is impeded. Blockade will occur when red blood cells become caught in the sinusoids. Such changes have been illustrated after large doses of the drug acetaminophen. A consequence of extensive sinusoidal blockade is that the liver becomes engorged with blood cells and the rest of the body goes into shock.

Progressive destruction of the endothelial wall of the sinusoid will lead to gaps and then ruptures of its barrier integrity, with entrapment of red blood cells. These disruptions of the sinusoid are considered the early structural features of the vascular disorder known as veno-occlusive disease, which occurs after exposure to pyrrolizidine alkaloids, which may be found in some herbal teas and chemotherapeutic agents.

Disruption of the Cytoskeleton—Phalloidin (from a mushroom) and microcystin (from blue-green algae) disrupt the integrity of hepatocyte cytoskeleton by affecting proteins that are vital to its dynamic nature, preventing disassembly of actin filaments. Phalloidin uptake into hepatocytes leads to an accentuated actin web of cytoskeleton and the canalicular lumen dilates.

Microcystin uptake into hepatocytes leads to hyperphosphorylation of cytoskeletal proteins. Reversible phosphorylations of cytoskeletal structural and motor proteins are critical to the dynamic integrity of the cytoskeleton. As depicted in Figure 13–4, extensive hyperphosphorylation produced by large amounts of microcystin leads to marked deformation of hepatocytes due to a unique collapse of the microtubular actin scaffold into a spiny central aggregate. Lower doses of microcystin interfere with vesicle transport by hyperphosphorylating the transport protein dynein.

Dynein is a mechanicochemical protein that drives vesicles along microtubules using energy from ATP hydrolysis; central to the hydrolysis of the dynein-bound ATP is a cycle of kinase phosphorylation and phosphatase dephosphorylation. Thus, hyperphosphorylation of dynein freezes this motor pump. Chronic exposure to low levels of microcystin has raised new concerns about the health effects of this water contaminant. Specifically, low levels of microcystin promote liver tumors and kill hepatocytes in the zone 3 region, where microcystin accumulates.

Fatty Liver—Fatty liver (steatosis) is defined biochemically as an appreciable increase in the hepatic lipid (mainly triglyceride) content, which is <5 wt% in the normal human liver. Currently, the most common cause of hepatic steatosis is insulin resistance due to central obesity and sedentary lifestyle.

when cells exceed their capacity to complex cadmium with the metal-binding protein metallothionein.

Hepatocytes contribute to the homeostasis of iron by extracting this essential metal from the sinusoid by a receptor-mediated process and maintaining a reserve of iron within the storage protein ferritin. Acute iron toxicity is most commonly observed in young children who accidently ingest iron tablets. The cytotoxicity of free iron is attributed to its function as an electron donor for the formation of reactive oxygen species, which initiate destructive oxidative stress reactions. Accumulation of excess iron beyond the capacity for its safe storage in ferritin leads to liver damage. Chronic hepatic accumulation of excess iron in cases of hemochromatosis is associated with a spectrum of hepatic disease including a greater than 200-fold risk for liver cancer.

Bioactivation and Detoxification—Hepatocytes have very high constitutive activity of the phase I enzymes that often convert xenobiotics to reactive electrophilic metabolites. Also, hepatocytes have a rich collection of phase II enzymes that add a polar group to a molecule and thereby enhance its removal from the body. Phase II reactions usually yield stable, nonreactive metabolites. In general, the balance between phase I and phase II reactions determines whether a reactive metabolite will initiate liver cell injury or be safely detoxified. Because the expression of phase I and II enzymes and of the hepatic transporters can be influenced by genetics (e.g., polymorphism of drug-metabolizing enzymes) and lifestyle (e.g., diet, consumption of other drugs and alcohol), the susceptibility to potential hepatotoxicants can vary markedly between individuals.

Acetaminophen—One of the most widely used analgesics acetaminophen (APAP) is a safe drug when used at therapeutically recommended doses. Overdose can cause severe hepatotoxicity, and certain acquired factors (e.g., diet, drugs, diabetes, and obesity) can enhance hepatotoxicity. Typical therapeutic doses of acetaminophen are not hepatotoxic, because most of the acetaminophen gets glucuronidated or sulfated with little drug bioactivation. Injury after large doses of acetaminophen is enhanced by fasting and other conditions that deplete glutathione and is minimized by treatments with *N*-acetylcysteine that enhance hepatocyte synthesis of glutathione.

Alcoholics are vulnerable to the hepatotoxic effects of acetaminophen at dosages within the high therapeutic range. This acquired enhancement has widely been attributed to accelerated bioactivation of acetaminophen to the electrophilic *N*-acetyl-*p*-benzoquinone imine (NAPQI) intermediate by ethanol induction of CYP2E1. Inducers of CYP3A including many drugs and dietary chemicals potentially influence acetaminophen toxicity.

Although many of the details of the mechanism for APAP-induced hepatotoxicity remain to be elucidated, newly gained insight into signaling events in response to APAP overdose suggests two fundamentally new developments. First, necrotic cell death is in most cases not caused by a single catastrophic event but can be the result of a cellular stress, which is initiated by metabolic activation and triggers sophisticated signaling mechanisms culminating in cell death (Figure 13–5). Second, the multitude of events following the initial stress offers many opportunities for therapeutic interventions at later time points. Because these events are not occurring in all cells to the same degree and at the same time, delayed interventions may not completely prevent cell damage but limit the area of necrosis enough to prevent liver failure.

Ethanol—Morbidity and mortality associated with the consumption of alcohol is mainly caused by the toxic effects of ethanol on the liver. This targeted toxicity is due to the fact that >90% of a dose of ethanol is metabolized in the liver. Three principal pathways of ethanol metabolism are known. In the primary pathway, ethanol is bioactivated by alcohol dehydrogenase to acetaldehyde, a reactive aldehyde, which is subsequently detoxified to acetate by aldehyde dehydrogenase. Both enzymes exhibit genetic polymorphisms that result in higher concentrations of acetaldehyde—a "fast" activity isozyme of alcohol dehydrogenase [ALD2*2] and a physiologically very "slow" mitochondrial isozyme of aldehyde dehydrogenase [ALDH2*2]. Approximately 50% of Asian populations but virtually no Caucasians have the slow aldehyde dehydrogenase; alcohol consumption by people with this slow polymorphism leads to uncomfortable symptoms of flushing and nausea due to high systemic levels of acetaldehyde.

The second major pathway involves the alcohol-inducible enzyme CYP2E1, which oxidizes ethanol to acetaldehyde. The enzyme is located predominantly in hepatocytes of the centrilobular region and requires oxygen and NADPH. Due to the nature of the enzyme, this reaction is most relevant for high doses of ethanol and for chronic alcoholism. The third pathway involves catalase in peroxisomes. In this reaction, ethanol functions as an electron donor for the reduction of hydrogen peroxide to water. Thus, the capacity of this pathway is limited due to the low levels of hydrogen peroxide. It is estimated that <2% of an ethanol dose is metabolized through this pathway.

Allyl Alcohol—An industrial chemical used in the production of resins, plastics, and fire retardants, allyl alcohol is also used as a model hepatotoxicant due to its preferential periportal (zone 1) hepatotoxicity. The alcohol is metabolized by alcohol dehydrogenase to acrolein, a highly reactive aldehyde, which is then further oxidized by aldehyde dehydrogenase to acrylic acid. The fact that the toxicity depends on depletion of hepatic glutathione levels is prevented by inhibitors of alcohol dehydrogenase but enhanced by inhibitors of aldehyde dehydrogenase suggests that acrolein formation is the critical event in liver injury. Age and gender differences in allyl alcohol hepatotoxicity can be explained by variations in the balance between alcohol dehydrogenase and aldehyde dehydrogenase expression. The preferential occurrence of allyl alcohol injury in zone 1 hepatocytes is caused by the predominant uptake of allyl alcohol in the periportal region and the oxygen dependence of the toxicity. Although protein binding of the reactive metabolite

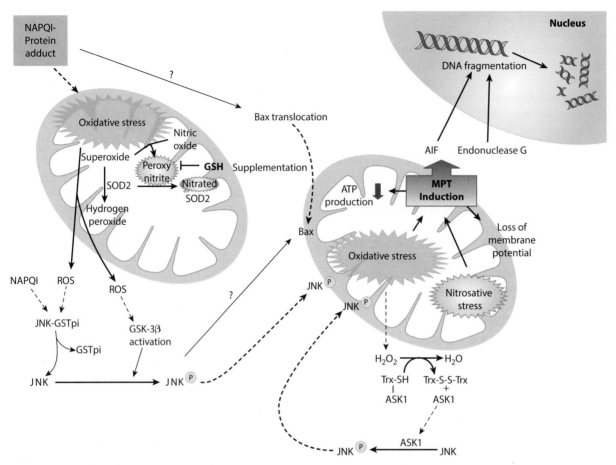

FIGURE 13–5 **Acetaminophen-induced mitochondrial oxidant stress and its influence on cellular signaling.** Metabolism of APAP results in the generation of the reactive intermediate, NAPQI, which forms protein adducts and induces mitochondrial oxidative stress. The increased generation of superoxide and its reaction with NO results in the production of peroxynitrite. The superoxide can be scavenged by SOD2 and converted into hydrogen peroxide, although the generation of peroxynitrite can interfere in this process by the nitration of SOD2. Mitochondrial oxidative stress and hydrogen peroxide can also activate the mitogen-activated protein kinase, JNK, by multiple pathways, resulting in its phosphorylation and translocation to the mitochondria. This then amplifies the mitochondrial oxidant stress, which, subsequently, leads to activation of the mitochondrial permeability transition, and translocation of mitochondrial proteins, such as AIF and endonuclease G, to the nucleus. This results in DNA fragmentation and, finally, oncotic necrosis. (Reproduced with permission from Jaeschke H, McGill MR, Ramachandra A: Oxidant stress, mitochondria, and cell death mechanisms in drug-induced liver injury: lessons learned from acetaminophen hepatotoxicity, *Drug Metab Rev*, 2012 Feb;44(1):88–106.)

acrolein and subsequent adduct formation appears to be the main cause of liver cell death, lipid peroxidation can become a relevant mechanism of cell injury under conditions of a compromised antioxidant status. Lipid peroxidation is caused by a reductive stress where the excessive NADH formation leads to mobilization of redox-active iron from storage proteins.

Carbon Tetrachloride—Cytochrome P450–dependent conversion of CCl_4 to $\cdot CCl_3$ and then to $CCl_3OO\cdot$ is the classic example of xenobiotic bioactivation to a free radical that initiates lipid peroxidation by abstracting a hydrogen atom from the polyunsaturated fatty acid of a phospholipid. Metabolic activation of CCl_4 primarily involves CYP2E1. CCl_4-induced lipid peroxidation increases the permeability of the plasma membrane to Ca^{2+}, leading to severe disturbances of the calcium homeostasis and necrotic cell death. Recent research

indicates that CCl_4 also induces significant mitochondrial damage, which is dependent on lipid peroxidation events and on CYP2E1 activity. In addition, the $\cdot CCl_3$ radical can directly bind to tissue macromolecules and some of the lipid peroxidation products are reactive aldehydes, e.g., 4-hydroxynonenal, which can form adducts with proteins. These events also cause the immune system to be involved, which can contribute to liver injury. Conditions in which cytochrome P450 is depleted lead to decreased liver damage when exposed to CCl_4.

Regeneration—The liver has a high capacity to restore lost tissue and function by regeneration. Loss of hepatocytes due to hepatectomy or cell injury triggers proliferation of all mature liver cells. This process is capable of restoring the original liver mass. However, regeneration is not just a response to cell death, but a process that actively determines the final injury after exposure to hepatotoxic chemicals. Stimulation of repair by exposure to a moderate dose of a hepatotoxicant strongly attenuates tissue damage of a subsequent high dose of the same chemical. Tissue repair is dose–responsive up to a threshold, after which the injury is too severe and cell proliferation is inhibited.

Inflammation and Immune Responses—The activation of resident macrophages (Kupffer cells), NK and NKT cells, and the migration of activated neutrophils, lymphocytes, and monocytes into regions of damaged liver are a well-recognized feature of the hepatotoxicity produced by many chemicals. The main reason for an inflammatory response is to remove dead and damaged cells. However, under certain circumstances, these inflammatory cells can aggravate the existing injury by release of directly cytotoxic mediators or by formation of pro- and anti-inflammatory mediators (Figure 13–6).

In addition to the activation of an inflammatory response, immune-mediated reactions may also lead to severe liver injury. Drugs and chemicals that have been suggested to cause immune-mediated injury mechanisms in the liver include halothane, tienilic acid, and dihydralazine. A delay in onset of the injury or the requirement for repeated exposure to the drug and the formation of antibodies against drug-modified hepatic proteins are characteristic features of immune reactions,

but the mechanisms are not well understood. Two proposed mechanisms of immune-mediated liver injury are the hapten hypothesis and the danger hypothesis (Figure 13–7).

The *hapten hypothesis* assumes that a reactive metabolite covalently binds to cellular proteins and the drug-modified protein is taken up by APCs, cleaved to peptide fragments, which are then presented within the major histocompatibility complex (MHC) to T cells. This hypothesis does not explain, however, why other drugs (e.g., APAP), which also form reactive metabolites and drug-modified proteins, do not trigger an immune response. The *danger hypothesis* (Figure 13–8) postulates that damaged cells release danger signals, which induce the upregulation of a peripheral protein B7 on activated antigen presenting cells (APCs), which when paired with CD28 on T cells generates a costimulatory signal. A cytotoxic immune response occurs only when the T-cell receptor stimulation with the antigen is accompanied by an independent costimulation of the T cell. In the absence of this costimulatory signal, the antigens derived from drug-modified proteins induce immune tolerance.

Activation of Sinusoidal Cells—Four kinds of observations, collectively, indicate roles for sinusoidal cell (immune cells present in the liver sinusoids) activation as primary or secondary factors in toxicant-induced injury to the liver:

1. Kupffer and Ito cells exhibit an activated morphology after acute and chronic exposure to hepatotoxicants.
2. Pretreatments that activate or inactivate Kupffer cells appropriately modulate the extent of damage produced by classic toxicants. Kupffer cell activation by vitamin A profoundly enhances the acute toxicity of carbon tetrachloride; this enhancement did not occur when animals were also given an inactivator of Kupffer cells.
3. Activated Kupffer cells secrete appreciable amounts of soluble cytotoxins, including reactive oxygen and nitrogen species.
4. Acute and chronic exposure to alcohol directly or indirectly affects sinusoidal cells.

Figure 13–8 summarizes information presented in this and earlier sections of this chapter about the multiplicity of toxicant-induced interactions with and between various liver cells. The effect on a given cell type can be direct or may result from a cascade of signals and responses between cell types.

Mitochondrial Damage—Mitochondrial DNA codes for several proteins in the mitochondrial electron transport chain. Nucleoside analog drugs for the therapy of hepatitis B and AIDS infections cause mitochondrial DNA damage directly, when incorporation of the analog base leads to miscoding or early termination of polypeptides. The severe hepatic mitochondrial injury produced by the nucleoside analog fialuridine is attributed to its higher affinity for the polymerase responsible for mitochondrial DNA synthesis than for the polymerases responsible for nuclear DNA synthesis. Mitochondrial DNA is also more vulnerable to miscoding (mutation) due to its limited capacity for repair.

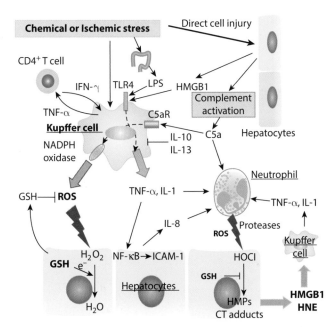

FIGURE 13–6 **Self-perpetuating inflammatory response after chemical or ischemic stress.** C5aR, C5a complement receptor; CT, chlorotyrosine protein adducts; GSH, reduced glutathione; HMGB1, high-mobility group box-1; HMPs, hypochlorous acid modified proteins; HNE, hydroxynonenal; HOCl, hypochlorous acid; ICAM-1, intercellular adhesion molecule-1; IFN-γ, interferon-γ; IL-1, interleukin-1; LPS, lipopolysaccharide; NF-κB, nuclear factor-κB; ROS, reactive oxygen species; TLR4, toll-like receptor-4; TNF, tumor necrosis factor.

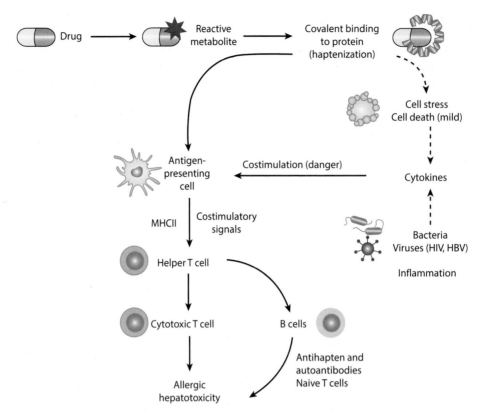

FIGURE 13-7 The danger hypothesis for immune-mediated idiosyncratic hepatotoxicity. Hapten formation leading to major histocompatibility complex class II (MHCII) presentation of haptenized peptide by antigen-presenting cells (APCs) along with costimulation of APC signaling molecules by mild injury, inflammation, or infection promotes helper T-cell activation leading to T-cell responses to the antigen. The cytotoxic T cells are then targeted against hepatocytes that express haptenized protein or MHCI presentation of haptenized peptides on the cell surface. Antibody to haptenized protein or concomitant autoantibodies could theoretically mediate and promote antibody-dependent cell-mediated hepatotoxicity. (Reproduced with permission from Kaplowitz N: Idiosyncratic drug hepatotoxicity. *Nat Rev Drug Discov*, 2005 June;4(6):489–499.)

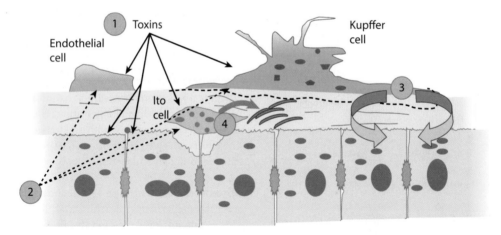

FIGURE 13-8 Schematic depicting the complex cascade of toxicant-evoked interactions between hepatocytes and sinusoidal cells. Sinusoidal cell responses to toxicants can lead to either injury or activation. A scenario could involve (1) toxicant injury to hepatocytes, (2) signals from the injured hepatocyte to Kupffer and Ito cells, followed by (3) Kupffer cell release of cytotoxins, and (4) Ito cell secretion of collagen. Activation of Kupffer cells is an important factor in the progression of injury evoked by many toxicants. Stimulation of collagen production by activated Ito cells is a proposed mechanism for toxicant-induced fibrosis.

TABLE 13–4 Examples of drugs with known idiosyncratic hepatotoxicity.

A. Immune-mediated (allergic) idiosyncratic hepatotoxicity
- Diclofenac (analgesic)
- Halothane (anesthetic)
- Nitrofurantoin (antibiotic)
- Phenytoin (anticonvulsant)
- Tienilic acid (diuretic)

B. Nonimmune-mediated (nonallergic) idiosyncratic hepatotoxicity
- Amiodarone (antiarrhythmic)
- Bromfenac (analgesic)—withdrawn from market
- Diclofenac (analgesic)
- Disulfiram (alcoholism)
- Isoniazid (antituberculosis)
- Ketoconazole (antifungal)
- Rifampicin (antimicrobial)
- Troglitazone (antidiabetes)—withdrawn from market
- Valproate (anticonvulsant)

Alcohol abuse causes mitochondrial injury by shifting the bioactivation/detoxification balance for ethanol, leading to an accumulation of its reactive acetaldehyde metabolite within mitochondria, because mitochondrial aldehyde dehydrogenase is the major enzymatic process for detoxification of acetaldehyde. Bioactivation of large amounts of ethanol by alcohol dehydrogenase hampers the detoxification reaction, since the two enzymes require the common, depletable cofactor nicotinamide adenine dinucleotide (NAD). Any type of ethanol-induced change that enhances the leakiness of the mitochondrial transport chain would lead to an increased release of reactive oxygen species capable of attacking nearby mitochondrial constituents.

Idiosyncratic Liver Injury—Idiosyncratic drug hepatotoxicity is a rare but potentially serious adverse event, which is not clearly dose-dependent, is at this point unpredictable, and affects only very few of the patients exposed to a drug or other chemicals. However, idiosyncratic toxicity is a leading cause for failure of drugs in clinical testing and it is the most frequent reason for posting warnings, restricting use, or even withdrawal of the drug from the market (Table 13–4). In addition, idiosyncratic hepatotoxicity is observed after consumption of herbal remedies and food supplements. Because idiosyncratic hepatotoxicity is a rare event for most drugs, it is likely that a combination of gene defects and adverse events need to be present simultaneously in an individual to trigger the severe liver injury. A detailed genomic analysis of patients with idiosyncratic responses to drug exposure may give additional insight as to what gene expression profile renders a patient susceptible.

FUTURE DIRECTIONS

Continued progress in the understanding of drug- and chemical-induced hepatotoxicity will depend on the use of relevant in vivo and in vitro models including human hepatocytes and analysis of human liver tissue. Traditional mechanistic investigations in combination with genomic and proteomic approaches have the greatest potential to yield important new insight into pathophysiologic mechanisms. Progress in the understanding of the liver's response to known hepatotoxicants and other adverse conditions will not only aid in the development of therapies to limit and reverse acute and chronic liver injury, but also improve the predictability of the potential hepatotoxicity of new drugs and other chemicals.

BIBLIOGRAPHY

Boyer TD, Manns MP, Sanyal AJ (eds.): *Zakim and Boyer's Hepatology: A Textbook of Liver Disease.* 6th ed. Philadelphia, PA: Saunders and Elsevier, 2012.

Crawford JM: *The Liver and the Biliary Tract.* In Kumar V, Abbas AK, Fausto N, Aster JC (eds.): *Robbins and Cotran: Pathologic Basis of Disease.* 8th ed. Philadelphia, PA: Saunders, 2010.

Kaplowitz N, Deleve LD (eds.): *Drug-induced Liver Disease.* 3rd ed. Waltham, MA: Academic Press/Elsevier, 2013.

Sahu S: *Hepatotoxicity: From Genomics to In Vitro and In Vivo Models.* Hoboken, NJ: John Wiley, 2007.

QUESTIONS

1. The impairment of hepatic function can have numerous negative consequences. Which of the following is likely NOT caused by impaired hepatic function?
   a. jaundice.
   b. hypercholesterolemia.
   c. hyperammonemia.
   d. hyperglycemia.
   e. hypoalbuminemia.

2. All of the following statements regarding the liver are true EXCEPT:
   a. The major role of the liver is to maintain metabolic homeostasis of the body.
   b. The liver encounters ingested nutrients before the heart does.
   c. Hepatic triads contain a branch of the hepatic portal vein, a branch of the hepatic artery, and a bile ductule.
   d. The liver manufactures and stores bile.
   e. The large fenestrae of hepatic sinusoids facilitate exchange of materials between the sinusoid and the hepatocyte.

3. Activation of which of the following cell types can result in increased secretion of collagen scar tissue, leading to cirrhosis?
   a. hepatocyte.
   b. Ito cell.
   c. Kupffer cell.
   d. endothelial cell.
   e. β-cell.

4. Wilson's disease is a rare genetic disorder characterized by the failure to export which of the following metals into bile?
   a. iron.
   b. zinc.
   c. silver.
   d. lead.
   e. copper.

5. Which of the following is NOT characteristic of apoptosis?
   a. cell swelling.
   b. nuclear fragmentation.
   c. lack of inflammation.
   d. programmed death.
   e. chromatin condensation.

6. A patient suffering from canalicular cholestasis would NOT be expected to exhibit which of the following?
   a. increased bile salt serum levels.
   b. jaundice.
   c. increased bile formation.
   d. dark brown urine.
   e. vitamin A deficiency.

7. Which of the following statements regarding liver injury is FALSE?
   a. Large doses of acetaminophen have been shown to cause a blockade of hepatic sinusoids.
   b. Hydrophilic drugs readily diffuse into hepatocytes because of the large sinusoidal fenestrations.
   c. There are sinusoidal transporters that take toxicants up into hepatocytes.
   d. Hepatocellular cancer has been associated with androgen abuse.
   e. In cirrhosis, excess collagen is laid down in response to direct injury or inflammation.

8. The inheritance of a "slow" aldehyde dehydrogenase enzyme would result in which of the following after the ingestion of ethanol?
   a. high ethanol tolerance.
   b. little response to low doses of ethanol.
   c. low serum levels of acetaldehyde.
   d. nausea.
   e. increased levels of blood ethanol compared to an individual with a normal aldehyde dehydrogenase.

9. Which of the following is not a common mechanism of hepatocellular injury?
   a. deformation of the hepatocyte cytoskeleton.
   b. mitochondrial injury.
   c. cholestasis.
   d. interference with vesicular transport.
   e. increased transcytosis between hepatocytes.

10. Ethanol is not known to cause which of the following types of hepatobiliary injury?
    a. fatty liver.
    b. hepatocyte death.
    c. fibrosis.
    d. immune-mediated responses.
    e. canalicular cholestasis.

Toxic Responses of the Kidney

Rick G. Schnellmann

The functional integrity of the mammalian kidney is vital to total body homeostasis because the kidney plays a principal role in the excretion of metabolic wastes and in the regulation of extracellular fluid volume, electrolyte composition, and acid–base balance. In addition, the kidney synthesizes and releases hormones, such as renin and erythropoietin, and metabolizes vitamin D_3 to the active 1,25-dihydroxyvitamin D_3 form. A toxic insult to the kidney therefore could disrupt any or all of these functions and could have profound effects on total body metabolism.

FUNCTIONAL ANATOMY

Gross examination of a sagittal section of the kidney reveals three clearly demarcated anatomical areas: the cortex, medulla, and papilla (Figure 14–1). The cortex constitutes the major portion of the kidney and receives a disproportionately higher percentage (90%) of blood flow compared with the medulla (~6% to 10%) or papilla (1% to 2%). Thus, when a bloodborne toxicant is delivered to the kidney, a high percentage of the material will be delivered to the cortex and will have a greater opportunity to influence cortical rather than medullary or papillary functions. However, medullary and papillary tissues are exposed to higher luminal concentrations of toxicants for prolonged periods of time, a consequence of the more concentrated tubular fluid and the more sluggish flow of blood and filtrate in these regions.

The functional unit of the kidney, the nephron, may be considered in three portions: the vascular element, the glomerulus, and the tubular element.

Renal Vasculature and Glomerulus

The renal artery branches successively into interlobar, arcuate, interlobular arteries and afferent arterioles that supply the glomerulus (Figure 14–1). Blood then leaves the glomerular capillaries via the efferent arterioles. Both the afferent and efferent arterioles control glomerular capillary pressure and glomerular plasma flow rate. These arterioles are innervated by the sympathetic nervous system and respond to nerve stimulation, angiotensin II, vasopressin (also called arginine vasopressin [AVP], anti-diuretic hormone [ADH]), endothelin, adenosine, and norepinephrine. The efferent arterioles draining the cortical glomeruli branch into a peritubular capillary network, whereas those draining the juxtamedullary glomeruli form a capillary loop, called the vasa recta (literally, straight vessels), supplying the medullary structures. These postglomerular capillary loops provide delivery of nutrients to the postglomerular tubular structures, delivery of wastes to the tubule for excretion, and return of reabsorbed electrolytes, nutrients, and water to the systemic circulation.

The glomerulus is a complex, specialized capillary bed composed primarily of endothelial cells that are characterized by an attenuated and fenestrated cytoplasm, visceral epithelial cells characterized by a cell body (podocyte) from which many trabeculae and pedicles (foot processes) extend, and a glomerular basement membrane (GBM), which is a trilamellar structure sandwiched between the endothelial and epithelial cells (Figure 14–2). A portion of the blood entering the glomerular capillary network is fractionated into a virtually protein-free and cell-free ultrafiltrate, which passes through Bowman's space and into the tubular portion of the nephron. The formation of such an ultrafiltrate is the net result of the balance between transcapillary hydrostatic pressure and colloid oncotic pressure. An additional determinant of ultrafiltration is the effective hydraulic permeability of the glomerular capillary wall, in other words, the ultrafiltration coefficient (K_f), which is determined by the total surface area available for filtration and the hydraulic permeability of the capillary wall. Consequently, chemically induced decreases in glomerular filtration rate (GFR) may be related to decreases in transcapillary hydrostatic pressure and glomerular plasma flow due to increased afferent arteriolar resistance or to decreases in the surface area available for filtration, resulting from decreases in the size and/or number of endothelial fenestrae or detachment or effacement of foot processes.

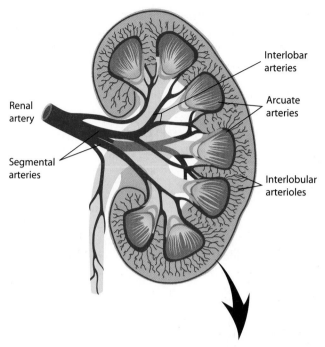

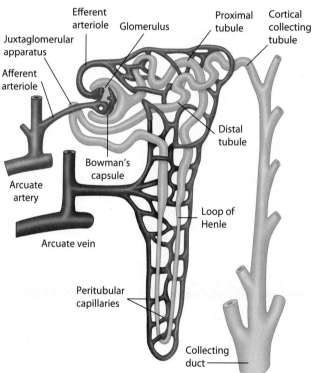

FIGURE 14–1 **Schematic of the human kidney showing the major blood vessels and the microcirculation and tubular components of each nephron.** (Reproduced with permission from Guyton AC, Hall JE: *Textbook of Medical Physiology*. 9th edition. Philadelphia, PA: Saunders/Elsevier; 1996.)

such as inulin (MW ~5 500), are freely filtered, whereas large molecules, such as albumin (MW 56 000–70 000), are restricted. Filtration of anionic molecules tends to be restricted compared to that of neutral or cationic molecules of the same size; this is primarily due to the charge-selective properties of the GBM (Figure 14–2).

Proximal Tubule

The proximal tubule consists of three discrete segments: the S_1 (pars convoluta), S_2 (transition between pars convoluta and pars recta), and S_3 (pars recta) segments. The formation of urine is a highly complex and integrated process in which the volume and composition of the glomerular filtrate is progressively altered as fluid passes through each of the different tubular segments. The proximal tubule is the workhorse of the nephron, as it reabsorbs approximately 60% to 80% of solute and water filtered at the glomerulus, mostly by numerous transport systems capable of driving the concentrative transport of many metabolic substrates. Toxicant-induced injury to the proximal

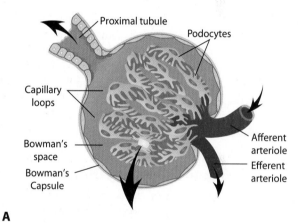

A

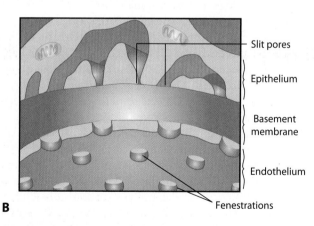

B

FIGURE 14–2 **Schematic of the ultrastructure of the glomerular capillary (A); cross section of the glomerular capillary membrane with the capillary epithelium, basement membrane and epithelium podocytes.** (Reproduced with permission from Guyton AC, Hall JE: *Textbook of Medical Physiology*. 9th edition. Philadelphia, PA: Saunders/Elsevier; 1996)

Although the glomerular capillary wall permits a high rate of fluid filtration (~20% of blood entering the glomerulus is filtered in a single pass), it provides a significant barrier to the transglomerular passage of macromolecules. Thus, small molecules, tubule therefore will have major consequences to water and solute balance.

The proximal tubule also reabsorbs virtually all the filtered low-molecular-weight proteins by specific endocytotic protein reabsorption processes. An important excretory function of the proximal tubule is secretion of weak organic anions and cations by specialized transporters that drive concentrative movement of these ions from postglomerular blood into proximal tubular cells, followed by secretion into tubular fluid. Toxicant-induced interruptions in the production of energy for any of these active transport mechanisms or the function of critical membrane-bound enzymes or transporters can profoundly affect proximal tubular and whole-kidney function.

Loop of Henle

The thin descending and ascending limbs and the thick ascending limb of the loop of Henle are critical to the processes involved in urinary concentration (Figure 14–1). Approximately 25% of the filtered Na^+ and K^+ and 20% of the filtered water are reabsorbed by the segments of the loop of Henle. The tubular fluid entering the thin descending limb is iso-osmotic to the renal interstitium; water is freely permeable and solutes, such as electrolytes and urea, may enter from the interstitium. In contrast, the thin ascending limb is relatively impermeable to water and urea, and Na^+ and Cl^- are reabsorbed by passive diffusion. The thick ascending limb is impermeable to water, and electrolytes are reabsorbed by the active $Na^+/K^+/2Cl^-$ cotransport mechanism, with the energy provided by the Na^+,K^+-ATPase.

Distal Tubule and Collecting Duct

The macula densa comprises specialized cells located between the end of the thick ascending limb and the early distal tubule, in close proximity to the afferent arteriole (Figure 14–1). Under normal physiologic conditions, increased solute delivery or concentration at the macula densa triggers a signal resulting in afferent arteriolar constriction leading to decreases in GFR (and hence decreased solute delivery). Thus, increases in fluid/solute out of the proximal tubule, due to impaired tubular reabsorption, will activate this feedback system, referred to as tubuloglomerular feedback (TGF) and resulting in decreases in the filtration rate of the same nephron. This regulatory mechanism is a volume-conserving mechanism, designed to decrease GFR and prevent massive losses of fluid/electrolytes due to impaired tubular reabsorption. Humoral mediation of TGF by the renin–angiotensin system has been proposed, and evidence suggests that other substances may be involved. The early distal tubule reabsorbs most of the remaining intraluminal Na^+, K^+, and Cl^- but is relatively impermeable to water.

The late distal tubule, cortical collecting tubule, and medullary collecting duct perform the final regulation and fine-tuning of urinary volume and composition. The remaining Na^+ is reabsorbed in conjunction with K^+ and H^+ secretion in the late distal tubule and cortical collecting tubule. The combination of medullary and papillary hypertonicity generated by countercurrent multiplication and the action of ADH serves to enhance water permeability of the medullary collecting duct. Chemicals that interfere with ADH action impair the concentrating ability of the distal nephron.

PATHOPHYSIOLOGIC RESPONSES OF THE KIDNEY

Acute Kidney Injury

One of the most common manifestations of nephrotoxic damage is acute renal failure (ARF) or acute kidney injury (AKI). AKI is characterized by an abrupt decline in GFR with resulting azotemia, or a buildup of nitrogenous wastes in the blood. AKI describes the entire spectrum of the disease and is defined as a complex disorder that comprises multiple causative factors with clinical manifestations ranging from minimal elevation in serum creatinine to anuric renal failure.

Any decline in GFR is complex and may result from prerenal factors (renal vasoconstriction, intravascular volume depletion, and insufficient cardiac output), postrenal factors (ureteral or bladder obstruction), and intrarenal factors (glomerulonephritis, tubular cell injury, death, and loss resulting in back-leak; renal vasculature damage; interstitial nephritis). Figure 14–3 illustrates the pathways that lead to diminished GFR following chemical exposure. Table 14–1 provides a partial list of chemicals that produce AKI through different mechanisms.

The maintenance of tubular integrity is dependent on cell-to-cell and cell-to-matrix adhesion (Figure 14–4). It has been hypothesized that after a chemical or hypoxic insult, adhesion of nonlethally damaged, apoptotic, and oncotic cells to the basement membrane is compromised, leading to gaps in the epithelial cell lining, potentially resulting in back-leak of filtrate and diminished GFR. These detached cells may aggregate in the tubular lumen (cell-to-cell adhesion) and/or adhere or reattach to adherent epithelial cells downstream, resulting in tubular obstruction.

Extensive evidence supports the idea that inflammatory cells play a role in ischemia-induced AKI. Injury to the renal vasculature endothelium results in chemokine and proinflammatory cytokine production and neutrophil adhesion, but the specific role of each inflammatory cell remains to be elucidated.

Adaptation Following Toxic Insult

The kidney has a remarkable ability to compensate for a loss in renal functional mass. Following a unilateral nephrectomy, GFR of the remnant kidney increases by approximately 40% to 60%. Compensatory increases in single-nephron GFR are accompanied by proportionate increases in proximal tubular water and solute reabsorption; glomerulotubular balance (i.e., constant fractional reabsorption of GFR by all segments of the nephron) is therefore maintained and overall renal function

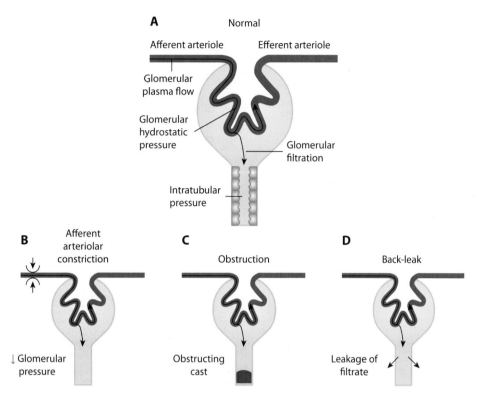

FIGURE 14–3 **Mechanisms of reduction of GFR. (A)** GFR depends on adequate blood flow to the glomerulus, adequate glomerular filtration pressure, glomerular permeability and low intratubular pressure. **(B)** Afferent arteriolar constriction decreases GFR by reducing blood flow, resulting in diminished capillary pressure. **(C)** Obstruction of the tubular lumen by cast formation increases tubular pressure; when tubular pressure exceeds glomerular capillary pressure, filtration decreases or ceases. **(D)** Back-leak occurs when the paracellular space between cells increases and the glomerular filtrate leaks into the extracellular space and bloodstream. (Reproduced with permission from Schrier RW: *Atlas of Diseases of the Kidney*. Philadelphia, PA: Current Medicine; 1999.)

appears normal by standard clinical tests. Consequently, chemically induced changes in renal function may not be detected until these compensatory mechanisms are overwhelmed by significant nephron loss and/or damage.

There are a number of cellular and molecular responses to a nephrotoxic insult. After a population of renal cells are exposed to a toxicant, a fraction of the cells will be severely injured and undergo cell death by apoptosis or oncosis (necrotic cell death). Those cells with nonlethal injuries

may undergo cell repair and/or adaptation, which contribute to the structural and functional recovery of the nephron (Figure 14–5). In addition, there is a population of uninjured cells that may undergo compensatory hypertrophy, cellular adaptation, and cellular proliferation. Tubular epithelial cells are primarily responsible for the structural and functional recovery of the nephron following injury by replacing dead and detached cells through de-differentiation, proliferation, migration, and re-differentiation.

TABLE 14–1 **Mechanisms of chemically induced acute kidney injury.**

Prerenal	Vasoconstriction	Crystalluria	Tubular Toxicity	Endothelial Injury	Glomerulopathy	Interstitial Nephritis
Diuretics	Nonsteroidal anti-inflammatory drugs	Sulfonamides	Aminoglycosides	Cyclosporine	Gold	Antibiotics
Angiotensin receptor antagonists	Radiocontrast agents	Methotrexate	Cisplatin	Mitomycin C	Penicillamine	Nonsteroidal anti-inflammatory drugs
Angiotensin converting enzyme inhibitors	Cyclosporine	Acyclovir	Vancomycin	Tacrolimus	Nonsteroidal anti-inflammatory drugs	Diuretics
	Tacrolimus	Triamterene	Pentamidine	Cocaine		
Antihypertensive agents	Amphotericin B	Ethylene glycol	Radiocontrast agents	Conjugated estrogens		
		Protease inhibitors	Heavy metals	Quinine		
			Haloalkane- and Haloalkene-cysteine conjugates			

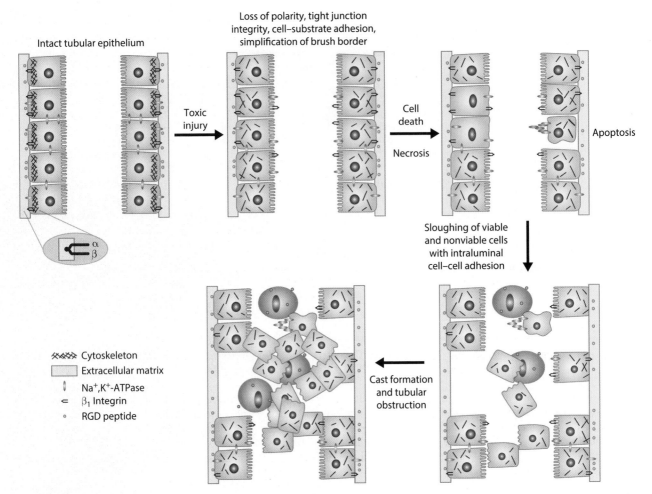

Intact tubular epithelium

Loss of polarity, tight junction integrity, cell–substrate adhesion, simplification of brush border

Toxic injury

Cell death

Necrosis

Apoptosis

Sloughing of viable and nonviable cells with intraluminal cell–cell adhesion

Cast formation and tubular obstruction

≈≈≈≈ Cytoskeleton
☐ Extracellular matrix
↕ Na$^+$,K$^+$-ATPase
⊂ β$_1$ Integrin
∘ RGD peptide

α
β

FIGURE 14–4 **After injury, alterations can occur in the cytoskeleton and in the normal distribution of membrane proteins such as Na$^+$,K$^+$-ATPase, and β1 integrins in sublethally injured renal tubular cells.** These changes result in loss of cell polarity, tight-junction integrity, and cell–substrate adhesion. Lethally injured cells undergo oncosis or apoptosis, and both dead and viable cells may be released into the tubular lumen. Adhesion of released cells to other released cells and to cells remaining adherent to the basement membrane may result in cast formation, tubular obstruction, and further compromise the GFR. (Reproduced with permission from Schrier RW: *Atlas of Diseases of the Kidney.* Philadelphia, PA: Current Medicine; 1999.)

Two of the most notable cellular adaptation responses are metallothionein induction and stress protein induction. The distribution of individual heat-shock proteins (Hsps) and glucose-regulated proteins (Grps) are two examples of stress protein families that are induced in response to a number of pathophysiologic states such as heat shock, anoxia, oxidative stress, toxicants, heavy metal exposure, and tissue trauma. The distribution of Hsps and Grps varies between different cell types in the kidney and within subcellular compartments. These proteins play important roles in protein folding, translocation of proteins across organelle membranes, prevention of aggregation of damaged proteins, and repair and degradation of damaged proteins, and thereby provide a defense mechanism against toxicity and/or for the facilitation of recovery and repair.

Chronic Kidney Disease

Progressive deterioration of renal function may occur with long-term exposure to various chemicals (e.g., analgesics,

lithium, and cyclosporine). Following nephron loss, adaptive increases in glomerular pressures and flows increase the single-nephron GFR of remnant viable nephrons, which serve to maintain whole-kidney GFR. With time, these alterations are maladaptive, and focal glomerulosclerosis eventually develops that may lead to tubular atrophy and interstitial fibrosis. Compensatory increases in glomerular pressures and flows of the remnant glomeruli may result in mechanical damage to the capillaries, leading to altered permeabilities.

SUSCEPTIBILITY OF THE KIDNEY TO TOXIC INJURY

Incidence and Severity of Toxic Nephropathy

A wide variety of drugs, environmental chemicals, and metals can cause site-specific nephrotoxicity (Table 14–1). The

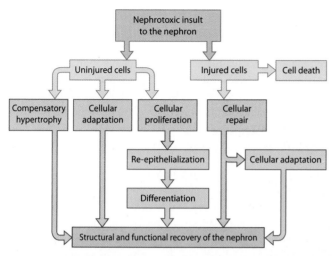

FIGURE 14–5 **The response of the nephron to a nephrotoxic insult.** After a population of cells is exposed to a nephrotoxicant, the cells respond; ultimately the nephron recovers function or, if cell death and loss are extensive, nephron function ceases. Terminally injured cells undergo cell death through oncosis or apoptosis. Cells injured sublethally undergo repair and adaptation in response to the nephrotoxicant. Cells not injured and adjacent to the injured area may undergo dedifferentiation, proliferation, migration or spreading, and differentiation. Cells not injured may also undergo compensatory hypertrophy in response to the cell loss and injury. Finally the uninjured cells also may undergo adaptation in response to a nephrotoxicant exposure. (Reproduced with permission from Schrier RW: *Atlas of Diseases of the Kidney*. Philadelphia, PA: Current Medicine; 1999.)

consequences of AKI vary from recovery to permanent renal damage, which may require dialysis or renal transplantation.

Reasons for the Susceptibility of the Kidney to Toxicity

Although the kidneys constitute only 0.5% of total body mass, they receive about 20% to 25% of the resting cardiac output. Consequently, any drug or chemical in the systemic circulation will be delivered to these organs in relatively high amounts. The processes involved in forming concentrated urine also serve to concentrate potential toxicants in the tubular fluid, thereby driving passive diffusion of toxicants into tubular cells. Therefore, a nontoxic concentration of a chemical in the plasma may reach toxic concentrations in the kidney and its tubules. Finally, renal transport, accumulation, and metabolism of xenobiotics contribute significantly to the susceptibility of the kidney to toxic injury.

In addition to intrarenal factors, the incidence and/or severity of chemically induced nephrotoxicity may be related to the sensitivity of the kidney to circulating vasoconstrictors (angiotensin II or ADH), whose actions are normally counterbalanced by the actions of increased vasodilatory prostaglandins. When prostaglandin synthesis is suppressed by nonsteroidal anti-inflammatory drugs (NSAIDs), renal blood flow (RBF)

declines markedly and AKI ensues due to the unopposed actions of vasoconstrictors. Another example of predisposing risk factors relates to the clinical use of angiotensin converting enzyme (ACE) inhibitors. Glomerular filtration pressure is dependent on angiotensin II–induced efferent arteriolar constriction. ACE inhibitors block this vasoconstriction, resulting in a precipitous decline in filtration pressure and AKI.

Site-Selective Injury

Many nephrotoxicants have their primary effects on discrete segments or regions of the nephron. The reasons underlying this site-selective injury are complex but can be attributed in part to site-specific differences in blood flow, transport and accumulation of chemicals, physicochemical properties of the epithelium, reactivity of cellular/molecular targets, balance of bioactivation/detoxification reactions, cellular energetics, and/or regenerative/repair mechanisms.

Glomerular Injury

The glomerulus is the initial site of chemical exposure within the nephron, and a number of nephrotoxicants produce structural injury to this segment. In certain instances, chemicals alter glomerular permeability to proteins by altering the size- and charge-selective functions.

Cyclosporine, amphotericin B, and gentamicin impair glomerular ultrafiltration without significant loss of structural integrity and decrease GFR. Amphotericin B decreases GFR by causing renal vasoconstriction and decreasing the glomerular capillary ultrafiltration coefficient (K_f). Gentamicin interacts with the anionic sites on the endothelial cells, decreasing K_f and GFR. Finally, cyclosporine not only causes renal vasoconstriction and vascular damage, but is also injurious to the glomerular endothelial cell.

Chemically induced glomerular injury may also be mediated by extrarenal factors. Circulating immune complexes may be trapped within the glomeruli (as could be the case in a type 3 hypersensitivity reaction). Neutrophils and macrophages are commonly observed within glomeruli in membranous glomerulonephritis, and the local release of cytokines and reactive oxygen species (ROS) may contribute to glomerular injury. Heavy metals, hydrocarbons, penicillamine, and captopril can produce this type of glomerular injury. A chemical may function as a hapten attached to some native protein or as a complete antigen and elicit an antibody response. Antibody reactions with cell-surface antigens (e.g., GBM) lead to immune deposit formation within the glomeruli, mediator activation, and subsequent injury to glomerular tissue.

Proximal Tubular Injury

The proximal tubule is the most common site of toxicant-induced renal injury. The reasons for this relate in part to the selective accumulation of xenobiotics into this segment of the nephron. The proximal tubule has a leaky epithelium, favoring the flux of compounds into proximal tubular cells. More importantly, tubular transport of organic anions and cations, low-molecular-weight proteins and peptides, GSH conjugates, and heavy metals is localized primarily if not exclusively to the proximal tubule. Thus, transport of these molecules will be greater in the proximal tubule than in other segments, resulting in proximal tubular accumulation and toxicity. Although correlations between proximal tubular transport, accumulation, and toxicity suggest that the site of transport is a crucial determinant of the site of toxicity, transport is unlikely to be the sole criterion.

In addition to segmental differences in transport, segmental differences in cytochrome P450 and cysteine conjugate β-lyase activity also are contributing factors to the enhanced susceptibility of the proximal tubule. Both enzyme systems are localized almost exclusively in the proximal tubule, with negligible activity in the glomerulus, distal tubules, or collecting ducts. Thus, nephrotoxicity requiring P450 and β-lyase-mediated bioactivation will most certainly be localized in the proximal tubule.

Finally, proximal tubular cells appear to be more susceptible to ischemic injury than distal tubular cells. Therefore, the proximal tubule will likely be the primary site of toxicity for chemicals that interfere with RBF, cellular energetics, and/or mitochondrial function.

Loop of Henle/Distal Tubule/Collecting Duct Injury

Functional abnormalities at distal nephron sites manifest primarily as impaired concentrating ability and/or acidification defects. Amphotericin B, cisplatin, and methoxyflurane induce an ADH-resistant polyuria, suggesting that the concentrating defect occurs at the level of the medullary thick ascending limb and/or the collecting duct.

Papillary Injury

The renal papilla is susceptible to the chronic injurious effects of abusive consumption of analgesics. The initial target of abusive consumption of analgesics is the medullary interstitial cells, followed by degenerative changes in the medullary capillaries, loops of Henle, and collecting ducts. High papillary concentrations of potential toxicants and inhibition of vasodilatory prostaglandins compromise RBF to the renal medulla/papilla and result in tissue ischemia.

ASSESSMENT OF RENAL FUNCTION

Both in vivo and in vitro methods are available for evaluation of the effects of a chemical on kidney function. Initially, nephrotoxicity can be assessed by evaluating serum and urine chemistries following treatment with the chemical in question. The standard battery of noninvasive tests includes measurement of urine volume and osmolality, pH, and urinary composition (e.g., electrolytes, glucose, and protein). Although specificity is often lacking in such an assessment, urinalysis provides a relatively easy and noninvasive assessment of overall renal functional integrity and can provide some insight into the nature of the nephrotoxic insult. The simultaneous analysis of cellular metabolites in sera and urine using nuclear magnetic analysis (metabonomics) has matured over the past few years and may provide an additional technology to identify and monitor nephrotoxicity.

Chemically induced increases in urine volume accompanied by decreases in osmolality may suggest an impaired concentrating ability, possibly via a defect in ADH synthesis, release, and/or action. Glucosuria may reflect chemically induced defects in proximal tubular reabsorption of sugars or be secondary to hyperglycemia. Urinary excretion of high-molecular-weight proteins, such as albumin, is suggestive of glomerular damage, whereas excretion of low-molecular-weight proteins, such as β_2-microglobulin, suggests proximal tubular injury. Urinary excretion of enzymes localized in the brush border (e.g., alkaline phosphatase and γ-glutamyl transferase) may reflect brush-border damage, whereas urinary excretion of other enzymes (e.g., lactate dehydrogenase) may reflect more generalized cell damage. Enzymuria is often a transient phenomenon, as chemically induced damage may result in an early loss of most of the enzyme available. Thus, the absence of enzymuria does not necessarily reflect an absence of damage.

GFR can be measured directly by determining creatinine or inulin clearance, both of which are essentially freely filtered and not reabsorbed or secreted. Therefore, the clearance of creatinine or inulin is about the same as the GFR. Creatinine is an endogenous compound released from skeletal muscle. Inulin is an exogenous compound. Creatinine or inulin clearance is determined by the following formula:

$$\text{Inulin clearance (mL/min)} = \frac{\text{Inulin concentration in urine (mg/L)} \times \text{Urine volume (mL/min)}}{\text{Inulin concentration in serum (mg/L)}}$$

Indirect markers of GFR are serial blood urea nitrogen (BUN) and serum creatinine concentrations. However, a 50% to 70% decrease in GFR must occur before increases in serum creatinine and BUN develop. Chemically induced increases in BUN and/or serum creatinine may not necessarily reflect renal damage, but rather may be secondary to dehydration, hypovolemia, and/or protein catabolism. Serum cystatin C levels may be more sensitive as a marker of mildly impaired GFR.

Histopathologic evaluation of the kidney following treatment is crucial in identifying the site, nature, and severity of the nephrotoxic lesion. Assessment of chemically induced nephrotoxicity therefore should include urinalysis, serum clinical chemistry, and histopathology to provide a reasonable profile of the functional and morphologic effects of a chemical on the kidney. Site-specific biomarkers for common nephrotoxicants are shown in Figure 14–6.

Various in vitro techniques may be used to elucidate underlying mechanisms of chemically induced nephrotoxicity.

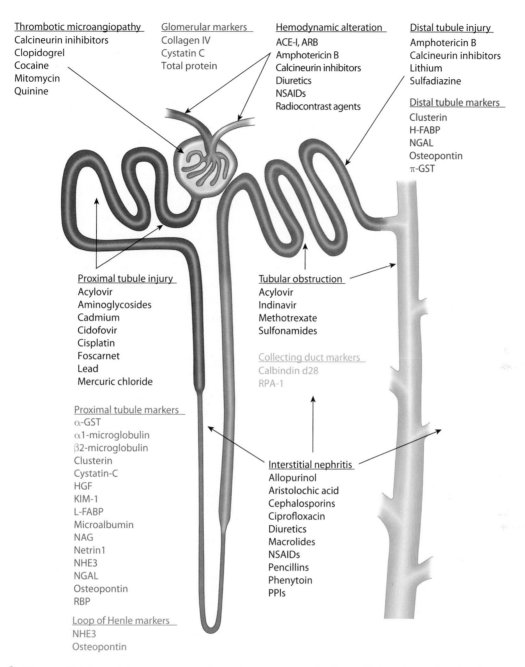

Thrombotic microangiopathy
Calcineurin inihibitors
Clopidogrel
Cocaine
Mitomycin
Quinine

Glomerular markers
Collagen IV
Cystatin C
Total protein

Hemodynamic alteration
ACE-I, ARB
Amphotericin B
Calcineurin inhibitors
Diuretics
NSAIDs
Radiocontrast agents

Distal tubule injury
Amphotericin B
Calcineurin inhibitors
Lithium
Sulfadiazine

Distal tubule markers
Clusterin
H-FABP
NGAL
Osteopontin
π-GST

Proximal tubule injury
Acylovir
Aminoglycosides
Cadmium
Cidofovir
Cisplatin
Foscarnet
Lead
Mercuric chloride

Proximal tubule markers
α-GST
α1-microglobulin
β2-microglobulin
Clusterin
Cystatin-C
HGF
KIM-1
L-FABP
Microalbumin
NAG
Netrin1
NHE3
NGAL
Osteopontin
RBP

Loop of Henle markers
NHE3
Osteopontin

Tubular obstruction
Acylovir
Indinavir
Methotrexate
Sulfonamides

Collecting duct markers
Calbindin d28
RPA-1

Interstitial nephritis
Allopurinol
Aristolochic acid
Cephalosporins
Ciprofloxacin
Diuretics
Macrolides
NSAIDs
Pencillins
Phenytoin
PPIs

FIGURE 14–6 Site-specific biomarkers, common nephrotoxicants, and mechanisms of injury. (Reproduced with permission from McQueen CA, Schnellmann (eds): *Comprehensive Toxicology*. Oxford, UK: Elsevier; 2010.)

Freshly prepared isolated perfused kidneys, kidney slices, and renal tubular suspensions and cells exhibit the greatest degree of differentiated functions and similarity to the in vivo situation, but these models have limited life spans of 2 to 24 h. In contrast, primary cultures of renal cells and established renal cell lines exhibit longer life spans (> 2 weeks). Once a mechanism has been identified in vitro, the postulated mechanism must be tested in vivo. Thus, appropriately designed in vivo and in vitro studies should provide a complete characterization of the biochemical, functional, and morphologic effects of a chemical on the kidney and an understanding of the underlying mechanisms in the target cell population(s).

BIOCHEMICAL MECHANISMS/ MEDIATORS OF RENAL CELL INJURY

Cell Death

Cell death may occur through either oncosis or apoptosis. Apoptosis is a tightly controlled, organized process that usually affects scattered individual cells, which break into small fragments that are phagocytosed by adjacent cells or macrophages without producing an inflammatory response. In contrast, oncosis often affects many contiguous cells; the cells rupture, releasing cellular contents and inflammation follows. With many toxicants, lower but injurious concentrations produce cell death through apoptosis. As the concentration of the toxicant increases, oncosis plays a predominant role.

Mediators of Toxicity

A chemical can initiate cell injury by various mechanisms (Figure 14–5). The chemical may initiate toxicity due to its intrinsic reactivity with cellular macromolecules, may require renal or extrarenal bioactivation to a reactive intermediate, or may initiate injury indirectly by inducing oxidative stress via increased production of ROS, such as superoxide anion, hydrogen peroxide, and hydroxyl radicals. ROS and reactive nitrogen species from nitric oxide, such as peroxynitrite ($ONOO^-$), can attack proteins, lipids, and DNA to induce cellular injury and death.

Cellular/Subcellular and Molecular Targets

A number of cellular targets have been identified to play a role in cell death. It is generally thought that an intracellular interaction (e.g., an alkylating agent or ROS with a macromolecule) initiates a sequence of events that leads to cell death. In the case of oncosis, a "point of no return" is reached in which the cell will die regardless of any intervention. The idea of a single sequence of events is probably simplistic for most toxicants, given the extensive number of targets available for alkylating species and ROS. Rather, multiple pathways, with both distinct and common sequences of events, may lead to cell death.

Many cellular processes depend on mitochondrial ATP and, thus, become compromised simultaneously with inhibition of respiration. Conversely, mitochondrial dysfunction may be a consequence of some other cellular process altered by the toxicant. Numerous nephrotoxicants cause mitochondrial dysfunction in different ways. Whether toxicants target mitochondria directly or indirectly, it is clear that mitochondria play a critical role in determining whether cells die by apoptosis or oncosis. It is thought that the mitochondrial permeability transition (MPT) occurs during cell injury and ultimately progresses to apoptosis if sufficient ATP is available, or to oncosis if ATP is depleted. Further, the release of apoptotic proteins, such as apoptosis inducing factor, cytochrome c, Smac/Diablo, Omi, and Endonuclease G following MPT play a key role in activating downstream caspases and executing apoptosis.

Ca^{2+} is a second messenger and plays a critical role in a variety of cellular functions. Sustained elevations or abnormally large increases in cytosolic free Ca^{2+} can exert a number of detrimental effects on the cell. For example, an increase in cytosolic free Ca^{2+} can activate a number of degradative Ca^{2+}-dependent enzymes, such as phospholipases and proteinases (e.g., calpains), and can produce aberrations in the structure and function of cytoskeletal elements. Release of endoplasmic reticulum (ER) Ca^{2+} stores may be a key step in initiating the injury process and increasing cytosolic free Ca^{2+} concentrations, because prior depletion of ER Ca^{2+} stores protects renal proximal tubules from extracellular Ca^{2+} influx and cell death

produced by mitochondrial inhibition and hypoxia. Mitochondria are known to accumulate Ca^{2+} in lethally injured cells through a low-affinity, high-capacity Ca^{2+} transport system. Although this system plays a minor role in normal cellular Ca^{2+} regulation, under injurious conditions the uptake of Ca^{2+} may facilitate ROS formation and damage.

Signaling kinases such as protein kinase C, mitogen-activated protein kinases (e.g., ERK1/2, p38, JNK/SAPK), protein kinase B (Akt), src, and phosphoinositide-3-kinase phosphorylate other proteins and, thereby, alter their activity, expression, or localization. Numerous recent studies reveal critical roles for signaling kinases in renal cell death and in the recovery of renal cells after toxicant injury.

Cell volume and ion homeostasis are tightly regulated and are critical for the reabsorptive properties of the tubular epithelial cells. Toxicants generally disrupt cell volume and ion homeostasis by either increasing ion permeability or inhibiting energy production. Loss of ATP results in the inhibition of membrane transporters that maintain the internal ion balance.

SPECIFIC NEPHROTOXICANTS

Heavy Metals

Many metals—including cadmium, chromium, lead, mercury, platinum, and uranium—are nephrotoxic. The nature and severity of metal nephrotoxicity varies with respect to its form. In addition, different metals have different primary targets within the kidney. Metals may cause renal cellular injury through their ability to bind to sulfhydryl groups of critical proteins within the cells and thereby inhibit their normal function.

Mercury—Humans and animals are exposed to elemental mercury vapor, inorganic mercurous and mercuric salts, and organic mercuric compounds through the environment. Administered elemental mercury is rapidly oxidized in erythrocytes or tissues to inorganic mercury, and thus the tissue distribution of elemental and inorganic mercury is similar. Due to its high affinity for sulfhydryl groups, virtually all of the Hg^{2+} found in blood is bound to albumin, other sulfhydryl-containing proteins, glutathione, and cysteine.

The kidneys are the primary target organs for accumulation of Hg^{2+}, and the S_3 segment of the proximal tubule is the initial site of toxicity, but the S_1 and S_2 segments may become affected as dose or duration increases. Renal uptake of Hg^{2+} is very rapid with as much as 50% of a nontoxic dose of Hg^{2+} found in the kidneys within a few hours of exposure. Considering the fact that virtually all of the Hg^{2+} found in blood is bound to an endogenous ligand, it is likely that the luminal and/or basolateral transport of Hg^{2+} into the proximal tubular epithelial cell is through cotransport of Hg^{2+} with an endogenous ligand such as glutathione, cysteine, or albumin, or through some plasma membrane Hg^{2+}-ligand complex.

The acute nephrotoxicity induced by $HgCl_2$ is characterized by proximal tubular necrosis and AKI within 24 to 48 h after administration. Early markers of $HgCl_2$-induced renal dysfunction include an increase in the urinary excretion of brush-border enzymes such as alkaline phosphatase and γ-glutamyl transferase. Subsequently, when tubular injury becomes severe, intracellular enzymes, such as lactate dehydrogenase and aspartate aminotransferase, increase in the urine. As injury progresses, tubular reabsorption of solutes and water decreases and there is an increase in the urinary excretion of glucose, amino acids, albumin, and other proteins. Also associated with the increase in injured proximal tubules is a decrease and progressive decline in the GFR.

Changes in mitochondrial morphology and function are very early events following $HgCl_2$ administration, supporting the hypothesis that mitochondrial dysfunction is an early and important contributor to inorganic mercury-induced cell death along the proximal tubule.

Cadmium—Chronic exposure of nonsmoking humans and animals to cadmium is primarily through food and results in nephrotoxicity. In the workplace, inhalation of cadmium-containing dust and fumes is the major route of exposure. Cadmium has a half-life of greater than 10 years in humans and thus accumulates in the body over time. Approximately 50% of the body's burden of cadmium can be found in the kidney. Cadmium produces proximal tubule dysfunction (S_1 and S_2 segments) and injury that may progress to a chronic interstitial nephritis.

Chemically Induced α_{2u}-Globulin Nephropathy

A diverse group of chemicals, including unleaded gasoline, jet fuels, D-limonene, 1,4-dichlorobenzene, decalin, tetrachloroethylene, and lindane, causes α_{2u}-globulin nephropathy or hyaline droplet nephropathy in male rats. Binding to α_{2u}-globulin decreases lysosomal proteases breakdown of α_{2u}-globulin. Chronic exposure to these compounds results in progression of these lesions and ultimately in chronic nephropathy.

Humans are not at risk because (1) humans do not synthesize α_{2u}-globulin; (2) humans secrete less proteins in general and in particular less low-molecular-weight proteins in urine than the rat; (3) the low-molecular-weight proteins in human urine are either not related structurally to α_{2u}-globulin, do not bind to compounds that bind to α_{2u}-globulin, or are similar to proteins in female rats, male Black Reiter rats, rabbits, or guinea pigs that do not exhibit α_{2u}-globulin nephropathy; and (4) mice excrete a low-molecular-weight urinary protein that is 90% homologous to α_{2u}-globulin, but they do not exhibit α_{2u}-globulin-nephropathy and renal tumors following exposure to α_{2u}-globulin-nephropathy-inducing agents.

Halogenated Hydrocarbons

Halogenated hydrocarbons are a diverse class of compounds and are used extensively as chemical intermediates, solvents, and pesticides. Consequently, humans are exposed to these compounds not only in the workplace but also through the environment. Numerous toxic effects have been associated with acute and chronic exposure to halogenated hydrocarbons, including nephrotoxicity.

Chloroform—The primary cellular target of chloroform is the proximal tubule, with no primary damage to the glomerulus or the distal tubule. Proteinuria, glucosuria, and increased BUN levels are all characteristic of chloroform-induced nephrotoxicity. The nephrotoxicity produced by chloroform is linked to its metabolism by renal cytochrome P450, which biotransforms chloroform to trichloromethanol, which is unstable and releases HCl to form phosgene, which injuriously reacts with cellular macromolecules.

Tetrafluoroethylene—Tetrafluoroethylene is conjugated with glutathione in the liver, and the GSH conjugate is secreted into the bile and small intestine where it is degraded to the cysteine S-conjugate (TFEC), reabsorbed, and transported to the kidney. Although several metabolites are formed, the cysteine S-conjugate is the penultimate nephrotoxicant. Following transport into the proximal tubule, the cysteine S-conjugate is a substrate for the cytosolic and mitochondrial forms of the enzyme cysteine conjugate β-lyase. The products of the reaction are ammonia, pyruvate, and a reactive thiol that is capable of binding covalently to cellular macromolecules causing cellular damage. Functionally, increases in urinary glucose, protein, cellular enzymes, and BUN are noted.

Bromobenzene—Biotransformation of bromobenzene and other halogenated benzenes is critical for their nephrotoxicity. Hepatic cytochrome P450 metabolizes bromobenzene and conjugates it to glutathione, and releases it as a form that can cause nephrotoxicity. The diglutathione conjugate of the hydroquinone is approximately 1000-fold more potent than bromobenzene in producing nephrotoxicity, producing the same pathologic changes in the S_3 segment, and increasing the amount of protein, glucose, and cellular enzymes in the urine.

Mycotoxins

Mycotoxins are products of molds and fungi, and a number of mycotoxins produce nephrotoxicity. Three examples of nephrotoxic mycotoxins will be discussed. Citrinin nephrotoxicity is characterized by decreased urine osmolality, GFR and RBF, glycosuria, and increased urinary enzyme excretion. Interestingly, the location of citrinin-induced tubular vacuolization and necrosis (proximal, distal) varies among species. Whereas the mechanism of citrinin toxicity to the tubules remains unresolved, citrinin enters the cells through the organic anion transporter and causes mitochondrial dysfunction.

Fumonisins B_1 and B_2 are commonly found on corn and corn products and they are known to produce nephrotoxicity in rats and rabbits. Histologic examination of the kidney revealed disruption of the basolateral membrane, mitochondrial swelling, increased numbers of clear and electron-dense vacuoles, and apoptosis in proximal tubular cells at the junction of the cortex and medulla. Changes in renal function included increased urine volume, decreased osmolality, and increased excretion of low- and high-molecular-weight proteins. The toxicity of fumonisins may be through increased sphinganine, reactive oxygen species, and apoptosis.

Aristolochic acids (AAs) and aristolactams are natural products found in the *Aristolochia* and *Asarum* genera. Despite the extensive use of *Aristolochia* as a herbal remedy for thousands of years, recent reports of its human toxicity include tubular dysfunction, proteinuria, and interstitial fibrosis. AAs form covalent DNA adducts, and are genotoxic and carcinogenic. Renal uptake of the penultimate toxicant, AA-I, involves mOat-mediated transport, and it is bioactivated through nitro-reduction to produce DNA and protein adducts.

Therapeutic Agents

Acetaminophen—Acetaminophen (APAP) nephrotoxicity is characterized by proximal tubular necrosis with increases in BUN and plasma creatinine, decreases in GFR and clearance of *para*-aminohippurate, increases in the fractional excretion of water, sodium, and potassium, and increases in urinary glucose, protein, and brush-border enzymes. Although renal cytochrome P450 plays a role in APAP activation and nephrotoxicity, glutathione conjugates of APAP may also contribute to APAP-induced nephrotoxicity.

Nonsteroidal Anti-inflammatory Drugs—NSAIDs such as aspirin, ibuprofen, naproxen, indomethacin, and cyclooxygenase-2 inhibitors (e.g., celecoxib) are extensively used as analgesics and anti-inflammatory drugs and produce their therapeutic effects through the inhibition of prostaglandin synthesis. At least three different types of nephrotoxicity have been associated with NSAID administration. AKI may occur within hours of a large dose of a NSAID, is usually reversible on withdrawal of the drug, and is characterized by decreased RBF and GFR and by oliguria. When normal production of vasodilatory prostaglandins (e.g., PGE_2, PGI_2) is inhibited by NSAIDs, vasoconstriction induced by circulating catecholamines and angiotensin II is unopposed, resulting in decreased RBF and ischemia.

In contrast, chronic consumption of NSAIDs and/or APAP (> 3 years) results in an often irreversible nephrotoxicity that is known as analgesic nephropathy. The primary lesion is papillary necrosis with chronic interstitial nephritis. The mechanism by which NSAIDs produce analgesic nephropathy is not known but may result from chronic medullary/papillary ischemia, secondary to renal vasoconstriction, or genesis of a reactive intermediate that, in turn, initiates an oxidative stress or binds covalently to critical cellular macromolecules.

The third albeit rare type of nephrotoxicity associated with NSAIDs is an interstitial nephritis. Patients normally present with elevated serum creatinine and proteinuria. If NSAIDs are discontinued, renal function improves in 1 to 3 months.

Aminoglycosides—The aminoglycoside antibiotics are so named because they consist of two or more amino sugars

joined in a glycosidic linkage to a central hexose nucleus. Although they are drugs of choice for many gram-negative infections, their use is primarily limited by their nephrotoxicity. Renal dysfunction by aminoglycosides is characterized by a nonoliguric renal failure with reduced GFR, an increase in serum creatinine and BUN, and polyuria. Within 24 h, increases in urinary brush-border enzymes, glucosuria, aminoaciduria, and proteinuria are observed. Histologically, lysosomal alterations are noted initially, followed by damage to the brush border, ER, mitochondria, and cytoplasm, ultimately leading to tubular cell necrosis. Interestingly, proliferation of renal proximal tubule cells can be observed early after the onset of nephrotoxicity.

The earliest lesion observed following clinically relevant doses of aminoglycosides is an increase in the size and number of lysosomes, which contain phospholipids. The renal phospholipidosis produced by the aminoglycosides is thought to occur through their inhibition of lysosomal hydrolases, such as sphingomyelinase and phospholipases.

Amphotericin B—Amphotericin B is an effective antifungal agent, causing nephrotoxicity characterized by ADH-resistant polyuria, renal tubular acidosis, hypokalemia, and either acute or chronic renal failure. The functional integrity of the glomerulus and of the proximal and distal portions of the nephron is impaired, leading to decreases in RBF and GFR secondary to renal arteriolar vasoconstriction or activation of tubuloglomerular feedback.

Cyclosporine—Cyclosporine is an important immunosuppressive agent and is widely used to prevent graft rejection in organ transplantation. Cyclosporine is a fungal cyclic polypeptide and acts by selectively inhibiting cyclophylin and, in turn, calcineurin and T-cell activation. Nephrotoxicity is a critical side effect of cyclosporine, with nearly all patients who receive the drug exhibiting some form of nephrotoxicity. Cyclosporine-induced nephrotoxicity may manifest as (1) acute reversible renal dysfunction, (2) acute vasculopathy, and (3) chronic nephropathy with interstitial fibrosis. Acute renal dysfunction is characterized by dose-related decreases in RBF and GFR and increases in BUN and serum creatinine. The decrease in RBF and GFR is related to marked vasoconstriction induced by cyclosporine.

Acute vasculopathy or thrombotic microangiopathy following cyclosporine treatment affects arterioles and glomerular capillaries, without an inflammatory component. The lesion consists of fibrin–platelet thrombi and fragmented red blood cells occluding the vessels.

Long-term treatment with cyclosporine can result in chronic nephropathy with interstitial fibrosis and tubular atrophy. Modest elevations in serum creatinine and decreases in GFR occur along with hypertension, proteinuria, and tubular dysfunction. Histologic changes are profound; they are characterized by arteriolopathy, global and segmental glomerular sclerosis, striped interstitial fibrosis, and tubular atrophy. These lesions may not be reversible if cyclosporine therapy is discontinued and may result in end-stage renal disease.

Cisplatin—Cisplatin is a valuable drug in the treatment of solid tumors, with nephrotoxicity limiting its clinical use. The kidney is not only responsible for the majority of cisplatin excreted but is also the primary site of accumulation. Cisplatin nephrotoxicity includes acute and chronic renal failure, renal magnesium wasting, and polyuria. Patients treated with cisplatin regimens permanently lose 10% to 30% of their renal function.

The nephrotoxicity of cisplatin can be grouped as (1) tubular toxicity, (2) vascular damage, (3) glomerular injury, and (4) interstitial injury. Early effects of cisplatin are decreases in RBF and polyuria that is concurrent with increased electrolyte excretion. GFR is produced by vasoconstriction and is followed by tubular injury with enzymuria. Although the primary cellular target associated with AKI is the proximal tubule S_3 segment in the rat, in humans the S_1 and S_2 segments, distal tubule, and collecting ducts can also be affected. Cisplatin may produce nephrotoxicity through its ability to inhibit DNA synthesis as well as transport functions. In addition, cisplatin is known to induce mitochondrial dysfunction and activates numerous pathways in the mitogen-activated protein kinase family.

Radiocontrast Agents—Iodinated contrast media used for the imaging of tissues have a very high osmolality (> 1200 mOsm/L) and are potentially nephrotoxic, particularly in patients with existing renal impairment, diabetes, or heart failure or who are receiving other nephrotoxic drugs. The newer nonionic contrast agents (e.g., iotrol and iopamidol) have lower nephrotoxicity. The nephrotoxicity of these agents is due to both hemodynamic alterations (vasoconstriction) and tubular injury (via ROS).

BIBLIOGRAPHY

Brenner BM, Rector FC (eds.): *Brenner and Rector's The Kidney*, 9th ed. Philadelphia, PA: Saunders Elsevier, 2011.

Fogo AB, Kashgarian M: *Diagnostic Atlas of Renal Pathology: Expert Consult*, 2nd ed. Philadelphia, PA: Elsevier Saunders, 2011.

Tarloff JB, Lash LH (eds.): *Toxicology of the Kidney*, 3rd ed. Boca Raton, FL: CRC Press, 2005.

QUESTIONS

1. The kidney is responsible for all of the following EXCEPT:
   a. synthesis of renin.
   b. acid–base balance.
   c. reabsorption of electrolytes.
   d. regulation of extracellular fluid.
   e. release of angiotensin.

2. Which of the following does NOT contribute to filtrate formation in the nephron?
   a. capillary hydrostatic pressure.
   b. positive charge of glomerular capillary wall.
   c. hydraulic permeability of glomerular capillary wall.
   d. colloid oncotic pressure.
   e. size of filtration slits.

3. Which of the following is NOT a characteristic of the loop of Henle?
   a. There is reabsorption of filtered Na^+ and K^+.
   b. Tubular fluid in the thin descending limb is iso-osmotic to the renal interstitium.
   c. Water is freely permeable in the thin ascending limb.
   d. Na^+ and Cl^- are reabsorbed in the thin ascending limb.
   e. The thick ascending limb is impermeable to water.

4. Although the kidneys constitute 0.5% of total body mass, approximately how much of the resting cardiac output do they receive?
   a. 0.5% to 1%.
   b. 5%.
   c. 10%.
   d. 20% to 25%.
   e. 50% to 60%.

5. Which of the following is most likely to occur after a toxic insult to the kidney?
   a. GFR will decrease in the unaffected kidney.
   b. Tight-junction integrity will increase in the nephron.
   c. The unaffected cells will undergo atrophy and proliferation.
   d. Clinical tests will likely show normal renal function.
   e. Glomerulotubular balance is lost.

6. Chronic renal failure does not typically result in:
   a. decrease in GFR of viable nephrons.
   b. glomerulosclerosis.
   c. tubular atrophy.
   d. increased glomerular pressures.
   e. altered capillary permeability.

7. All of the following statements regarding toxicity to the kidney are true EXCEPT:
   a. Concentration of toxins in tubular fluid increase the likelihood that the toxin will diffuse into tubular cells.
   b. Drugs in the systemic circulation are delivered to the kidneys at relatively high amounts.
   c. The distal convoluted tubule is the most common site of toxicant-induced renal injury.
   d. Immune complex deposition within the glomeruli can lead to glomerulonephritis.
   e. Antibiotics and/or antifungal drugs affect the functioning of the nephron at multiple locations.

8. Which of the following test results is NOT correctly paired with the underlying kidney problem?
   a. increased urine volume—defect in ADH synthesis.
   b. glucosuria—defect in reabsorption in the proximal convoluted tubule.
   c. proteinuria—glomerular damage.
   d. proteinuria—proximal tubular injury.
   e. brush-border enzymuria—glomerulonephritis.

9. Renal cell injury is NOT commonly mediated by which of the following mechanisms?
   a. loss of membrane integrity.
   b. impairment of mitochondrial function.
   c. increased cytosolic Ca^{2+} concentration.
   d. increased Na^+,K^+-ATPase activity.
   e. caspase activation.

10. Which of the following statements is FALSE with respect to nephrotoxicants?
    a. Mercury poisoning can lead to proximal tubular necrosis and acute renal failure.
    b. Cisplatin may cause nephrotoxicity because of its ability to inhibit DNA synthesis.
    c. Chronic consumption of NSAIDs results in nephrotoxicity that is reversible with time.
    d. Amphotericin B nephrotoxicity can result in ADH-resistant polyuria.
    e. Acetaminophen becomes nephrotoxic via activation by renal cytochrome P450.

Toxic Responses of the Respiratory System

George D. Leikauf

Toxic substances can disrupt the respiratory system and distant organs after chemicals enter the body by means of inhalation. Pathological changes in the respiratory tract also can be a target of blood-borne agents. *Inhalation toxicology* refers to the route of exposure, whereas *respiratory toxicology* refers to target organ toxicity. Lung tissue can be injured directly or secondarily by metabolic products from organic compounds. However, the most important effect of many toxic inhalants is to place an undue oxidative burden on the lungs.

RESPIRATORY TRACT STRUCTURE AND FUNCTION

Oronasal Passages

Structure—The respiratory tract is divided into the upper respiratory tract (extrathoracic airway passages above the neck) and lower respiratory track (airway passages and lung parenchyma below the pharynx) (Figure 15–1). The upper respiratory track reaches from the nostril or mouth to the pharynx and functions to conduct, heat, humidify, filter, and chemosense incoming air. Leaving the nasal passage, air is warmed to about 33°C and humidified to about 98% water saturation. Air is filtered in the nasal passages with highly water-soluble gases being absorbed efficiently. The nasal passages also filter particles, which may be deposited by impaction or diffusion on the nasal mucosa.

Sensory Functions—In addition to conducting, conditioning, and filtering air to the lower respiratory tract, a major function of the oronasal passage is chemosensory. Nasal epithelia can metabolize many foreign compounds by cytochrome P450 and other enzymes. Humans can distinguish between more than 5000 odors. The detection of odor can be protective and can induce avoidance behaviors. Odorant can be added to the otherwise colorless and almost odorless gas used by consumers (e.g., mercaptans to methane), to assist in detecting leaks and thereby preventing fires or explosions.

Chemosensory function of the nasal passages is accomplished by a wide variety of specialized receptors in major subtypes including (1) olfactory receptors, (2) trace amine–associated receptors (TAARs), (3) membrane guanylyl cyclase GC-D receptors, (4) vomeronasal receptors, and (5) formyl peptide receptors (FPRs).

The olfactory epithelium contains specialized chemosensory olfactory neurons located in the superior portion of the nasal passage. Airflow in this region of the nasal passage is typically low, thus sniffing can increase perception. TAARs detect trace amines, with fishy or putrid odor, that are found in foods and can also be generated during fermentation or decay. GC-D receptors are located in the cilia of olfactory sensory neurons and detect the natriuretic peptides, uroguanylin (found in urine) and guanylin. In rodents, these receptors detect carbon dioxide, which is odorless in humans and other primates. Vomeronasal receptors are separate from, but adjacent to, olfactory neurons. They can detect higher molecular weight stimuli, including nonvolatile chemicals. FPRs are also a part of the vomeronasal system and detect bacterial or mitochondrial formylated peptides, which are thought to identify pathogens or pathogenic states.

Irritant, Thermosensory, and Mechanosensory Functions—In addition to the detection of odor, the detection of irritant chemicals, cold and hot temperatures, or mechanical stress can be a protective mechanism that may limit exposure. The main nerve endings that perceive irritants, the chemical nociceptors also discern temperature and mechanical stress. Two protein families, the transient receptor potential (TRP) channels and the taste (TAS) receptors, perform these functions in the upper respiratory tract. TRP channels are ion channels that are permeable to cations, including calcium, magnesium, and sodium. These receptors are sensitive to a variety of natural ingredients, pain stimuli, and heat. Taste buds, which contain TAS, determine salt, sour, sweet, umami (glutamate and nucleotides), and bitter.

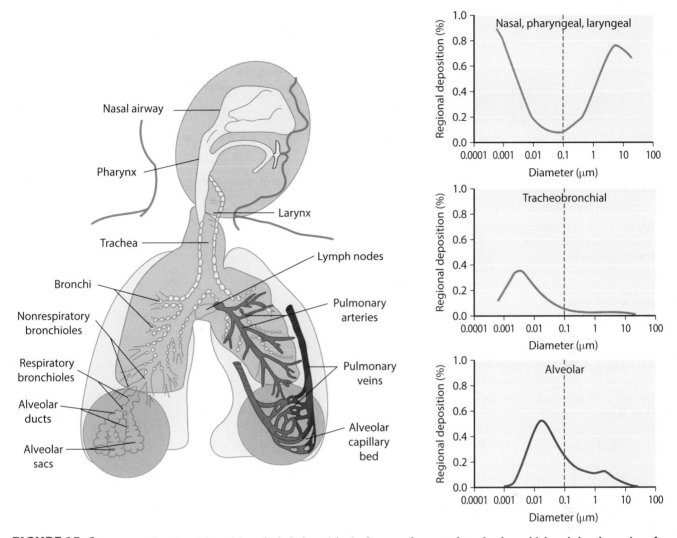

FIGURE 15–1 Predicted fractional deposition of inhaled particles in the nasopharyngeal, tracheobronchial, and alveolar region of the human respiratory tract during nose breathing. (Used with permission of J. Harkema.) (Reproduced with permission from Oberdorster G, Oberdorster E, Oberdorster J: Nanotoxicology: an emerging discipline evolving from studies of ultrafine particles, *Environ Health Perspect*, 2005 Jul;113(7):823–839.)

Conducting Airways

Structure—At the beginning of the lower respiratory track is the larynx, which is responsible for speech (phonation). The conducting airways of the lower respiratory tract can be divided into proximal (trachea and bronchi) and distal regions (bronchioles). Conducting airways have a bifurcating structure, with successive airway generations containing about twice the number of bronchi progressively decreasing in internal diameter. Eventually a transition zone is reached where cartilaginous bronchi give way to noncartilaginous bronchioles, which in turn give way to gas exchange regions, respiratory bronchioles, and alveoli. In the bronchiolar epithelium, mucus-producing cells and glands give way to bronchiolar secretoglobin cells (BSCs). One way in which airflow is altered is by smooth muscle that surrounds the airways and is under autonomic innervation via the vagus nerve.

Mucociliary Clearance and Antimicrobial Functions—

In humans, the proximal airway and a portion of the nasal passage are covered by a pseudostratified respiratory epithelium that contains a number of specialized cells including ciliated, mucous, and basal cells (Figure 15–2). These cells work together to form a mucous layer that traps and removes inhaled material via mucociliary clearance. For mucociliary clearance in the airways to function optimally, regulation of ion transport, fluid, and mucus must be coordinated. Chloride ion channels and the cystic fibrosis transmembrane regulator are needed to move fluid into the airway lumen and sodium channels are needed to move water out of the lumen.

Ciliated cells have microtubule-based protrusions, cilia, of which there are two types: motile and primary. Motile cilia exert mechanical force through continuous motion to propel harmful inhaled material out of the nose and lung. Motile cilia

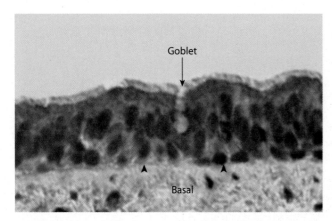

FIGURE 15–2 **Pseudo stratified respiratory epithelium lines the nasal cavity, trachea, and bronchi.** The surface includes mainly ciliated epithelial cells that may or may not touch the basement membrane, (arrow) surface mucous (goblet) cell, and (arrowhead) basal cells. (Modified with permission from the Human Protein Atlas (www.proteinatlas.org).)

also exhibit mechanosensory and chemosensory functions and can respond to mechanical stress, heat, acidic pH, and endogenous and synthetic agonists. Primary cilia often serve as sensory organelles.

Serous cells contain and secrete a less viscous fluid, and are also enriched in antimicrobial proteins including lysozyme and lactotransferin. These cells also contain the antimicrobial protein, BPIF2 (aka SPLUNC2). Secretory leukocyte proteinase inhibitor (SLPI) is a serine proteinase inhibitor that is produced locally in the lung by cells of the submucosal bronchial glands and by nonciliated epithelial cells. The main function of SLPI is the inhibition of neutrophil elastase and other proteinases, and may also have antimicrobial functions.

Another airway secretory cell is the bronchiolar secretoglobin cell (BSC), previously called the Clara cell. The role of secretoglobins is not fully understood in the lung, but they are known to inhibit phospholipase A2 and limit inflammation. In humans, BSCs are found mainly in the distal airways and can act as tissue stem cells.

Gas Exchange Region

Structure—The gas exchange region consists of terminal bronchioles, respiratory bronchioles, alveolar ducts, alveoli, blood vessels, and lung interstitium (Figure 15–3). Gas exchange occurs in the alveoli, which comprise ~85% of the total parenchymal lung volume. Adult human lungs contain an estimated 300 to 500 million alveoli. Capillaries, blood plasma, and formed blood elements are separated from the air space by a thin layer of tissue formed by epithelial, interstitial, and endothelial components.

The alveolar epithelium consists of two cells, the alveolar type I and type II cell (Figure 15–4). Alveolar type I cells cover

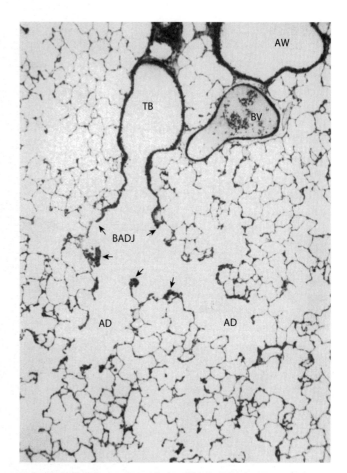

FIGURE 15–3 **Centriacinar region (ventilatory unit) of the lung.** An airway (AW) and a blood vessel (BV) (arteriole) are in close proximity to the terminal bronchiole (TB). The terminal bronchiole leads to the bronchiole–alveolar duct junction (BADJ) and the alveolar duct (AD). A number of the (arrows) alveolar septal tips close to the BADJ are thickened after a brief (4-h) exposure to asbestos fibers, indicating localization of fiber deposition. Other inhalants, such as ozone, produce lesions in the same locations. (Used with permission of Dr Kent E. Pinkerton, University of California, Davis.)

~95% of the alveolar surface and therefore are susceptible to damage by noxious agents that penetrate to the alveolus. Alveolar type I cells have an attenuated cytoplasm to enhance gas exchange. Alveolar type II cells produce and secrete surfactant, a mixture of lipids, and four surfactant associated proteins and can undergo mitotic division and replace damaged type I cells. Surfactant protein B and C are amphipathic and aid in spreading secreted lipids which form a monolayer that reduces surface tension. Surfactant proteins A1, A2, and D are members of the subfamily of C-type lectins called collectins, which defend against pathogens. Surfactant proteins A1 and A2 do not alter lipid structure but do bind lipopolysaccharides (LPS) and various microbial pathogens, enhancing their clearance from the lung. Surfactant protein D is also necessary in the suppression of pulmonary inflammation and in host defense against viral, fungal, and bacterial pathogens.

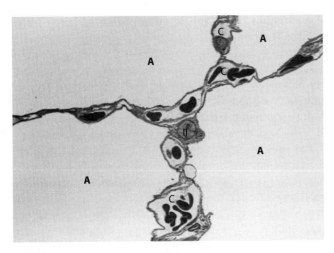

FIGURE 15-4 **Alveolar region of the lung.** The (A) alveolus is separated by the thin air-to-blood tissue barrier of the alveolar septal wall, which is composed of flat alveolar type I cells and occasional rounded (II) alveolar type II cells. A small interstitial space separates the epithelium and endothelium that form the (C) capillary wall. During lung injury the interstitial space enlarges and interferes with gas exchange. (Used with permission of Dr Kent E. Pinkerton, University of California, Davis.)

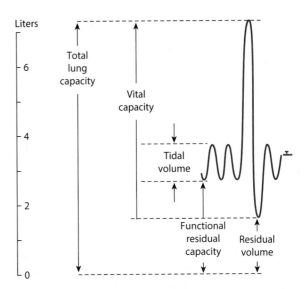

FIGURE 15-5 **A spirometer reading of lung volumes.** The total lung capacity is the total volume of air in an inflated human lung. After a maximum expiration, the lung retains a small volume of air, which is the residual volume. The air volume moved into and out of the lung during maximal inspiratory and expiratory movement, which is called the vital capacity. The tidal volume is typically moved into and out of the lung during each breathe. The functional residual capacity and residual volume cannot be measured with spirometer.

Function

Ventilation—The principal function of the lung is gas exchange, which consists of ventilation, perfusion, and diffusion. During inhalation, fresh air is moved into the lung through the upper respiratory tract and conducting airways and into the terminal respiratory units when the thoracic cage enlarges and the diaphragm moves downward; the lung passively follows this expansion. After diffusion of oxygen into the blood and that of CO_2 from the blood into the alveolar spaces, the air (now enriched in CO_2) is expelled by exhalation. Relaxation of the chest wall and diaphragm diminishes the internal volume of the thoracic cage, the elastic fibers of the lung parenchyma recoil, and air is expelled from the alveolar zone through the airways. Any interference with the elastic properties of the lung, e.g., the alteration of elastic fibers that occurs in emphysema, adversely affects ventilation, as do the decrease in the diameters of, or blockage of, the conducting airways, as in asthma.

Lung function changes with age and disease and can be measured with a spirometer (Figure 15–5). The total lung capacity (TLC) is the total volume of air in an inflated human lung, 4 to 5 L (women) and 6 to 7 L (men). After a maximum expiration, the lung retains 1.1 L (women) and 1.2 L (men), which is the residual volume (RV). The vital capacity is the air volume moved into and out of the lung during maximal inspiratory and expiratory movement and typical is 3.1 L (women) and 4.8 L (men). Only a small fraction of the VC, the tidal volume (TV), is typically moved into and out of the lung during quiet breathing. In resting humans, the TV measures ~0.5 L with each breath. The respiratory frequency is 12 to 20 breaths per minute (thus the resting ventilation is about 6–8 L/min).

Spirometry is a test in which an individual inhales maximally and then exhales as rapidly as possible. The volume of air expired in one second, called the forced expiratory volume 1 second (FEV1), and the total amount expired, forced vital capacity (FVC), and the ratio of FEV1/FVC, are good measures of the recoil capacity and airway obstruction of the lung. In a healthy individual the FEV1/FVC = ~80%.

Perfusion—The lung receives the entire output from the right ventricle, ~75 mL of blood per heartbeat. Blood with high CO_2 and low O_2 travels to the lung via the pulmonary artery and leaves the lung with high O_2 and low CO_2 via the pulmonary vein. The bronchi also have independent circulation with O_2-enriched blood supplied by an artery. Substantial amounts of toxic chemicals carried in the blood can be delivered to the lung. A chemical placed onto or deposited under the skin (subcutaneous injection) or introduced directly into a peripheral vein (intravenous injection) travels through the venous system to the right ventricle and comes into contact with the lungs before distribution to other organs or tissues in the body.

Diffusion—Gas exchange takes place across the entire alveolar surface, meaning contact with an airborne toxic chemical occurs over an area of ~140 m². This surface area is second only to the small intestine (~250 m²) and is considerably larger than the skin (~2 m²). Oxygen normally diffuses, unhindered, across the pulmonary capillary and into erythrocytes. Acute events that can disrupt this process may include collection of liquid in the alveolar or interstitial space and disruption of the pulmonary surfactant system. Chronic toxicity can impair diffusion due to abnormal alveolar architecture or abnormal formation and deposition of extracellular substances such as collagen in the interstitium.

BIOTRANSFORMATION IN THE RESPIRATORY TRACT

Often overlooked as an organ involved in metabolism of chemicals, in favor of the liver, the lung has substantial capabilities for biotransformation (see Chapter 6). Total lung cytochrome P450 (CYP) activity is roughly one-tenth to one-third of that in the liver. However, when specific activity in a few cell types is considered, the difference is only twofold for many enzymes, and in the case of nasal mucosa, higher enzyme activity is reported per cell. Metabolic competence in the lung and nasal tissues is concentrated in a few cell types and these have a defined, and sometimes limited, distribution in the respiratory tract that can vary substantially by species.

The CYP monooxygenase system is concentrated into a few lung cells: BSCs, alveolar type II cells, macrophages, and endothelial cells. Of these cell types, BSCs have the most CYP, followed by the type II cells. The total amount of total lung CYP contributed by BSCs is species-dependent, as are the CYP isoforms present and their location along the respiratory tract. Most species have CYPs in nasal tissue and some are predominantly expressed in the olfactory mucosa, which may play a role in providing or preventing access of inhalants directly to the brain.

Phase II enzymes include glutathione S-transferases (GSTs) (alpha, mu, and pi), glucuronosyl transferases, and sulfotransferases (SULTs). GSTs (and glutathione) play a major role in the modulation of both acute and chronic chemical toxicity in the lung. These enzyme systems work in concert with one another and it is the combined action of all these enzymes that determines toxicity. The regulation of many of these enzymes is under coordinated control of the transcription factor nuclear factor, erythroid-derived 2, -like 2 (aka Nrf2).

A major determinant of the potential for detoxification may also be the cellular localization of, and the ability to synthesize, glutathione in the lung. The distribution of GST isoforms varies by lung region and their activity is 5% to 15% of that in the rodent liver and about 30% of that in the human liver. Polymorphisms in glutathione transferase genes have been associated with a possible increase in risk of developing lung cancer, particularly in smokers.

GENERAL PRINCIPLES IN THE PATHOGENESIS OF LUNG DAMAGE CAUSED BY CHEMICALS

Toxic Inhalants, Gases, and Dosimetry

In inhalation toxicology, exposure is measured as a concentration (compound mass per unit of air). Typically highly toxic compounds can produce adverse effects in a concentration of mg/m^3 or μg/m^3. For reference, 1 m^3 is 1 000 L. For gases, concentration may also be expressed as volume to volume of air, that is, parts per million (ppm) or parts per billion (ppb). This can be calculated from the mass per unit air by using the ideal gas law to determine the gas's volume. It is important to note that exposure does not equate to dose (compound mass per unit), which requires a measure of organ, cell, or subcellular target.

The sites of deposition of gases in the respiratory tract define the pattern of toxicity of those gases. Solubility, diffusivity, and metabolism/reactivity in respiratory tissues and breathing rate are the critical factors in determining how deeply a given gas penetrates into the lung. Highly soluble gases such as SO$_2$ or formaldehyde do not penetrate farther than the nose (during nasal breathing) unless doses are very high, and are therefore relatively nontoxic to the lung of rats (which are obligatory nasal breathers). Relatively insoluble gases such as ozone and NO$_2$ penetrate deeply into the lung and reach the smallest airways and the alveoli (centriacinar region), where they can elicit toxic responses. Very insoluble gases such as CO and H$_2$S efficiently pass through the respiratory tract and are taken up by the pulmonary blood supply to be distributed throughout the body. Mathematical models of gas entry and deposition in the lung predict sites of lung lesions fairly accurately. These models may be useful for extrapolating findings made in laboratory animals to humans.

Regional Particle Deposition

Particle size is a critical factor in determining the region of the respiratory tract in which a particle will be deposited. In respiratory toxicology, aerosols (solid or liquid particles dispersed into air) include dusts, fumes, smoke, mists, fog, or smog (ranging from ≥ 1.0 μm for dusts to ≥ 0.01–50 μm for smog). Smaller aerosols include submicrometer particles, nanometer particles or nanoparticles. All these distinguishing forms are included in the term "aerosol" or "particle."

The upper respiratory tract is very efficient in removing particles that are very large (> 10 μm) or very small (< 0.01 μm) (Figure 15–1). During nasal breathing, 1 to 10 μm particles are usually deposited in the upper nasopharyngeal region or the first five generations of large conducting airways. During oral breathing, deposition of these particles can increase in the tracheobronchial airways and alveolar region. Smaller particles (0.001–0.1 μm) can also be deposited in the tracheobronchial region. Particles ranging from 0.003 to 5 μm can be transported to the smaller airways and deposited in the alveolar region.

Patterns of breathing can change the site of deposition of a particle of a given size. The size of a particle may change during inspiration before deposition in the respiratory tract. Materials that are hygroscopic (i.e., those that readily absorb moisture), such as sodium chloride, sulfuric acid, and glycerol, take on water and grow in size in the warm, saturated atmosphere of the upper and lower respiratory tract.

Deposition Mechanisms

In the respiratory tract, particles deposit by impaction, interception, sedimentation, diffusion, and electrostatic deposition (for positively charged particles only) (Figure 15–6). Impaction occurs in the upper respiratory tract and large proximal airways where the airflow is faster than in the small distal airways because the cumulative diameter is smaller than in the proximal airways. In humans, most $> 10\,\mu m$ particles are deposited in the nose or oral pharynx and cannot penetrate tissues distal to the larynx. For 2.5 to $10\,\mu m$ particles, impaction continues to be the mechanism of deposition in the first generations of the tracheobronchial region.

Interception occurs when the trajectory of a particle brings it near enough to a surface so that an edge of the particle contacts the airway surface. Although fiber diameter determines the probability of deposition by impaction and sedimentation, interception is dependent on fiber length. Thus, a fiber with a diameter of $1\,\mu m$ and a length of $200\,\mu m$ will be deposited in the bronchial tree primarily by interception rather than impaction. Interception is also important for submicrometer particles in the tracheobronchial region where inertial airflow directs a disproportionately large fraction of the flow volume toward the surface of small airway bifurcations.

Sedimentation controls deposition in the smaller bronchi, the bronchioles, and the alveolar spaces, where the airways are small and the velocity of airflow is low. Air resistance and buoyancy act on a particle in an upward direction while gravity acts on a particle in a downward direction. These forces eventually balance as a particle travels through air, causing the particle to settle. Sedimentation is not a significant route of particle deposition when the aerodynamic diameter is $\leq 0.5\,\mu m$. Sedimentation is dependent on the time a particle is in a compartment (i.e., an alveolus) and can be increased by breath holding.

Diffusion of a particle within the air is an important factor in the deposition of submicrometer particles. The distance a particle travels within a gas depends upon the ratio of the particle's mass to the momentum of the colliding gas molecules such that large particles are hardly moved and nanoparticles are moved extensively. Diffusion is an important deposition mechanism in the nose, airways, and alveoli for particles $\leq 0.5\,\mu m$. Nanometer particles ($0.1\,\mu m$ and smaller) are also trapped relatively efficiently in the upper airways by diffusion. Particles that penetrate beyond the upper airways are available to be deposited in the bronchial region and the deep-lying airways.

Electrostatic deposition is a minor deposition mechanism for positively charged particles. The surface of the airways is negatively charged and attracts positively charged particles. Freshly fractured mineral dust particles and laboratory-generated aerosols from evaporation of aqueous droplets can have substantial electrostatic mobilities.

During quiet breathing, in which the TV is only two to three times the volume of the anatomic dead space (i.e., the volume of the conducting airways where gas exchange does not occur), a large proportion of the inhaled particles may be exhaled. During exercise, when larger volumes are inhaled at higher velocities,

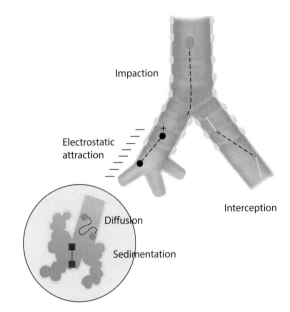

FIGURE 15–6 **Mechanism of particle deposition in the respiratory tract.** Impaction occurs in the upper respiratory tract and large proximal airways where fast airflow imparts momentum to the inhaled particle. The particle's inertia causes it to continue to travel along its original path and deposit on the airway surface. Interception occurs when the trajectory of a particle brings it near enough to a surface so that an edge of the particle contacts the airway surface. Sedimentation controls deposition in the smaller bronchi, the bronchioles, and the alveolar spaces, where the airways are small and the velocity of airflow is low. Sedimentation is dependent on the time a particle is in a compartment (i.e., an alveolus) and can be increased by breath holding. Diffusion is an important factor in the deposition of submicrometer particles. Electrostatic deposition is a minor deposition mechanism for positively charged particles. The surface of the airways is negatively charged and attracts positively charged particles. (Adapted with permission from Lippmann M (ed): *Environmental toxicants human exposures and their health effects.* 3rd edition. New York, NY: Wiley; 2009.)

impaction in the large airways and sedimentation and diffusion in the smaller airways and alveoli increase. Breath holding also increases deposition from sedimentation and diffusion. Cigarette smoke is hydroscopic aerosol of nicotine-laden particles that grow to a median diameter of about 0.5 to $1.0\,\mu m$. Thus, a smoker's respiratory pause at the end of inhalation increases alveolar sedimentation and thereby nicotine delivery to the alveolar surface and to the blood upon absorption.

Factors that modify the diameter of the conducting airways can alter particle deposition. In patients with chronic bronchitis or pneumonia, the airway lining fluid can greatly thicken and may partially block the airways in some areas. Sonic jets (e.g., during wheezing and rales) formed by high air flowing through such partially occluded airways have the potential to increase the deposition of particles by impaction and diffusion in the small airways. Irritant materials that produce bronchoconstriction tend to increase the proximal tracheobronchial deposition of particles.

Particle Clearance

Lung defense is dependent on particle clearance, wherein rapid removal lessens the time available to cause damage to the pulmonary tissues or permit local absorption. However, it is important to remember that particle clearance is not equivalent to clearance from the body.

Nasal Clearance—Particles deposited in the anterior portion of the nose are removed by extrinsic actions such as wiping and blowing. Particles deposited in the posterior portion of the nose are removed by mucociliary clearance that propels mucus toward the glottis, after which the particles are swallowed. Soluble particles may dissolve and enter the epithelium and/or blood before they can be mechanically removed.

Tracheobronchial Clearance—Particles deposited in the tracheobronchial tree are also removed by mucociliary clearance. In addition to deposited particles, particle-laden macrophages are also moved upward to the oropharynx, where they are swallowed.

Alveolar Clearance—Particles deposited in the alveolar region are removed by specialized cells, the alveolar macrophage. Lung defense involve both the innate and adaptive and immune systems (see Chapter 12). Macrophages are the primary effector of innate lung immunity and their ability to accomplish phagocytosis depends on the recognition of foreign or damage cells by a variety of macrophage surface macromolecules and receptors. Phagocytosis requires (1) particle binding to the membrane specifically via recognition molecule–receptor interactions or nonspecifically by electrostatic forces (inert materials), (2) receptor activation that initiates cell signaling, (3) actin polymerization and coordinated cytoskeletal movements that leads to extension of membranes, and (4) vesicular membrane closure closely apposed to the particle or the fiber ingested forming a phagosome shaped by the material ingested.

ACUTE RESPONSES OF THE LUNG TO INJURY

Trigeminally Mediated Airway Reflexes

Certain gases and vapors stimulate nerve endings in the nose, particularly those of the trigeminal nerve. The result is holding of the breath or changes in breathing patterns, to avoid or reduce further exposure. Transient receptor potential channel receptors may be activated by many irritants causing tickling, itching, and painful nasal sensations. Subfamily A receptors are activated by several irritants including acrolein, allyl isothiocyanate (wabasi), allicin (garlic), cinamaldehyde, chlorine, ozone, and hydrogen peroxide.

If continued exposure cannot be avoided, many acidic or alkaline irritants produce cell necrosis and increased permeability of the alveolar walls. Other inhaled agents can be more insidious; inhalation of high concentrations of HCl, NO_2, NH_3, or phosgene may at first produce very little apparent damage in the respiratory tract. The epithelial barrier in the alveolar zone, after a latency period of several hours, begins to leak, flooding the alveoli and producing a delayed pulmonary edema that is often fatal.

A different pathogenetic mechanism is typical of highly reactive molecules such as ozone. It is unlikely that ozone as such can penetrate beyond the layer of fluid covering the cells of the lung. Instead, ozone lesions are propagated by a cascade of secondary reaction products and by reactive oxygen species arising from free radical reactions.

Bronchoconstriction, Airway Hyperreactivity, and Neurogenic Inflammation

Large diameter airways are surrounded by bronchial smooth muscles, which help maintain airway tone and diameter during expansion and contraction of the lung. Bronchial smooth muscle tone is normally regulated by the autonomic nervous system. Bronchoconstriction can be provoked by irritants (acrolein), cigarette smoke, air pollutants, cholinomimetic drugs (acetylcholine), histamine, various prostaglandins and leukotrienes, substance P, and nitric oxide. Bronchoconstriction causes a decrease in airway diameter and a corresponding increase in resistance to airflow. Characteristic symptoms include wheezing, coughing, a sensation of chest tightness, and dyspnea. Exercise potentiates these problems. Because the major component of airway resistance usually is contributed by large bronchi, inhaled chemicals that cause reflex bronchoconstriction are generally irritant gases with moderate solubility.

Acute Lung Injury (Pulmonary Edema)

Acute lung injury (adult or infant respiratory distress syndrome) is marked by alveolar epithelial and endothelial cell perturbation and inflammatory cell influx that leads to surfactant disruption, pulmonary edema, and atelectasis. Toxic pulmonary edema represents an acute, exudative phase of lung injury that alters ventilation–perfusion relationships and limits diffusive transfer of O_2 and CO_2 even in otherwise structurally normal alveoli. Acrolein, HCl, NO_2, NH_3, or phosgene may compromise alveolar barrier function several hours after exposure to low concentrations, and immediate alveolar damage and death with high concentrations.

CHRONIC RESPONSES OF THE LUNG TO INJURY

Chronic Obstructive Pulmonary Disease

Characterized by a progressive airflow obstruction, chronic obstructive pulmonary disease involves airway (bronchitis) and alveolar pathology. Chronic bronchitis is defined by the presence of sputum production and cough for at least three months. In emphysema, destruction of the gas-exchanging surface area results in a distended, hyperinflated lung that no

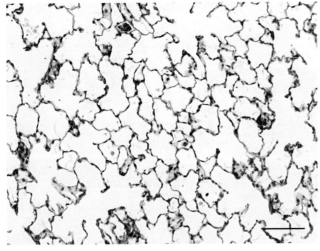

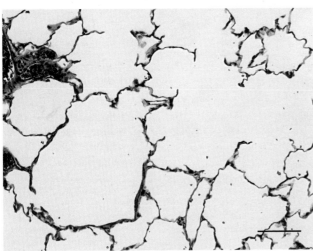

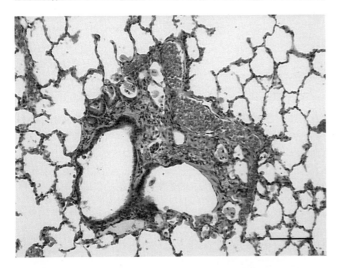

FIGURE 15-7 **Airspace enlargement induced by tobacco smoke and pulmonary fibrosis induced by asbestos in rat lung.** *Top panel*: Normal rat lung. *Middle panel*: Extensive distention of the alveoli (emphysema) in rat lung following inhalation of tobacco smoke (90 mg/m³ of total suspended particulate material). *Bottom panel*: Lung of a rat one year after exposure to chrysotile asbestos. Note accumulation of connective tissue around blood vessel and airways (fibrosis). Bar length: 100 μm. (Used with permission of Dr Kent E. Pinkerton, University of California, Davis.)

longer effectively exchanges oxygen and carbon dioxide as a result of both loss of tissue and air trapping (Figure 15–7). The major cause of human emphysema is, by far, cigarette smoke inhalation, although other toxicants also can elicit this response. A feature of toxicant-induced emphysema is severe or recurrent inflammation.

The pathogenesis of emphysema involves a proteinase–antiprotease imbalance that leads to the remodeling of the supportive connective tissue in the parenchyma and separate lesions that coalesce to destroy lung tissue. Alpha$_1$-antiprotease (also called alpha$_1$-antitrypsin) is one of the body's main defenses against uncontrolled proteolytic digestion by this class of elastolytic enzymes, which includes elastase. Studies in smokers led to the hypothesis that neutrophil (and perhaps alveolar macrophage) elastases can break down lung elastin and thus cause emphysema; these elastases usually are kept in check by alpha$_1$-antiprotease that diffuses into the lung from the blood. As the individual ages, an accumulation of random elastolytic events can cause the emphysematous changes in the lungs that are normally associated with aging. Toxicants that cause inflammatory cell influx and thus increase the burden of neutrophil elastase can accelerate this process.

Lung Cancer

Lung cancer is now the leading cause of death from cancer among men and women. Retrospective and prospective epidemiologic studies unequivocally show an association between tobacco smoking and lung cancer. Average smokers have a 10-fold and heavy smokers a 20-fold increased risk of developing lung cancer compared with nonsmokers. Many other agents also cause lung cancer (see Table 15–1).

Human lung cancers may have a latency period of 20 to 40 years, making the relationship to specific exposures difficult to establish. Two major forms are non-small-cell lung cancer, which accounts for about 85% of all lung cancers, and may be characterized as squamous cell carcinoma, adenocarcinoma, and large-cell lung cancer. Small-cell lung cancers account for about 15% of lung cancers. Compared with cancer in the lung, cancer in the upper respiratory tract is less common.

The potential mechanisms of lung carcinogenesis center on damage to DNA. An activated carcinogen or its metabolic product may interact with DNA. DNA damage caused by active oxygen species is another potentially important mechanism. Ionizing radiation leads to the formation of superoxide. Cigarette smoke contains high quantities of active oxygen species and other free radicals. Critical genetic and epigenetic changes include DNA mutations, loss of heterozygosity, and promoter methylation. Global transcriptome changes can include stimulation of mitogenic pathways and suppression of apoptosis.

Asthma

Asthma is characterized clinically by attacks of shortness of breath, which is caused by narrowing of the large conducting

TABLE 15–1 Agents that produce lung injury and disease.

Toxicant	Disease	Exposure	Acute Effect	Chronic Effect
Acrolein	Acute lung injury, chronic obstructive pulmonary disease	Biomass or hot oil cooking, fire fighters, environmental tobacco smoke, biocide water treatment	Cough, shortness of breath, extreme oronasal irritation, pulmonary edema, airway hyperreactivity	Chronic obstructive pulmonary disease, possibly asthma or lung cancer
Aluminum abrasives	Shaver disease, corundum smelter's lung, bauxite lung	Abrasives manufacturing, smelting	Alveolar edema	Interstitial fibrosis, emphysema
Aluminum dust	Aluminosis	Aluminum, firework, ceramic, paint, electrical good, and abrasive manufacturing	Cough, shortness of breath	Interstitial fibrosis
Ammonia		Farming, refrigeration operations, ammonia, fertilizer, chemical, and explosive manufacturing	Oronasal and bronchial irritation, pulmonary edema	Acute lung injury, chronic bronchitis
Arsenic		Pesticide, pigment, glass, and alloy manufacturing	Bronchitis	Laryngitis, bronchitis, and lung cancer
Asbestos	Asbestosis	Mining, construction, shipbuilding, brake repair, vermiculite contaminant		Fibrosis, pleural calcification, lung cancer, mesothelioma
Aspergillus	Framer lung, composte lung, malt worker's lung	Working with moldy hay, compost, or barley	Bronchoconstriction, cough, chest tightness	Extrinsic allergic alveolitis (hypersensitivity pneumonitis)
Avian protein	Bird fancier's lung	Bird handling and farming with exposure to bird droppings	Bronchoconstriction, cough, chest tightness	Extrinsic allergic alveolitis (hypersensitivity pneumonitis)
Beryllium	Berylliosis	Mining, alloy, and ceramic manufacturing, Milling beryllium	Pulmonary edema, pneumonia	Interstitial granulomatosis, progressive dyspnea, cor pulmonarle, fibrosis, and lung cancer
Cadmium		Welding, smelting, and electrical equipment, battery, alloy, and pigment manufacturing	Cough, pneumonia	Emphysema, cor pulmonale
Carbides of tungsten, titanium, or tantalum	Hard metal disease	Metal cutting and manufacturing	Bronchial epithelial hyper- and metaplasia	Peribronchial and perivascular fibrosis
Chlorine		Paper, plastics, chlorinated product manufacturing	Cough, hemoptysis, dyspnea, bronchitis, pneumonia	
Chromium (VI)		Chromium compound, paint, pigment, chromite ore reduction manufacturing	Oronasal and bronchial irritation	Fibrosis, lung cancer
Coal dust	Coal worker's pneumoconiosis	Coal mining		Fibrosis with emphysema
Cotton dust	Byssinosis	Textile manufacturing	Chest tightness, wheezing, dyspnea	Restrictive lung disease, chronic bronchitis
Hydrogen fluoride		Chemical, photograph film, solvent and plastic manufacturing	Airway irritation, hemorrhagic pulmonary edema	

TABLE 15-1 **Agents that produce lung injury and disease.** (*Continued*)

Toxicant	Disease	Exposure	Acute Effect	Chronic Effect
Iron oxides	Siderotic lung disease, silver finisher's lung, hematite miner's lung, arc welder's lung	Welding, steel and jewelry manufacturing, foundry work, hematite mining	Cough	Silver finisher's lung with subpleural and perivascular macrophage aggregates; hematite miner's lung with diffuse fibrosis-like pneumoconiosis; arc welder's lung with bronchitis
Isocyanates		Auto painting, and plastic and chemical manufacturing	Airway irritation, cough, dyspnea	Asthma
Kaolin	Kaolinosis	Pottery making		Fibrosis
Manganese	Manganese pneumonia	Chemical and metal manufacturing	Acute pneumonia (often fatal)	Recurrent pneumonia
Nickel		Nickel mining, smelting, electroplating, battery manufacturing, fossil fuel combustion	Delayed pulmonary edema, skin allergy	Acute lung injury, chronic bronchitis, non- small-cell lung cancer, nasal cancer
Nitrogen oxides	Silo-filler's diseases	Silo filling, welding, explosive manufacturing	Immediate or delayed pulmonary edema	Bronchiolitis obliterans, emphysema in experimental animals
Nontuberculous mycobacteria	Metalworking fluid hypersensitivity	Working with metal cutting fluid contain water and contaminated with mycobacteria	Bronchoconstriction, cough, chest tightness	Extrinsic allergic alveolitis (hypersensitivity pneumonitis)
Organic (sugar cane) dust (possibly contaminated with thermophilic actinomycete)	Bagassosis	Sugarcane and molasses manufacturing (bagasse is the fibrosis residue from sugar extraction)	Bronchoconstriction, cough, chest tightness	Extrinsic allergic alveolitis (hypersensitivity pneumonitis)
Ozone		Welding, photocopying, bleaching flour, water treatment, deordorizing	Substernal pain, exacerbation of asthma, bronchitis, pulmonary edema	Fibrosis (including airways)
Perchloroethylene		Dry cleaning, metal degreasing, grain fumigation	Edema	Hepatic and lung cancer
Phosgene		Plastic, pesticide, and chemical manufacturing	Severe pulmonary edema	Bronchitis and fibrosis
Silica	Silicosis, pneumoconiosis	Mining, stone cutting, sand blasting, farming, quarry mining, tunneling	Acute silicosis (inflammation)	Fibrosis, silicotuberculosis
Sulfur dioxide		Chemical manufacturing, refrigeration, bleaching, fumigation	Bronchoconstriction, cough, chest tightness	Chronic bronchitis
Talc	Talcosis	Mining, rubber manufacturing, cosmetics	Cough	Fibosis
Thermophilic actinomycete	Farmer's lung, mushroom worker's lung, penguin humidifier lung	Farming (hay or grain degradation)	Bronchoconstriction, cough, chest tightness	Extrinsic allergic alveolitis (hypersensitivity pneumonitis)
Tin		Mining, tin processing		Widespread mottling in chest X-ray often without clinical impairment
Vanadium		Metal cutting and manufacturing, specialty steel manufacturing	Airway irritation and mucus production	Chronic bronchitis

airways (bronchi). The clinical hallmark of asthma is increased airway reactivity of the bronchial smooth muscle in response to exposure to irritants. There may be common mechanisms between asthma and pulmonary fibrosis, with regard to the role of recurrent or chronic inflammation in disease pathogenesis. Agents that can induce asthma are listed in Table 15–1.

Pulmonary Fibrosis

Fibrotic lungs from humans with acute or chronic pulmonary fibrosis contain increased amounts of collagen. In lungs damaged by toxicants, the response resembles adult or infant respiratory distress syndrome. Excess lung collagen is usually observed not only in the alveolar interstitium, but also throughout the alveolar ducts and respiratory bronchioles (Figure 15–7).

Types I and III collagen are major interstitial components and are found in an approximate ratio of 2:1. There is an increase in type I collagen relative to type III collagen in patients with idiopathic pulmonary fibrosis and patients dying of acute respiratory distress syndrome. It is not known whether shifts in collagen types, compared with absolute increases in collagen content, account for the increased stiffness of fibrotic lungs. Because type III collagen is more compliant than type I, increasing type I relative to type III collagen may result in a stiffer lung. Changes in collagen cross-linking in fibrotic lungs also may contribute to the increased stiffness.

AGENTS KNOWN TO PRODUCE LUNG INJURY IN HUMANS

There are over 7 900 unique chemicals that are commonly used in industry, many of which represent hazards to the respiratory tract. Exposure prevention is one of the most effective approaches to prevent lung injury and disease, and many values and exposure limits exist to aid prevention. Nonetheless, given the large morbidity and mortality associated with current acute and chronic lung disease, a great need exists to develop additional preventative and therapeutic strategies based on the knowledge of the cellular and molecular events that determine lung injury and repair. Table 15–1 lists a portion of the respiratory toxicants that can produce acute and chronic lung injury in humans.

EVALUATION OF TOXIC LUNG DAMAGE

Human Studies

Although the lung is susceptible to multiple toxic injuries, it is also amenable to a number of tests that allow evaluation of proper functioning. Commonly used tests include measurement of FEV1, FVC, and airway resistance. Additional tests evaluate the maximal flow rates and different lung volumes, diffusion capacity, oxygen, and carbon dioxide content of the arterial and venous blood, distribution of ventilation, and lung and chest wall compliance.

Diffusion defects (i.e., defects in gas exchange across the pulmonary capillary) can be evaluated by measuring the arterial partial pressure of both oxygen and CO_2. In general, blood gas analysis is a comparatively insensitive assay for disturbed ventilation because of the organisms' buffering and reserve capacities, but may be a useful tool in clinical medicine. Measurement of diffusion capacity with CO, a gas that binds with 250 times higher affinity to hemoglobin than does oxygen, is more sensitive. Proper lung function in humans can be evaluated with several additional techniques, including computed tomography (CT), molecular content analysis, fiberoptic bronchoscopy.

Animal Studies

The toxicology of inhaled materials has been and continues to be extensively studied in experimental animals. Obviously, selecting animals with a respiratory system similar to that of humans is particularly desirable (e.g., monkey). However, rodents are widely used despite fundamental differences to combat cost and ethical considerations.

Inhalation Exposure Systems—In inhalation studies, animals are kept within a chamber that is ventilated with a defined test atmosphere. Generation of such an atmosphere is comparatively easy for gases that are available in high purity in a compressed tank (e.g., SO_2, O_2, NO_2). Gas concentration within the chamber is measured continuously, and is usually within 5% of the targeted concentration. More challenging is the generation of particles or complex mixtures (e.g., tobacco smoke, diesel, and gasoline exhaust or residual oil fly ash), particularly because of the possibility of interactions between individual mixture constituents and the possibility of formation of artifacts.

Pulmonary Function Tests in Experimental Animals— Conducting pulmonary function tests in experimental animals poses distinct challenges, especially in small rodents. Experimental animals cannot be made to maximally inhale or exhale at the investigator's will, for instance. Analysis of pressure–volume curves, which provides an indication of lung compliance, is comparatively easy to perform in animals in that it does not require a specialized apparatus. Another pulmonary function test is the analysis of airway resistance, which can be measured via restrained plethysmography, unrestrained video-assisted plethysmography, or unrestrained acoustic plethysmography. Analysis of breathing pattern can also be used and may differentiate between upper airway and lower airway irritants. In rodents, upper airway ("sensory") irritants produce a breathing pattern of decreased respiratory frequency with increased tidal volume, whereas lower airway ("pulmonary") irritants produce a breathing pattern of increased respiratory frequency and decreased minute volume (i.e., the total volume of air breathed in 1 minute).

Morphological Techniques—The pathology of acute and chronic injury may be examined by gross inspection and under the microscope and should include the nasal passages, larynx, major bronchi, and the lung parenchyma.

Regional distribution of lesions in nasal passages can be assessed after fixation and decalcification. Various regions of the nasal passages can then be examined by obtaining cross sections at multiple levels, staining the tissue to highlight particular structures, and examining the tissue under a microscope. This permits semiquantitative or quantitative measurements to be made.

Additional tools for the study of toxic lung injury include immunohistochemistry, in situ hybridization, and analysis of cell kinetics. Transcriptome, proteome, and metabolome profiling are additional valuable tools to assess the lung in health and disease.

Pulmonary Lavage and Pulmonary Edema—Pulmonary edema and/or pulmonary inflammation are early events in acute and chronic lung injury. The fluid lining the pulmonary epithelium can be recovered by the medical procedure, bronchoalveolar lavage. Analysis of the lavage fluid is a useful tool to detect respiratory tract toxicity. Influx of neutrophils or other leukocytes such as lymphocytes or eosinophils into the lavage fluid is the most sensitive sign of inflammation. Measurements of lung injury include total protein and/or albumin. Additional measurements include secretory products of macrophages and epithelial cells include fribronectin, chemokines, and other cytokines (e.g., TNF or IL1B). Reduced glutathione levels may be an indicator of oxidative stress. Lactate dehydrogenase activity (and its substituent isozymes), N-acetylglucosaminidase, acid or alkaline phosphatase, other lysosomal hydrolases, and sialic acid add additional information. In addition pulmonary edema can be assessed by determining lung wet:dry ratio or injection of Evan blue dye albumin.

In Vitro Studies

In vitro systems with materials originally obtained from either human tissues or experimental animals are particularly suited for the study of mechanisms that cause lung injury. The methods include isolated perfused lung, microdissection/organotypic tissue culture systems, and cell type–specific cell culture.

Isolated Perfused Lung—The isolated perfused lung method is applicable to lungs from many laboratory species (e.g., mouse, rat, guinea pig, or rabbit). The lung is perfused with blood or a blood substitute through the pulmonary arterial bed. At the same time, the lung is actively (through rhythmic inflation–deflation cycles with positive pressure) or passively (by creating negative pressure with an artificial thorax in which the lung is suspended) ventilated. Toxic agents can be introduced into the perfusate or the inspired air. Repeated sampling of the perfusate allows one to determine the rate of metabolism of drugs and the metabolic activity of the lung.

Airway Microdissection and Organotypic Tissue Culture Systems—Many inhalants act in specific regions of the respiratory tract. Microdissection of the nasal passage and airways consists of stripping away surrounding tissue or parenchyma while maintaining the airway structure and exposing the epithelium. Microdissected airways can be studied in culture for up to one week, can be used to study site-specific gene expression, morphological changes in toxicant injury and repair, or can be used for biochemical analyses including enzyme activity measurements and determination of antioxidant concentrations (such as glutathione).

Tissue culture systems have been developed in which epithelial cells maintain their polarity, differentiation, and normal function similar to what is observed in vivo. Epithelial cell surfaces are exposed to air (or a gas phase containing an airborne toxic agent), while the basal portion is bathed by a tissue culture medium.

Lung Cell Culture—Many lung-specific cell types have been isolated and can be maintained as cell culture. Human and animal alveolar or interstitial macrophages can be obtained from lavage or lung tissue. Their function can be examined in vitro with or without exposure to appropriate toxic stimuli. Type II alveolar epithelial cells can be isolated and primary cell cultures maintained in culture for short periods. Direct isolation of type I epithelial cells has also been successful.

BIBLIOGRAPHY

Gardner DE (ed): *Toxicology of the Lung*, 4th ed. Boca Raton, FL: CRC Press/Taylor & Francis, 2006.

Morris JB, Shusterman DJ: *Toxicology of the Nose and Upper Airways*, New York: Informa, 2010.

Salem H, Katz SA: *Inhalation Toxicology*, 3rd ed., Boca Raton, FL: CRC Press, 2015.

QUESTIONS

1. Which of the following statements is FALSE regarding the role of mucus in the conducting airways?
   a. Pollutants trapped by mucus can be eliminated via expectoration or swallowing.
   b. Mucus is of a basic pH.
   c. The beating of cilia propels mucus out of the lungs.
   d. Mucus plays a role promoting oxidative stress.
   e. Free radical scavenging is believed to be a role of mucus.

2. Respiratory distress syndrome sometimes affects premature neonates due to lack of surfactant production by which of the following cell types?
   a. lung fibroblasts.
   b. type II pneumocytes.
   c. endothelial cells.
   d. alveolar macrophages.
   e. type I pneumocytes.

3. In a situation where there is an increased metabolic demand for oxygen, which of the following volume measurements will greatly increase?
   a. total lung capacity (TLC).
   b. residual volume (RV).
   c. functional residual capacity (FRC).
   d. tidal volume (TV).
   e. vital capacity (VC).

4. The free radicals that inflict oxidative damage on the lungs are generated by all of the following EXCEPT:
   a. tobacco smoke.
   b. neutrophils.
   c. ozone.
   d. monocytes.
   e. SO_2.

5. Which of the following gases would most likely pass all the way through the respiratory tract and diffuse into the pulmonary blood supply?
   a. O_3 (ozone).
   b. NO_2.
   c. H_2O.
   d. CO.
   e. SO_2.

6. All of the following statements regarding particle deposition and clearance are true EXCEPT:
   a. One of the main modes of particle clearance is via mucociliary escalation.
   b. Diffusion is important in the deposition of particles in the bronchial regions.
   c. Larger volumes of inspired air increase particle deposition in the airways.
   d. Sedimentation results in deposition in the bronchioles.
   e. Swallowing is an important mechanism of particle clearance.

7. Which of the following is not a common location to which particles are cleared?
   a. stomach.
   b. lymph nodes.
   c. pulmonary vasculature.
   d. liver.
   e. GI tract.

8. Pulmonary fibrosis is marked by which of the following?
   a. increased type I collagen.
   b. decreased type III collagen.
   c. increased compliance.
   d. elastase activation.
   e. decreased overall collagen levels.

9. Activation of what enzyme(s) is responsible for emphysema?
   a. antitrypsin.
   b. epoxide hydrolase.
   c. elastase.
   d. hyaluronidase.
   e. nonspecific proteases.

10. Which of the following measurements would NOT be expected from a patient with restrictive lung disease?
    a. decreased FRC.
    b. decreased RV.
    c. increased VC.
    d. decreased FEV_1.
    e. impaired ventilation.

Toxic Responses of the Nervous System

Virginia C. Moser, Michael Aschner, Rudy J. Richardson, and Martin A. Philbert

OVERVIEW OF THE NERVOUS SYSTEM

Several generalities that allow a basic understanding of the actions of neurotoxicants include (1) the privileged status of the nervous system (NS) with the maintenance of a biochemical barrier between the brain and the blood; (2) the importance of the high energy requirements of the brain; (3) the spatial extensions of the NS as long cellular processes and the requirements of cells with such a complex geometry; (4) the maintenance of an environment rich in lipids; (5) the transmission of information across extracellular space at the synapse; (6) the distances over which electrical impulses must be transmitted, coordinated, and integrated; and (7) development and regenerative patterns of the NS.

Blood–Brain Barrier

The NS is protected from the adverse effects of many potential toxicants by an anatomical barrier between the blood and the brain, or a "blood–brain barrier" (BBB). Most of the brain, spinal cord, retina, and peripheral NS (PNS) maintain this barrier with the blood, with selectivity similar to the interface between cells and the extracellular space. To gain entry to the NS, molecules must pass into the cell membranes of endothelial cells of the brain rather than between endothelial cells, as they do in other tissues (Figure 16–1). The principal basis of the blood–brain barrier is thought to be specialized endothelial cells in the brain's microvasculature, aided, at least in part, by interactions with glia. In addition to this interface with blood, the

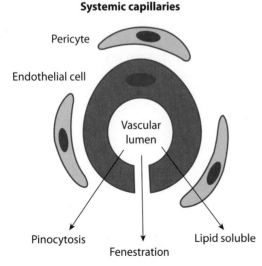
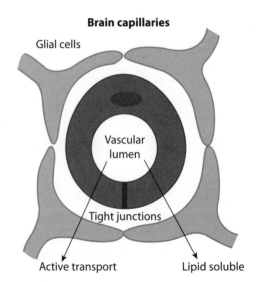

FIGURE 16–1   Schematic diagram of the blood–brain barrier. Systemic capillaries are depicted with intercellular gaps, or fenestrations, which permit the passage of molecules incapable of crossing the endothelial cell. There is also more abundant pinocytosis in systemic capillaries, in addition to the transcellular passage of lipid-soluble compounds. In brain capillaries, tight junctions between endothelial cells and the lack of pinocytosis limit transport to compounds with active transport mechanisms or those that pass through cellular membranes by virtue of their lipid solubility.

brain, spinal cord, and peripheral nerves are also completely covered with a continuous lining of specialized cells that limits the entry of molecules from adjacent tissue. In the brain and spinal cord, this is the meningeal surface; in peripheral nerves, each fascicle of nerve is surrounded by perineurial cells. Among the unique properties of endothelial cells in the NS is the presence of tight junctions between cells. Thus, molecules must pass through membranes of endothelial cells, rather than between them, as they do in other tissues.

The blood–brain barrier also contains xenobiotic transporters that transport some xenobiotics that have diffused through endothelial cells back into the blood. If not actively transported into the brain, the penetration of toxicants or their metabolites is largely related to their lipid solubility and to their ability to pass through the plasma membranes of cells forming the barrier. However, spinal ganglia, autonomic ganglia, and a small number of other sites within the brain are not protected by blood–tissue barriers. This discontinuity of the barrier is the basis for the selective neurotoxicity of some compounds. The blood–brain barrier is incompletely developed at birth and even less so in premature infants. This predisposes the premature infant to brain injury by toxicants that are excluded from the NS later in life.

Energy Requirements

Neurons (and cardiac myocytes) are highly dependent on aerobic metabolism because they must use this energy to maintain proper ion gradients. The brain is extremely sensitive to even brief interruptions in the supply of oxygen or glucose. Exposure to toxicants that inhibit aerobic respiration (e.g., cyanide) or to conditions that produce hypoxia (e.g., CO poisoning) leads to early signs of neuronal dysfunction. Damage to the NS under these conditions is a combination of direct toxic effects on neurons and secondary damage from systemic hypoxia or ischemia.

Axonal Transport

Impulses are conducted over great distances at rapid speed, providing information about the environment to the organism in a coordinated manner that allows an organized response to be carried out at a specific site. However, the intricate organization of such a complex network places an unparalleled demand on the cells of the NS. Single cells, rather than being spherical and a few micrometers in diameter, are elongated and may extend over 1 m in length. Two immediate demands placed on the neuron are the maintenance of a much larger cellular volume, requiring more protein synthesis, and the transport of intracellular materials over great distances using various mechanisms. These demands require ATP.

Axonal transport moves protein products from the cell body to the appropriate site in the axon. *Fast axonal transport* carries a large number of proteins from their site of synthesis in the cell body into the axon. Many proteins associated with vesicles migrate through the axon at a rate of 400 mm/day (Figure 16–2). This process is dependent on microtubule-associated ATPase activity and the microtubule-associated motor proteins (kinesin and dynein) that provide both the mechanochemical force in the form of a microtubule-associated ATPase and the interface between microtubules as the track and vesicles as the cargo. Vesicles are transported rapidly in an anterograde direction by kinesin, and they are transported in a retrograde direction by dynein. This mechanism of cytoplasmic transport is amplified within the NS, compared with other cells, by the distances encompassed by the axonal extensions of neurons.

The transport of some organelles, including mitochondria, constitutes an intermediate component of axonal transport, moving at 50 mm/day. The slowest component of axonal transport represents the movement of the cytoskeleton itself (Figure 16–2). The cytoskeleton is composed of microtubules formed by the association of tubulin subunits and

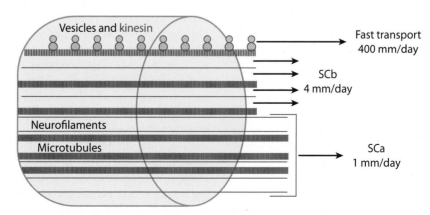

FIGURE 16–2 Schematic diagram of axonal transport. Fast axonal transport is depicted as spherical vesicles moving along microtubules with intervening microtubule-associated motors. The slow component A (SCa) represents the movement of the cytoskeleton, composed of neurofilaments and microtubules. Slow component B (SCb) moves at a faster rate than SCa and includes soluble proteins, which are apparently moving between the more slowly moving cytoskeleton.

neurofilaments formed by the association of three neurofilament protein subunits.

Neurofilaments and microtubules move at a rate of approximately 1 mm/day and make up the majority of SCa, which is the slowest moving component of axonal transport. Moving at only a slightly more rapid rate of 2 to 4 mm/day in an anterograde direction is SCb, which is composed of many proteins. Included in SCb are several structural proteins, such as the component of microfilaments (actin) and several microfilament-associated proteins (M2 protein and fodrin), as well as clathrin and many soluble proteins.

This continual transport of proteins from the cell body through the various components of anterograde axonal transport is the mechanism through which the neuron provides the distal axon with its complement of functional and structural proteins. Some vesicles are also moving in a retrograde direction and undoubtedly provide the cell body with information concerning the status of the distal axon.

Axonal Degeneration

When the neuronal cell body has been lethally injured, it degenerates, in a process called *neuronopathy*. This is characterized by the loss of the cell body and all of its processes, with no potential for regeneration. However, when the injury is at the level of the axon, the axon may degenerate while the neuronal cell body continues to survive, a condition known as an *axonopathy*. In this setting, there is a potential for regeneration and recovery from the toxic injury as the axonal stump sprouts and regenerates (Figure 16–3).

The result of axotomy (transection of an axon) is that the distal axon is destined to degenerate, a process known as axonal degeneration, which is unique to the NS. The cell body of the neuron responds to the axotomy as well and undergoes a process of chromatolysis. The sequence of events that occurs in the distal stump of an axon following transection is referred to as *Wallerian degeneration*. Because the axonal degeneration associated with chemicals and some disease states is thought to occur through a similar sequence of events, it is often referred to as *Wallerian-like* axonal degeneration.

Following axotomy, there is degeneration of the distal nerve stump, followed by generation of a microenvironment supportive of regeneration and involving the distal axon, ensheathing glial cells and the blood nerve barrier. Initially there is a period during which the distal stump survives and maintains relatively normal structural, transport, and conduction properties. The duration of survival is proportional to the length of the axonal stump, and this relationship appears to be maintained across species.

Terminating the period of survival is an active proteolysis that digests the axolemma and axoplasm, leaving only a myelin sheath surrounding a swollen degenerate axon. Digestion of the axon appears to be an all-or-none event effected through endogenous proteases that are activated through increased levels of intracellular free Ca^{2+}.

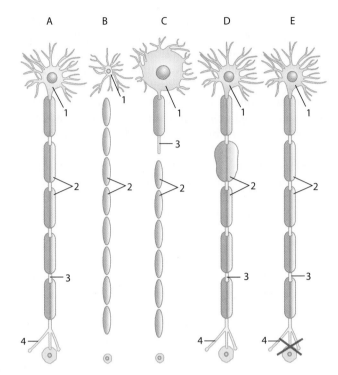

FIGURE 16–3 **Patterns of neurotoxic injury. (A)** Normal neuron showing (1) cell body and dendrites, (2) myelinating cells, encircling the (3) axon, and (4) synapse. **(B)** A neuronopathy resulting from the death of the entire neuron. Astrocytes often proliferate in response to the neuronal loss, creating both neuronal loss and gliosis. **(C)** An axonopathy occurs when the axon is the primary site of injury, the axon degenerates, and the surviving neuron shows only chromatolysis with margination of its Nissl substance and nucleus to the cell periphery. **(D)** Myelinopathy resulting from disruption of myelin or selective injury to the myelinating cells. To prevent cross-talk between adjacent axons, myelinating cells divide and cover the denuded axon rapidly; however, the process of remyelination is much less effective in the CNS than in the PNS. **(E)** Some forms of toxicity are due to interruption of the process of neurotransmission, either through blocking excitation or by excessive stimulation, rather than actual cell death.

In the PNS, Schwann cells respond to loss of axons by decreasing synthesis of myelin lipids, down-regulating genes encoding myelin proteins, and dedifferentiating to a premyelinating mitotic Schwann cell phenotype. The proliferating Schwann cells create a tubular structure around the axon (referred to as a band of Bungner), providing physical guidance for regenerating axons. These tubes also provide trophic support from nerve growth factor (NGF), brain-derived neurotrophic factor, insulin-like growth factor, and corresponding receptors produced by the associated Schwann cells. Resident macrophages distributed along the endothelium within the endoneurium and the denervated Schwann cells assist in clearing myelin debris, but the recruitment of hematogenous macrophages accounts for the removal of the majority of myelin. Another essential role of recruited, circulating macrophages is the production of interleukin-1 (IL-1), which is responsible for stimulating production of NGF by Schwann cells.

A critical difference exists between axonal degeneration in the CNS compared with that in the PNS: peripheral axons can regenerate, whereas central axons cannot. Main factors contributing to the inability of the CNS to regenerate include inhibitory factors secreted by oligodendrocytes, astrocyte scarring, and glial interference. Interestingly, experiments involving cellular transplants of Schwann cells to the CNS or CNS neurons to the PNS show that the regenerative capability of CNS neurons depends on both the microenvironment and the properties of mature neurons.

Wallerian degeneration was long thought to be a passive process that proceeded inexorably after separating the axon from the trophic support provided by the cell body. However, we now know from several lines of evidence that Wallerian degeneration is an active process mediated by the axon itself, and that it is possible to slow or even halt its progression. Moreover, although axonal degeneration can be initiated by many different means, including physical, genetic, or toxic, the mechanisms of degeneration converge into common regulated pathways that are potentially subject to pharmacological intervention.

Myelin Formation and Maintenance

Myelin is formed in the CNS by oligodendrocytes and in the PNS by Schwann cells. Both of these cell types form concentric layers of lipid-rich myelin by the progressive wrapping of their cytoplasmic processes around the axon in successive loops (Figure 16–4). These cells exclude cytoplasm from the inner

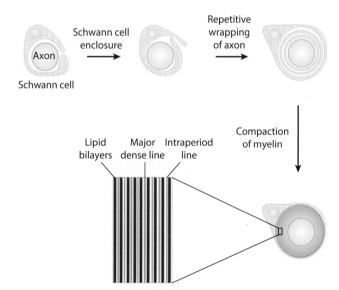

FIGURE 16–4   Process of myelination. Myelination begins when a myelinating cell encircles an axon, either Schwann cells in the peripheral nervous system or oligodendrocytes in the CNS. Simple enclosure of the axon persists in unmyelinated axons. Myelin formation proceeds by a progressive wrapping of multiple layers of the myelinating cell around the axon, with extrusion of the cytoplasm and extracellular space to bring the lipid bilayers into close proximity. The intracellular space is compressed to form the major dense line of myelin, and the extracellular space is compressed to form the intraperiod line.

surface of their membranes to form the major dense line of myelin. In a similar process, the extracellular space is reduced on the extracellular surface of the bilayers, and the lipid membranes stack together.

The maintenance of myelin is dependent on a number of membrane-associated proteins and on metabolism of specific lipids present in myelin bilayers. Some toxic compounds interfere with this complex process of the maintenance of myelin and result in the toxic "myelinopathies" (Figure 16–3). In general, the loss of myelin with the preservation of axons is referred to as *demyelination*.

Neurotransmission

Intercellular communication is achieved in the NS through the synapse. Neurotransmitters released from one neuron act as the first messenger. Binding of the transmitter to the postsynaptic receptor is followed by modulation of an ion channel or activation of a second-messenger system, leading to changes in the responding cell. Various therapeutic drugs and toxic compounds impact the process of neurotransmission.

Neurotoxicity expresses itself in terms of altered conduction and propagation of nerve impulses and changes in functions such as behavior, performance, and conditioning. Chemicals acting on neurotransmission may interrupt the transmission of impulses, block or accentuate transsynaptic communication, block reuptake of neurotransmitters or precursors, or interfere with second-messenger systems.

In terms of toxicity, many side effects of neurological drugs may be viewed as short-term interactions that are reversible with time or that may be counteracted by the use of appropriate antagonists. However, some of the toxicity associated with long-term exposures may be irreversible. Excessive stimulation of neurotransmitter systems may also have long-term consequences; e.g., excitatory system (e.g., glutamate) produces excitotoxicity that is manifest as CNS diseases and nerve cell death.

Development of the Nervous System

The NS begins development during gestation and continues through adolescence. Proliferation, migration, differentiation, synaptogenesis, apoptosis, and myelination are the basic processes that underlie development of the NS, and these occur in a tightly choreographed sequence that depends on the region, cell type, and neurotrophic signals. The proliferation and migration of neurons and glia occur in waves that are specific for brain regions, but in general, the brain develops in a caudal to rostral direction (with cerebellar development being a notable exception). During differentiation (phenotype expression) and synaptogenesis (formation of functional synaptic connections), the circuitry of the NS is established. Chemicals such as nerve growth factors, adhesive molecules, and neurotransmitters serve as morphogenic signals; neurotransmitter developmental signals are separate from their synaptic transmission function. Selected cells are also removed during ontogeny via apoptosis (programmed cell death), which results in the appropriate cell types in the correct regions. The glial supportive cells develop last, and myelination is protracted.

The immature NS is especially vulnerable to certain agents and there are several factors that make the developing NS uniquely susceptible. Cell sensitivity differs with the developmental stage, leading to critical windows of vulnerability. Chemicals that alter the timing and formation of neural connections could result in permanent malformations, the consequences of which may be quite unlike the chemical's effects in the adult NS. Furthermore, while synaptogenesis can continue throughout life, proliferation cannot; therefore, the CNS is unique in that damaged neural cells are not readily replaced. Finally, there are physiological and kinetic differences in the developing organism that may profoundly influence its sensitivity, including the slow formation of the blood–brain barrier and lack of key metabolic enzymes to protect the brain and eliminate toxicants.

Factors Relevant to Neurodegenerative Diseases

A classic example of toxicant-induced neurodegeneration is exposure to 1-methyl-4-phenyl-1,2,3,6-tetrahydropyridine (MPTP), which is a by-product of the opioid analgesic, MPPP. Exposure to a sufficient amount of MPTP can lead to immediate parkinsonism, a disease in which dopaminergic neurons of the substantia nigra are lost. Exposure to an amount of MPTP insufficient to cause immediate parkinsonism leads to early signs of the disease years later. It does not seem likely that an early sublethal injury to dopaminergic neurons later becomes lethal. Rather, smaller exposures to MPTP may cause a decrement in the population of dopaminergic neurons and leave the individual vulnerable to further loss of dopaminergic neurons.

Epidemiological studies also implicate exposure to herbicides, pesticides, and metals as risk factors for Parkinson's disease (PD). Several studies suggest that dithiocarbamates also play an important role. Interestingly, some studies suggest that cigarette smoking may have a protective effect against both Alzheimer's disease and PD.

Environmental chemicals may cause heritable alterations in gene expression in the absence of changes in genome sequences. The study of epigenetics has established two categories of mechanisms affecting gene expression: DNA methylation and histone posttranslational modifications. In most instances, methylation of the promotor region results in transcriptional repression of the gene. Histone posttranslational modifications are characterized by lysine acetylation, arginine and lysine methylation, serine phosphorylation, lysine ubiquitylation, etc.

Finally, it is necessary to recognize that microRNAs (miRNAs) provide regulatory control over gene expression. mRNAs can control developmental timing, cell proliferation, cell death, and patterning of the NS, thus providing extensive regulatory networks with a complexity comparable to that of transcription factors. More than 250 miRNAs have been already identified, but their mRNA targets and functions have yet to be

fully appreciated. Emerging studies also suggest that miRNAs may be targeted by neurotoxicants, thus potentially affecting a broad spectrum of functions, encompassing cell differentiation and migration, neurogenesis, as well as synaptic function, to name a few.

FUNCTIONAL MANIFESTATIONS OF NEUROTOXICITY

Functions of the NS include motor, sensory, autonomic, and cognitive capabilities. Functional assessment uses a battery of tests as a means for screening potentially neurotoxic compounds. Specific behavioral methods include functional observational batteries (FOBs), Irwin screens, tests of motor activity, and expanded clinical observations. These tests have the advantage over biochemical and pathological measures in that they permit evaluation of a single animal over longitudinal studies to determine the onset, progression, duration, and reversibility of a neurotoxic injury.

Some functional tests are more specific than observations and motor activity, and many of these functions have a clinical or behavioral correlate in humans. Electrophysiological tests provide sensory-specific information on nerve conduction velocity and integrity, and have been used to complement behavioral evaluations. Measures of sensory function tap specific neuronal pathways that govern stimuli-dependent reflexes. Autonomic function includes evaluations of cardiovascular status and cholinergic/adrenergic balance.

Deficits in cognitive function, especially in the context of developmental toxicity, represent an end point of great public concern and rhetoric. In most cases, deficits in human cognitive function may be detected in laboratory animals as well, although the affected cognitive domain may vary. Ultimately, neurotoxicants identified by behavioral methods are also evaluated at a cellular and molecular level to provide an understanding of the events in the NS that cause the neurological dysfunction.

MECHANISMS OF NEUROTOXICITY

Individual neurotoxic compounds typically have one of four targets: the neuron, the axon, the myelinating cell, or the neurotransmitter system.

Neuronopathies

Certain toxicants are specific for neurons, resulting in their injury or death. Neuron loss is irreversible and includes degeneration of all of its cytoplasmic extensions, dendrites and axons, and the myelin ensheathing the axon (Figure 16–3). Unique features of the neuron that place it at risk for the action of cellular toxicants include a high metabolic rate, a long cellular process that is supported by the cell body, and an excitable membrane that is rapidly depolarized and repolarized.

Although a large number of compounds are known to result in toxic neuronopathies (Table 16–1), all of these toxicants

TABLE 16–1 Chemicals associated with neuronal injury (neuronopathies).

Neurotoxicant	Neurologic Findings	Cellular Basis of Neurotoxicity
Aluminum	Dementia, encephalopathy (humans), learning deficits	Spongiosis cortex, neurofibrillary aggregates, degenerative changes in cortex
6-Amino-nicotinamide	Not reported in humans; hind limb paralysis (experimental animals)	Spongy (vacuolar) degeneration in spinal cord, brainstem, cerebellum; axonal degeneration of the peripheral nervous system (PNS)
Arsenic	Encephalopathy (acute), peripheral neuropathy (chronic)	Brain swelling and hemorrhage (acute); axonal degeneration in PNS (chronic)
Azide	Insufficient data (humans); convulsions, ataxia (primates)	Neuronal loss in cerebellum and cortex
Bismuth	Emotional disturbances, encephalopathy, myoclonus	Neuronal loss, basal ganglia, and Purkinje cells of cerebellum
Carbon monoxide	Encephalopathy, delayed parkinsonism/dystonia	Neuronal loss in cortex, necrosis of globus pallidus, focal demyelination; blocks oxygen-binding site of hemoglobin and iron-binding sites of brain
Carbon tetrachloride	Encephalopathy (secondary to liver failure)	Enlarged astrocytes in striatum, globus pallidus
Chloramphenicol	Optic neuritis, peripheral neuropathy	Neuronal loss (retina), axonal degeneration (PNS)
Cyanide	Coma, convulsions, rapid death; delayed parkinsonism/dystonia	Neuronal degeneration, cerebellum, and globus pallidus; focal demyelination; blocks cytochrome oxidase/ATP production
Doxorubicin	Insufficient data (humans); progressive ataxia (experimental animals)	Degeneration of dorsal root ganglion cells, axonal degeneration (PNS)
Ethanol	Mental retardation, hearing deficits (prenatal exposure)	Microcephaly, cerebral malformations
Lead	Encephalopathy (acute), learning deficits (children), neuropathy with demyelination (rats)	Brain swelling, hemorrhages (acute), axonal loss in PNS (humans)
Manganese	Emotional disturbances, parkinsonism/dystonia	Degeneration of striatum, globus pallidus
Mercury, inorganic	Emotional disturbances, tremor, fatigue	Insufficient data in humans (may affect spinal tracts; cerebellum)
Methanol	Headache, visual loss or blindness, coma (severe)	Necrosis of putamen, degeneration of retinal ganglion cells
Methylazoxymethanol acetate (MAM)	Microcephaly, retarded development (rats)	Developmental abnormalities of fetal brain (rats)
Methyl bromide	Visual and speech impairment; peripheral neuropathy	Insufficient data
Methyl mercury (organic mercury)	Ataxia, constriction of visual fields, paresthesias (adult) Psychomotor retardation (fetal exposure)	Neuronal degeneration, visual cortex, cerebellum, ganglia Spongy disruption, cortex, and cerebellum
1-Methyl-4-phenyl-1,2,3,6-tetrahydropyridine (MPTP)	Parkinsonism, dystonia (acute exposure) Early onset parkinsonism (late effect of acute exposure)	Neuronal degeneration in substantia nigra Neuronal degeneration in substantia nigra
3-Nitropropionic acid	Seizures, delayed dystonia/grimacing	Necrosis in basal ganglia
Phenytoin (diphenyl-hydantoin)	Nystagmus, ataxia, dizziness	Degeneration of Purkinje cells (cerebellum)
Quinine	Constriction of visual fields	Vacuolization of retinal ganglion cells
Streptomycin (aminoglycosides)	Hearing loss	Degeneration of inner ear (organ of Corti)
Thallium	Emotional disturbances, ataxia, peripheral neuropathy	Brain swelling (acute), axonal degeneration in PNS
Trimethyltin	Tremors, hyperexcitability (experimental animals)	Loss of hippocampal neurons, amygdala pyriform cortex

share certain features. Each toxic condition is the result of a cellular toxicant that has a predilection for neurons. The initial injury to neurons is followed by apoptosis or necrosis, leading to permanent loss of the neuron. These agents tend to be diffuse in their action, although they may show some selectivity in the degree of injury of different neuronal subpopulations. The expression of these cellular events is often a diffuse encephalopathy, with global dysfunctions.

Doxorubicin—Doxorubicin (Adriamycin), a quinone-containing anthracycline antibiotic, is one of the most effective antimitotics in cancer chemotherapy. Unfortunately, clinical application of doxorubicin is greatly limited by its acute and chronic cardiotoxicity. Doxorubicin injures neurons in the PNS, specifically those of the dorsal root ganglia and autonomic ganglia by intercalating with DNA and interfering with transcription. Other important mechanisms of action of doxorubicin include its interaction with topoisomerase II, which forms a DNA-cleavable complex and generation of reactive oxygen species (ROS) by enzymatic electron reduction of doxorubicin by variety of oxidases, reductases, and dehydrogenases. The vulnerability of sensory and autonomic neurons appears to reflect the lack of protection of these neurons by a blood–tissue barrier within ganglia.

Methyl Mercury—Methyl mercury (MeHg) exposure occurs primarily from eating fish in which the substance has accumulated. In addition, mercury is a common pollutant in hazardous waste sites in the United States. The clinical picture of MeHg poisoning varies with both the severity of exposure and the age of the individual at the time of exposure. In adults, the most dramatic sites of injury are the neurons of the visual cortex and the small internal granular cell neurons of the cerebellar cortex, whose massive degeneration results in blindness and marked ataxia. In children, developmental disabilities, retardation, and cognitive deficits occur. It has been suggested that these differences are caused by an immature blood–brain barrier causing a more generalized distribution of mercury in the developing brain. Recent studies in rats show that the neurons that are most sensitive to the toxic effects of MeHg are those that reside in the dorsal root ganglia, perhaps again reflecting the vulnerability of neurons not shielded by blood–tissue barriers. The mechanism of MeHg toxicity has been the subject of intense investigation and it remains unknown whether the ultimate toxicant is MeHg itself or the liberated mercuric ion. A variety of aberrations in cellular function have been noted, including impaired glycolysis, nucleic acid biosynthesis, aerobic respiration, protein synthesis, and neurotransmitter release. In addition, there is evidence for enhanced oxidative injury and altered calcium homeostasis. Exposure to MeHg leads to widespread neuronal injury and subsequently to a diffuse encephalopathy.

Trimethyltin—Organotins are used industrially as plasticizers, antifungal agents, or pesticides. Intoxication with trimethyltin has been associated with a potentially irreversible limbic-cerebellar syndrome in humans and similar behavioral changes in primates. Trimethyltin gains access to the NS where, by an undefined mechanism, it leads to diffuse neuronal injury. Several hypotheses are suggested for the mechanism of trimethyltin neurotoxicity, however, including energy deprivation and excitotoxic damage.

Axonopathies

The neurotoxic disorders termed *axonopathies* are those in which the primary site of toxicity is the axon itself. The axon degenerates, and with it the myelin surrounding that axon; however, the neuron cell body remains intact (Figure 16–5). The toxicant results in a "chemical transection" of the axon at some point along its length, and the axon distal to the transection degenerates.

A critical difference exists in the significance of axonal degeneration in the CNS compared with that in the PNS: peripheral axons can regenerate, whereas central axons cannot. In the PNS, glial cells and macrophages support axonal regeneration. In the CNS, release of inhibitory factors from damaged myelin and astrocyte scarring actually interferes with regeneration. The clinical relevance of the disparity between the CNS and PNS is that partial to complete recovery can occur after axonal degeneration in the PNS, whereas the same event is irreversible in the CNS.

Axonopathies can be considered to result from a chemical transection of the axon. The number of axonal toxicants is large and increasing in number (Table 16–2). As the axons degenerate, sensations and motor strength are first impaired in the most distal extent of the axonal processes (e.g., the hands and feet), resulting in a "glove-and-stocking" neuropathy. With time and continued injury, the deficit progresses to involve more proximal areas of the body and the long axons of the spinal cord.

Gamma-diketones—Humans develop a progressive sensorimotor distal axonopathy when exposed to high concentrations of a simple alkane, *n*-hexane, day after day in work settings or after repeated intentional inhalation of hexane-containing glues. An identical axonopathy can be produced by methyl-*n*-butyl ketone (2-hexanone).

The ω-1 oxidation of *n*-hexane results in the γ-diketone, 2,5-hexanedione (HD), which reacts with amino groups in all tissues to form pyrroles that derivatize and cross-link neurofilaments, leading to development of neurofilament aggregates of the distal, subterminal axon (Figure 16–5). The neurofilament-filled axonal swellings distort nodal anatomy and impair axonal transport. The pathologic processes of neurofilament accumulation and degeneration of the axon are followed by the emergence of a clinical peripheral neuropathy.

Carbon Disulfide—The most significant exposures of humans to CS_2 have occurred in the vulcan rubber and viscose rayon industries. High-level exposures of humans to CS_2 cause a distal axonopathy that is identical pathologically to that caused by hexane. Covalent cross-linking of neurofilaments also occurs and it is known that CS_2 is itself the ultimate toxicant.

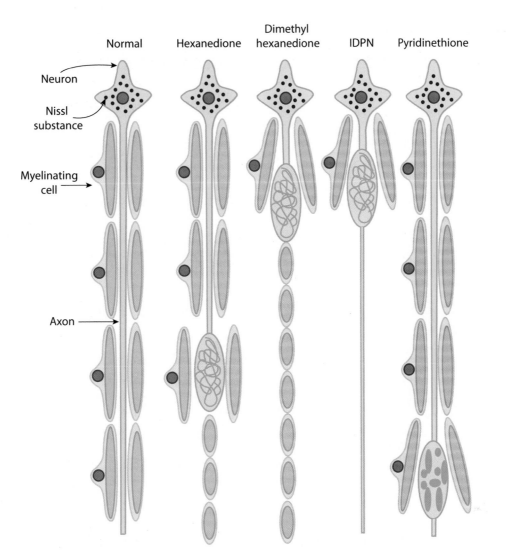

FIGURE 16–5 **Diagram of axonopathies.** Whereas 2,5-hexanedione results in the accumulation of neurofilaments in the distal regions of the axon, 3,4-dimethyl-2,5-hexanedione results in identical accumulation within the proximal segments. These proximal neurofilamentous swellings are quite similar to those that occur in the toxicity of β,β′-iminodipropionitrile (IDPN), although the distal axon does not degenerate in IDPN axonopathy but becomes atrophic. Pyridinethione results in axonal swellings that are distended with tubulovesicular material, followed by distal axonal degeneration.

The clinical effects of exposure to CS_2 in the chronic setting are very similar to those of hexane exposure, with the development of sensory and motor symptoms occurring initially in a glove-and-stocking distribution. In addition to this chronic axonopathy, CS_2 can also lead to aberrations in mood and signs of diffuse encephalopathic disease.

β,β′-Iminodipropionitrile (IDPN)—IDPN is a synthetic, bifunctional nitrile that causes a bizarre "waltzing syndrome" in rats and other mammals, although human exposure has never been documented. Features of this syndrome include excitement, circling, head twitching, and overalertness, which appears to result from degeneration of the vestibular sensory hair cells. In addition, administration of IDPN leads to accumulation of neurofilaments in the proximal axon, leading to

swelling without degeneration in most animals. These neurofilament swellings are similar to those observed in carbon disulfide or γ-diketone toxicity.

Repeated exposure to IDPN leads to demyelination and onion bulb formation (Figure 16–5), and eventually can produce distal axonal atrophy due to a reduction in anterograde neurofilament transport to the distal axon. This impairment of axonal transport results from the disruption of the association between microtubules and neurofilaments by IDPN, causing neurofilament accumulation. This leads to complete disturbance of the cytoskeleton of the axon.

Acrylamide—Acrylamide is a man-made vinyl monomer used widely in water purification, paper manufacturing, mining, and waterproofing. It is also used extensively in

TABLE 16–2 Chemicals associated with axonal injury (axonopathies).

Neurotoxicant	Neurologic Findings	Basis of Neurotoxicity
Acrylamide	Peripheral neuropathy (often sensory)	Axonal degeneration, axon terminal affected in earliest stages
p-Bromophenylacetyl urea	Peripheral neuropathy	Axonal degeneration in the peripheral nervous system (PNS) and central nervous system (CNS)
Carbon disulfide	Psychosis (acute), peripheral neuropathy (chronic)	Axonal degeneration, early stages include neurofilamentous swelling
Chlordecone (Kepone)	Tremors, in coordination (experimental animals)	Insufficient data (humans); axonal swelling and degeneration
Chloroquine	Peripheral neuropathy, weakness	Axonal degeneration, inclusions in dorsal root ganglion cells; also vacuolar myopathy
Clioquinol	Encephalopathy (acute), subacute myelooptic neuropathy (subacute)	Axonal degeneration, spinal cord, PNS, optic tracts
Colchicine	Peripheral neuropathy	Axonal degeneration, neuronal perikaryal filamentous aggregates; vacuolar myopathy
Dapsone	Peripheral neuropathy, predominantly motor	Axonal degeneration (both myelinated and unmyelinated axons)
Dichlorophenoxyacetate	Peripheral neuropathy (delayed)	Insufficient data
Dimethylaminopropionitrile	Peripheral neuropathy, urinary retention	Axonal degeneration (both myelinated and unmyelinated axons)
Ethylene oxide	Peripheral neuropathy	Axonal degeneration
Glutethimide	Peripheral neuropathy (predominantly sensory)	Insufficient data
Gold	Peripheral neuropathy (may have psychiatric problems)	Axonal degeneration, some segmental demyelination
n-Hexane	Peripheral neuropathy, severe cases have spasticity	Axonal degeneration, early neurofilamentous swelling, PNS, and spinal cord
Hydralazine	Peripheral neuropathy	Insufficient data
β,β′-Iminodipropionitrile	No data in humans; excitatory movement disorder (rats)	Proximal axonal swellings, degeneration of olfactory epithelial cells, vestibular hair cells
Isoniazid	Peripheral neuropathy (sensory), ataxia (high doses)	Axonal degeneration
Lithium	Lethargy, tremor, ataxia (reversible)	Insufficient data
Methyl n-butyl ketone	Peripheral neuropathy	Axonal degeneration, early neurofilamentous swelling, PNS, and spinal cord
Metronidazole	Sensory peripheral neuropathy, ataxia, seizures	Axonal degeneration, mostly affecting myelinated fibers; lesions of cerebellar nuclei
Misonidazole	Peripheral neuropathy	Axonal degeneration
Nitrofurantoin	Peripheral neuropathy	Axonal degeneration
Organophosphorus compounds (NTE inhibitors)	Abdominal pain (acute); peripheral neuropathy	Axonal degeneration
Paclitaxel (taxoids)	Delayed peripheral neuropathy (motor), spasticity	Axonal degeneration (delayed after single exposure), PNS, and spinal cord
Platinum (cisplatin)	Peripheral neuropathy	Axonal degeneration; microtubule accumulation in early stages
Pyridinethione (pyrithione)	Movement disorders (tremor, choreoathetosis)	Axonal degeneration (variable)
Vincristine (vinca alkaloids)	Cranial (most often trigeminal) neuropathy Peripheral neuropathy, variable autonomic symptoms	Insufficient data Axonal degeneration (PNS), neurofibrillary changes (spinal cord, intrathecal route)

biochemical laboratories, and is present in many foods prepared at high temperatures. Although it can be dangerous if not handled carefully, most toxic events in humans have been observed as peripheral neuropathies in factory workers exposed to high doses.

Studies of acrylamide neuropathy revealed a distal axonopathy characterized by multiple axonal swellings. A single large dose is sufficient to produce these swellings; however, repeated dosing results in a more proximal axonopathy, in a "dying back" process. These changes are caused by accumulations of neurofilaments at the nerve terminal. Recently it has been observed that nerve terminal degeneration occurs prior to development of axonopathy, suggesting that this degeneration is the primary lesion.

Organophosphorus Compounds—Organophosphorus (OP) compounds are used as insecticides, chemical warfare agents, chemical intermediates, flame retardants, fuel additives, hydraulic fluids, lubricants, pharmaceuticals, and plasticizers. The OP insecticides and nerve agents are designed to inhibit AChE, thereby causing accumulation of acetylcholine in cholinergic synapses resulting in cholinergic toxicity and death. Some OP compounds, such as tri-o-cresyl phosphate (TOCP), can cause a severe sensorimotor central peripheral distal axonopathy called OP compound–induced delayed neurotoxicity (OPIDN) without inducing cholinergic poisoning.

Many OP compounds are lipophilic and readily enter the NS, where they can phosphorylate neural target proteins. When the principal target is AChE, cholinergic toxicity can ensue, either because of suprathreshold levels of inhibition or inhibition plus aging. When *aging* of inhibited AChE also occurs (i.e., net loss of a ligand from the phosphorus of the OP-enzyme conjugate, leaving a negatively charged phosphoryl moiety attached to the active site), the qualitative nature of the toxicity does not change. Instead, the inhibited AChE becomes intractable to reactivation. When the principal target is neuropathy target esterase (neurotoxic esterase, NTE), OPIDN can result only if both suprathreshold (>70%) inhibition occurs *and* the inhibited enzyme undergoes aging. Thus, in the case of NTE and OPIDN, inhibition alone is insufficient to precipitate toxicity. Neuropathic (aging) inhibitors of NTE include compounds from the phosphate, phosphonate, and phosphoramidate classes of OP compounds.

Axonal degeneration does not commence immediately after acute exposure to a neuropathic OP compound but is delayed for at least eight days between the acute high-dose exposure and clinical signs of axonopathy. Some effective regeneration of axons occurs in the PNS while axonal degeneration is progressive and persistent in the long tracts of the spinal cord.

Human cases of OPIDN are now rare and usually arise from intentional ingestion of massive doses of OP insecticides in suicide attempts. Nevertheless, the fact remains that OPIDN is a debilitating and incurable condition. While the preceding discussion was limited to organic compounds of pentacovalent phosphorus, organic compounds of trivalent phosphorous also produce axonal degeneration in the CNS and PNS albeit in a different form than classical OPIDN.

Pyridinethione—This compound is a chelating agent that is usually encountered as the zinc complex, called zinc pyridinethione (ZPT), which has antibacterial and antifungal properties and is a component of shampoos that are effective in the treatment of seborrhea and dandruff. Although the compound is applied to the human scalp in antidandruff shampoos, dermal absorption of ZPT is minimal and exposure primarily occurs orally. Only the pyridinethione moiety is absorbed following ingestion, with the majority of zinc eliminated in the feces. Pyridinethione appears to interfere with the fast axonal transport systems, impairs the turnaround of rapidly transported vesicles, and slows the retrograde transport of vesicles. Aberration of the fast axonal transport systems most likely contributes to the accumulation of tubular and vesicular structures in the distal axon (Figure 16–5). As these materials accumulate in one region of the axon, the axon degenerates in its more distal regions beyond the accumulated structures. The earliest signs are diminished grip strength and changes of the axon terminal, leading to a peripheral neuropathy.

Microtubule-associated Neurotoxicity—A number of plant alkaloids alter the assembly and depolymerization of microtubules in nerve axons, causing neurotoxicity. The oldest known of these are colchicine and the vinca alkaloids, which bind to tubulin and cause depolymerization of microtubules. Colchicine is an alkaloid pharmaceutical used in the treatment of gout, familial Mediterranean fever, and other disorders. Vincristine and vinblastine are two vinca alkaloids used as chemotherapeutic agents. Both colchicine and the vinca alkaloids produce a similar peripheral axonal neuropathy. Hallmarks of this neuropathy include paresthesia (tingling) of the fingers, generalized weakness, and clumsiness.

Paclitaxel (Taxol), another plant alkaloid, has become a popular chemotherapeutic drug used to treat a variety of neoplasms. However, side effects include a predominantly sensory neuropathy, beginning in the hands and feet. Like colchicine and the vinca alkaloids, paclitaxel binds to tubulin; however, instead of leading to depolymerization, it promotes the formation of microtubules. Once formed, these microtubules remain stabilized by paclitaxel even in conditions that normally lead to dissociation of tubulin subunits, including cold temperatures or the presence of calcium.

The pathologies of the axon induced by these drugs are different. Although colchicine leads to atrophy of the axon and a decrease in the number of microtubules, paclitaxel causes the aggregation to form a matrix that may inhibit fast axonal transport, which has been demonstrated with both colchicine and paclitaxel.

Myelinopathies

Myelin provides electrical insulation of neuronal processes, and its absence leads to a slowing of conduction and aberrant conduction of impulses between adjacent processes. Toxicants exist that result in the separation of the myelin lamellae, termed *intramyelinic edema*, and in the selective loss of myelin, termed *demyelination*. Intramyelinic edema may be caused by alterations in the transcript levels of myelin basic protein mRNA, and early in its evolution is reversible. Demyelination may result from progressive intramyelinic edema or from direct toxicity to the myelinating cell. Remyelination in the CNS occurs to only a limited extent after demyelination. However, Schwann cells in the PNS are capable of remyelinating the axon. All the compounds in Table 16–3 lead to a myelinopathy.

Hexachlorophene—Hexachlorophene, or 2,2′-methylenebis-(3,4,6-trichlorophenol), caused neurotoxicity when newborn infants were bathed with the compound to avoid staphylococcal skin infections. Following skin absorption of this hydrophobic compound, hexachlorophene enters the NS and results in intramyelinic edema, which leads to the formation of vacuoles creating a "spongiosis" of the brain. Hexachlorophene causes intramyelinic edema that leads to segmental demyelination. Swelling of the brain causes increased intracranial pressure, axonal degeneration, along with degeneration of photoreceptors in the retina. Humans exposed acutely to hexachlorophene may have generalized weakness, confusion, and seizures. Progression may occur, to include coma and death.

Tellurium—Although exposures have not been reported in humans, the neurotoxicity of tellurium in young rats alters the synthesis of myelin lipids in Schwann cells, because of various lipid abnormalities. As biochemical changes occur, lipids accumulate in Schwann cells, which eventually lose their ability to maintain myelin in the PNS.

Lead—Lead exposure in animals results in a peripheral neuropathy with prominent segmental demyelination. In young children, acute massive exposures to lead result in severe cerebral edema, perhaps from damage to endothelial cells. Children absorb lead more readily, and the very young do not have the protection of the blood–brain barrier. Chronic lead intoxication in adults results in peripheral neuropathy, gastritis, colicky abdominal pain, anemia, and the prominent deposition of lead in particular anatomical sites, creating lead lines in the gums and in the epiphyses of long bones in children. Lead in the peripheral nerve of humans slows nerve conduction. The basis of lead encephalopathy is unclear, although an effect on the membrane structure of myelin and myelin membrane fluidity has been shown.

Astrocytes

Astrocytes perform and regulate a wide range of physiologic functions in the CNS. The astrocyte appears to be a primary means of defense in the CNS following exposure to neurotoxicants, as a spatial buffering system for osmotically active ions, and as a depot for the sequestration and metabolic processing of endogenous molecules and xenobiotics.

Ammonia—At high CNS concentrations, ammonia produces seizures, resulting from its depolarizing action on cell membranes, whereas at lower concentrations, ammonia produces

TABLE 16–3 Chemicals associated with injury of myelin (myelinopathies).

Neurotoxicant	Neurologic Findings	Basis of Neurotoxicity
Acetylethyltetramethyl tetralin (AETT)	Not reported in humans; hyperexcitability, tremors (rats)	Intramyelinic edema; pigment accumulation in neurons
Amiodarone	Peripheral neuropathy	Axonal degeneration and demyelination; lipid-laden lysosomes in Schwann cells
Cuprizone	Not reported in humans; encephalopathy (experimental animals)	Status spongiosis of white matter, intramyelinic edema (early stages); gliosis (late)
Disulfiram	Peripheral neuropathy, predominantly sensory	Axonal degeneration, swellings in distal axons
Ethidium bromide	Insufficient data (humans)	Intramyelinic edema, status spongiosis of white matter
Hexachlorophene	Irritability, confusion, seizures	Brain swelling, intramyelinic edema in CNS and PNS, late axonal degeneration
Lysolecithin	Effects only on direct injection into PNS or CNS (experimental animals)	Selective demyelination
Perhexilene	Peripheral neuropathy	Demyelinating neuropathy, membrane-bound inclusions in Schwann cells
Tellurium	Hydrocephalus, hind limb paralysis (experimental animals)	Demyelinating neuropathy, lipofuscinosis (experimental animals)
Triethyltin	Headache, photophobia, vomiting, paraplegia (irreversible)	Brain swelling (acute) with intramyelinic edema, spongiosis of white matter

stupor and coma, consistent with its hyperpolarizing effects. Ammonia intoxication is associated with astrocytic swelling and morphological changes. Increased intracellular ammonia concentrations have also been implicated in the inhibition of neuronal glutamate precursor synthesis, resulting in diminished glutamatergic neurotransmission, changes in neurotransmitter uptake (glutamate), and changes in receptor-mediated metabolic responses of astrocytes to neuronal signals.

Nitrochemicals—Organic nitrates are used for peripheral vasodilatation and reduction of blood pressure (nitroglycerine) in treatment of cardiovascular disease. The dinitrobenzenes are important synthetic intermediates in the industrial production of dyes, plastics, and explosives. The neurotoxic compound, 1,3-dinitrobenzene (DNB), produces gliovascular lesions that specifically target astrocytes in the periaqueductal gray matter of the brainstem and deep cerebellar roof nuclei. Metronidazole, a 5-nitroimidazole [1-(2-hydroxyethyl)-2-methyl-5-nitroimidazole], is an antimicrobial, antiprotozoal agent that is commonly used for the treatment of a wide variety of infections. Prolonged treatment with metronidazole is associated with a peripheral neuropathy characterized by paraesthesias, dysaesthesias, headaches, glossitis, urticaria, and pruritus in addition to other somatosensory disorders.

Methionine Sulfoximine—Methionine sulfoximine (MSO) is an irreversible inhibitor of the astrocyte-specific enzyme, glutamine synthase. Ingestion of large amounts of MSO leads to neuronal cell loss in the hippocampal fascia dentata and pyramidal cell layer, in the short association fibers and lower layers of the cerebral cortex, and in cerebellar Purkinje cells. MSO also leads to large increases of glycogen levels, primarily within astrocytic cell bodies, as well as swollen and damaged astrocytic mitochondria.

Fluoroacetate and Fluorocitrate—The Krebs cycle inhibitor fluorocitrate (FC) and its precursor fluoroacetate (FA) are preferentially taken up by glia. FA occurs naturally in a number of plants, and is available commercially as a rodenticide (Compound 1080). Exposure to FA may also occur via exposure to the anti-cancer drug 5-fluorouracil. Ingestion of large amounts of FA results in ionic convulsions, with onset of seizures within minutes of consumption; those surviving these episodes frequently die later on due to respiratory arrest or heart failure. The actions of FC and FA have been attributed both to the disruption of carbon flux through the Krebs cycle and to impairment of ATP production.

Neurotransmission-associated Neurotoxicity

A wide variety of naturally occurring toxins, as well as synthetic chemicals, alter specific mechanisms of intercellular communication (Table 16–4). Although neurotransmitter-associated

TABLE 16–4 Chemicals associated with neurotransmitter-associated toxicity.

Neurotoxicant	Neurologic Findings	Basis of Neurotoxicity
Amphetamine and methamphetamine	Tremor, restlessness (acute); cerebral infarction and hemorrhage; neuropsychiatric disturbances	Bilateral infarcts of globus pallidus, abnormalities in dopaminergic, serotonergic, cholinergic systems Acts at adrenergic receptors (PNS)
Atropine	Restlessness, irritability, hallucinations	Blocks cholinergic receptors (anticholinergic)
Cocaine	Increased risk of stroke and cerebral atrophy (chronic users); increased risk of sudden cardiac death; movement and psychiatric abnormalities, especially during withdrawal Decreased head circumference (fetal exposure)	Infarcts and hemorrhages; alteration in striatal dopamine neurotransmission Structural malformations in newborns
Domoic acid	Headache, memory loss, hemiparesis, disorientation, seizures	Neuronal loss, hippocampus and amygdala, layers 5 and 6 of neocortex Kainate-like pattern of excitotoxicity
Kainate	Insufficient data in humans; seizures in animals (selective lesioning compound in neuroscience)	Degeneration of neurons in hippocampus, olfactory cortex, amygdala, thalamus Binds AMPA/kainate receptors
β-N-Methylamino-L-alanine (BMAA)	Weakness, movement disorder (monkeys)	Degenerative changes in motor neurons (monkeys) Excitotoxic probably via NMDA receptors
Muscarine (mushrooms)	Nausea, vomiting, headache	Binds muscarinic receptors (cholinergic)
Nicotine	Nausea, vomiting, convulsions	Binds nicotinic receptors (cholinergic) low-dose stimulation; high-dose blocking
β-N-Oxalylamino-L-alanine (BOAA)	Seizures	Excitotoxic probably via AMPA class of glutamate receptors

actions may be well understood for some agents, the specificity of the mechanisms should not be assumed.

Nicotine—Widely available in tobacco products and in certain pesticides, nicotine has diverse pharmacological actions and may be the source of considerable toxicity. Nicotine exerts its effects by binding to a subset of nicotinic cholinergic receptors. Smoking and "pharmacologic" doses of nicotine accelerate heart rate, elevate blood pressure, and constrict blood vessels within the skin as a result of stimulation of the ganglionic sympathetic NS.

The rapid rise in circulating levels of nicotine after acute overdose leads to excessive stimulation of nicotinic receptors, a process that is followed rapidly by ganglionic paralysis. Initial nausea, rapid heart rate, and perspiration are followed shortly by marked slowing of heart rate with a fall in blood pressure. Somnolence and confusion may occur, followed by coma; if death results, it is often the result of paralysis of the muscles of respiration.

Acute poisoning with nicotine fortunately is uncommon; however, exposure to lower levels for longer duration is very common. In humans, it has been difficult to separate the effects of nicotine from those of other components of cigarette smoke. The complications of smoking include cardiovascular disease, cancers (especially malignancies of the lung and upper airway), chronic pulmonary disease, and attention deficit disorders in children of women who smoke during pregnancy.

An increased propensity for platelets to aggregate is seen in smokers, and this platelet abnormality correlates with the level of nicotine. Nicotine also places an increased burden on the heart through its acceleration of heart rate and blood pressure, suggesting that nicotine may play a role in the onset of myocardial ischemia. In addition, nicotine also inhibits apoptosis and may play a direct role in tumor promotion and tobacco-related cancers.

Cocaine and Amphetamines—Cocaine blocks the reuptake of dopamine (DA), norepinephrine (NE), and serotonin (5-HT) at the nerve terminal in the CNS, and also causes release of DA from storage vesicles. The primary event responsible for the addictive properties and euphoric feeling when intoxicated is a block on the DA reuptake transporter (DAT).

Cocaine abuse also puts individuals at risk for cerebrovascular defects, cerebral atrophy, stroke, and intracranial hemorrhage. Cerebrovascular resistance has also been found to be higher in cocaine abusers. In chronic cocaine users, neurodegenerative disorders have been observed, similar to those observed with amphetamine use.

Amphetamines affect catecholamine neurotransmission in the CNS and have the potential to damage monoaminergic cells directly. Amphetamines, including methylenedioxymethamphetamine (MDMA, or "ecstasy"), have become popular with young adults in recent decades due to the belief that it is a "safe" drug, and its ability to increase energy and sensation in adults. Similar to cocaine, the most pronounced effect of amphetamines is on the DAergic neurons, but they can also damage

5-HT axons and axon terminals. The result is a distal axotomy of DA and 5-HT neurons.

The exact mechanism of amphetamine neurotoxicity is still unknown, but it seems that oxidative stress plays a key role. DA is oxidized to produce free radicals, and chronic use can affect superoxide dismutase (SOD) and catalase balance in rodents. In support of this hypothesis, studies have shown amphetamine neurotoxicity is attenuated by antioxidants.

Excitatory Amino Acids—Glutamate and certain other acidic amino acids are excitatory neurotransmitters. The toxicity of glutamate can be blocked by certain glutamate antagonists, and the concept has emerged that the toxicity of excitatory amino acids may be related to such conditions as hypoxia, epilepsy, and neurodegenerative diseases.

Glutamate is the main excitatory neurotransmitter of the brain, and its effects are mediated by several subtypes of receptors (Figure 16–6) called *excitatory amino acid receptors* (EAARs). The two major subtypes of glutamate receptors are those that are ligand-gated directly to ion channels (ionotropic) and those that are coupled with G proteins (metabotropic). Ionotropic receptors may be further subdivided by their specificity for binding kainate, quisqualate, α-amino-3-hydroxy-5-methylisoxazole-4-propionic acid (AMPA), and N-methyl-D-aspartate (NMDA). The entry of glutamate into the CNS is regulated at the blood–brain barrier, and glutamate exerts its effects in the circumventricular organ of the brain in which the blood–brain barrier is least developed. Within this site of limited access, glutamate injures neurons, apparently by opening glutamate-dependent ion channels, ultimately leading to neuronal swelling and neuronal cell death. The only known related human condition is the "Chinese restaurant syndrome,"

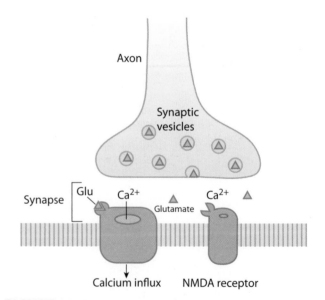

FIGURE 16–6 Schematic diagram of a synapse. Synaptic vesicles are transported to the axonal terminus, and released across the synaptic cleft to bind to the postsynaptic receptors. Glutamate, as an excitatory neurotransmitter, binds to its receptor and opens a calcium channel, leading to the excitation of the postsynaptic cell.

in which consumption of large amounts of monosodium gluta-mate (MSG) as a seasoning may lead to a burning sensation in the face, neck, and chest.

The cyclic glutamate analog kainate, isolated from a seaweed in Japan, is extremely potent as an excitotoxin, being a 100-fold more toxic than glutamate, and is selective at a molecular level for the kainate receptor. Like glutamate, kainate selec-tively injures dendrites and neurons and shows no substantial effect on glia or axons. Injected into a region of the brain, it can destroy the neurons of that area without disrupting all of the fibers that pass through the same region. Kainate has become a tool for neurobiologists to explore the anatomy and function of the NS. Kainate, through its selective action on neuronal cell bodies, has provided a greater understanding of the functions of cells within a specific region of the brain, whereas previous lesioning techniques addressed only regional functions. This void in understanding and the epidemiologic evidence that some neurodegenerative diseases may have environmental contributors inspire a heightened desire to appreciate more fully the effects of elements of our environment on the NS.

Development of permanent neurologic deficits occurred in individuals accidentally exposed to high doses of the EAAR agonist domoic acid, an analog of glutamate. The acute illness most commonly presented as gastrointestinal disturbance, severe headache, and short-term memory loss. A subset of the more severely afflicted patients had chronic memory defi-cits and motor neuropathy. Neuropathologic investigation of patients who died within 4 months of intoxication showed neurodegeneration that was most prominent in the hippocam-pus and amygdala.

Models of Neurodegenerative Disease

MPTP—A contaminant formed during meperidine synthe-sis, 1-methyl-4-phenyl-1,2,3,6-tetrahydropyridine (MPTP) (Figure 16–7), produces over hours to days the signs and symp-toms of irreversible Parkinson's disease. Autopsy studies have demonstrated marked degeneration of dopaminergic neurons in the substantia nigra, with degeneration continuing many years after exposure. It appears that MPTP is metabolized by two 2-electron oxidation reactions to the pyridinium ion, MPP+, which enters the dopaminergic neurons of the substan-tia nigra, resulting in their deaths by blocking mitochondrial respiration at complex I. Although not identical, MPTP neu-rotoxicity and Parkinson's disease produce symptomatology of masked facies, difficulties in initiating and terminating move-ments, resting "pill-rolling" tremors, rigidity, and bradykinesias.

Manganese—As an essential trace metal that is found in all tissues, manganese (Mn) is required for normal metabo-lism of amino acids, proteins, lipids, and carbohydrates, act-ing as a cofactor of synthesis enzymes. Excessive exposure to Mn produces neurotoxicity. The most common commercial sources of Mn include the fuel additive methylcyclopentadienyl

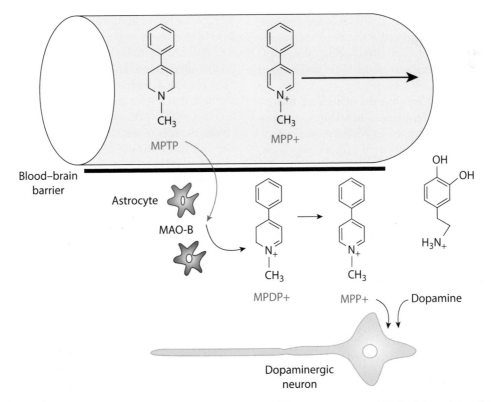

FIGURE 16–7 MPTP toxicity. MPP+, either formed elsewhere in the body following exposure to MPTP or injected directly into the blood, is unable to cross the blood–brain barrier. In contrast, MPTP gains access and is oxidized in situ to MPDP+ and MPP+. The same transport system that carries dopamine into the dopaminergic neurons also transports the cytotoxic MPP+.

manganese tricarbonyl (MMT), pesticides such as Maneb, steel factories, welding, and mining plants. Occupational exposure to toxic levels of Mn in industrial workers results in psychologic and neurologic disturbances, including delusions, hallucinations, depression, disturbed equilibrium, compulsive or violent behavior, weakness, and apathy, followed by extrapyramidal motor system defects such as tremors, muscle rigidity, ataxia, bradykinesia, and dystonia. Mn toxicity causes a loss of DA neurons in the substantia nigra, and as in Parkinson's disease, oxidative stress appears to play a significant role in the disorder.

Developmentally Neurotoxic Chemicals

Replication, migration, differentiation, myelination, and synapse formation are the basic processes that occur in specific spatial and temporal patterns and underlie development of the NS. There are a variety of insults known to disrupt NS development, the outcomes of which may be very different depending on the time of exposure, including exposures to certain metals, solvents, antimetabolites, persistent organic pollutants, pesticides, pharmaceuticals, and ionizing radiation. Multiple mechanisms of action may be present, producing a wide array of effects in the offspring. The impact on the developing NS may be very different, and often cannot be predicted, from effects observed in adults. A number of neurodevelopmental disorders have been, at least partially, attributed to exposures to neurotoxicological agents during the fetal, infant, or childhood periods.

Ethanol exposure during pregnancy can result in abnormalities in the fetus, including abnormal neuronal migration and facial development, and diffuse abnormalities in the development of neuronal processes, especially the dendritic spines. The clinical result of fetal alcohol exposure is often mental retardation, with malformations of the brain and delayed myelination of white matter.

MeHg exposure leads to developmental disabilities, including cerebral palsy, mental retardation, and seizures, in many children at birth. Children exposed to MeHg in utero show widespread neuronal loss, disruption of cellular migration, profound mental retardation, and paralysis.

There is considerable evidence that chronic exposure to nicotine has effects on the developing fetus. Along with decreased birth weights, attention deficit disorders are more common in children whose mothers smoke cigarettes during pregnancy, and nicotine has been shown to lead to analogous neurobehavioral abnormalities in animals exposed prenatally to nicotine.

Cocaine is able to cross the placental barrier and the fetal blood–brain barrier, and also causes reduced blood flow in the uterus. In severe events at large doses taken by the mother, the fetus may develop hypoxia, leading to a higher rate of birth defects. Maternal cocaine use is associated with low–birth weight and behavioral defects, including a decreased awareness of the surroundings and altered response to stress and pain sensitivity.

Several epidemiological studies have reported deficits in neurodevelopment and psychological performance in children exposed to polychlorinated biphenyls (PCBs) and/or dioxins. These persistent pollutants produce endocrine disruptions, cognitive deficits, and changes in activity levels in exposed offspring; however, the specific outcomes depend on the congener or mixture tested as well as the timing of exposure. Changes in estrogen or thyroid hormone, neurotransmitter function, and second messenger systems have been proposed as cellular bases for PCB toxicity. Another persistent class of hydrocarbons, polybrominated diphenyl ethers (PBDEs), have shown similarities in altering thyroid hormone metabolism and cholinergic function, and it has thus been proposed that this chemical class would also be developmentally neurotoxic.

CHEMICALS THAT INDUCE DEPRESSION OF NERVOUS SYSTEM FUNCTION

Generalized depression of CNS function is produced by a variety of volatile solvents, including ethanol, organics, and anesthetics. These solvents include several chemical classes—aliphatic and aromatic hydrocarbons, halogenated hydrocarbons, ketones, esters, alcohols, and ethers—that are small, lipophilic molecules. They are widely found in industry, medicine, and commercial products. Human exposure ranges from chronic low level to occupational to high levels occurring with solvent abuse. Recent research has implicated interactions with ligand-gated ion channels as well as voltage-gated calcium channels as the mechanism of generalized depression.

IN VITRO AND OTHER ALTERNATIVE APPROACHES TO NEUROTOXICOLOGY

The goal for future studies of neurotoxicology is to replace standard in vivo assessments with high-throughput in vitro assays and quantitative structure–activity relationships (QSARs) to predict adverse outcomes. The use of tiered testing schemes has been proposed, where the first tiers rely on high-throughput methods that test for chemical actions on key biological receptors that initiate pathways of changes that lead to adverse outcomes, in order to identify chemicals for future testing. Second tier tests could involve the use of alternative species, such as small fish or invertebrate species, that will allow more moderate throughput, but in an intact or developing NS. Chemicals identified as having neurotoxic properties could then be tested in intact mammalian models as necessary. The extraordinary conservation of both genomic/epigenomic elements and differentiation processes between mammals and nonmammals, which has been revealed during the last two decades, makes more feasible the use of these alternative models.

BIBLIOGRAPHY

Berent S, Albers JW: *Neurobehavioral Toxicology: Neuropsychological and Neurological Perspectives*. New York: Taylor & Francis, 2005.

Dobbs MR, Rusyniak DE: *Frontiers in Clinical Neurotoxicology, an Issue of Neurologic Clinics*. 1st ed. Philadelphia, PA: Saunders Elsevier, 2011.

Harry GJ, Tilson HA: *Neurotoxicology*. 3rd ed. New York: Informa, 2010.

Webster LR: *Neurotoxicity Syndromes*. New York: Nova Biomedical, 2012.

QUESTIONS

1. Which of the following statements regarding axons and/or axonal transport is FALSE?
   a. Single nerve cells can be over 1 m in length.
   b. Fast axonal transport is responsible for movement of proteins from the cell body to the axon.
   c. Anterograde transport is accomplished by the protein kinesin.
   d. The motor proteins, kinesin and dynein, are associated with microtubules.
   e. A majority of the ATP in nerve cells is used for axonal transport.

2. Which of the following statements is not characteristic of Schwann cells in Wallerian degeneration?
   a. Schwann cells provide physical guidance needed for the regrowth of the axon.
   b. Schwann cells release trophic factors that stimulate growth.
   c. Schwann cells act to clear the myelin debris with the help of macrophages.
   d. Schwann cells increase synthesis of myelin lipids in response to axonal damage.
   e. Schwann cells are responsible for myelination of axons in the peripheral nervous system.

3. Prenatal exposure to ethanol can result in mental retardation and hearing deficits in the newborn. What is the cellular basis of the neurotoxicity?
   a. neuronal loss in cerebellum.
   b. acute cortical hemorrhage.
   c. microcephaly.
   d. loss of hippocampal neurons.
   e. degeneration of the basal ganglia.

4. Which of the following characteristics is LEAST likely to place a neuron at risk of toxic damage?
   a. high metabolic rate.
   b. ability to release neurotransmitters.
   c. long neuronal processes supported by the soma.
   d. excitable membranes.
   e. large surface area.

5. The use of meperidine contaminated with MPTP will result in a Parkinson's disease-like neurotoxicity. Where is the most likely site in the brain that MPTP exerts its toxic effects?
   a. cerebellum.
   b. cerebral cortex.
   c. brainstem.
   d. substantia nigra.
   e. hippocampus.

6. Which of the following statements regarding the PNS and the CNS is TRUE?
   a. Nerve impulse transduction is much faster in the CNS than in the PNS.
   b. PNS axons can regenerate, whereas CNS axons cannot.
   c. Remyelination does not occur in the CNS.
   d. Oligodendrocytes perform remyelination in the PNS.
   e. In the CNS, oligodendrocyte scarring interferes with axonal regeneration.

7. Platinum (cisplatin) results in which of the following neurologic problems?
   a. peripheral neuropathy.
   b. trigeminal neuralgia.
   c. spasticity.
   d. gait ataxia.
   e. tremor.

8. Which of the following is NOT characteristic of axonopathies?
   a. There is degeneration of the axon.
   b. The cell body of the neuron remains intact.
   c. Axonopathies result from chemical transaction of the axon.
   d. A majority of axonal toxicants cause motor deficits.
   e. Sensory and motor deficits are first noticed in the hands and feet following axonal degeneration.

9. All of the following statements regarding lead exposure are true EXCEPT:
   a. Lead exposure results in peripheral neuropathy.
   b. Lead slows peripheral nerve conduction in humans.
   c. Lead causes the transection of peripheral axons.
   d. Segmental demyelination is a common result of lead ingestion.
   e. Lead toxicity can result in anemia.

10. Regarding excitatory amino acids, which of the following statements is FALSE?
    a. Glutamate is the most common excitatory amino acid in the CNS.
    b. Excitotoxicity has been linked to conditions such as epilepsy.
    c. Overconsumption of monosodium glutamate (MSG) can result in a tingling or burning sensation in the face and neck.
    d. An ionotropic glutamate receptor is coupled to a G protein.
    e. Glutamate is toxic to neurons.

Toxic Responses of the Ocular and Visual System[1]

Donald A. Fox and William K. Boyes

[1]This chapter has been reviewed by the National Health and Environmental Effects Research Laboratory, U.S. EPA, and approved for publication.

- Toxic chemicals and systemic drugs can affect all parts of the eye, including cornea, iris, ciliary body, lens retina, and optic nerve.
- Ophthalmologic procedures for evaluating the health of the eye include routine clinical screening evaluations using a slit-lamp biomicroscope and ophthalmoscope, and an examination of the pupillary light reflex.

- Most electrophysiologic or neurophysiologic procedures for testing visual function after toxicant exposure involve stimulating the eyes with visual stimuli and electrically recording potentials generated by visually responsive neurons.

INTRODUCTION TO OCULAR AND VISUAL SYSTEM TOXICOLOGY

Environmental and occupational exposure to toxic chemicals, gases, and vapors as well as side effects resulting from therapeutic drugs frequently result in structural and functional alterations in the eye and central visual system. The retina and central visual system are especially vulnerable to toxic insult.

EXPOSURE TO THE EYE AND VISUAL SYSTEM

Ocular Pharmacodynamics and Pharmacokinetics

Toxic chemicals and systemic drugs can affect all parts of the eye (Figure 17–1; Tables 17–1 and 17–2). Factors determining whether a chemical can reach a particular ocular site of action include physiochemical properties of the chemical, concentration and duration of exposure, and movement across ocular compartments and barriers. The cornea, conjunctiva, and eyelids are often exposed directly to chemicals, gases, drugs, and particles. The first site of action is the tear film, a three-layered structure with both hydrophobic and hydrophilic properties. The outermost thin tear film layer is secreted by the meibomian (sebaceous) glands. This superficial lipid layer protects the underlying thicker aqueous layer that is produced by the lacrimal glands. The third layer is the very thin mucoid layer that is secreted by the goblet cells of the conjunctiva and acts as an interface between the hydrophilic layer of the tears and the hydrophobic layer of the corneal epithelial cells.

The avascular cornea is considered the external barrier to the internal ocular structures. Greater systemic absorption occurs through contact with the vascularized conjunctiva (Figure 17–2). The human cornea has several distinct layers through which a chemical must pass in order to reach the anterior chamber. The first is the corneal epithelium of stratified squamous, nonkeratinized cells with tight junctions. The permeability of the corneal epithelium is low and only lipid-soluble chemicals readily pass through this layer. Bowman's membrane separates the epithelium from the stroma. The corneal stroma comprises 90% of the corneal thickness and is composed of

water, collagen, and glycosaminoglycans, which permits hydrophilic chemicals to easily dissolve in this thick layer. The inner edge of the corneal stroma is bounded by a thin basement membrane, called Descemet's membrane, which is secreted by the corneal endothelium. The innermost layer of the cornea, the corneal endothelium, is composed of a single layer of cells that are surrounded by lipid membranes. The permeability of the corneal endothelial cells to ionized chemicals is relatively low.

There are two separate vascular systems in the eye: (1) the uveal blood vessels, which include the vascular beds of the iris, ciliary body, and choroid, and (2) the retinal vessels. In the anterior segment of the eye, there is a blood–aqueous barrier that has relatively tight junctions between the endothelial cells of the iris capillaries and nonpigmented cells of the ciliary epithelium. The major function of the ciliary epithelium is to produce aqueous humor from the plasma filtrate present in the stroma of the ciliary processes.

In humans and several widely used experimental animals (e.g., monkeys, pigs, dogs, rats, and mice), the retina has a dual circulatory supply: choroidal and retinal. The retina consists of the outer plexiform layer (OPL), inner nuclear layer (INL), inner plexiform layer (IPL), and ganglion cell layer (GCL). The endothelial cells of capillaries of the retinal vessels have tight junctions forming the blood–retinal barrier. However, at the level of the optic disk, the blood–retinal barrier is lacking and thus hydrophilic molecules can enter the optic nerve (ON) head by diffusion from the extravascular space and cause selective damage at this site of action. The outer or distal retina, which consists of the retinal pigment epithelium (RPE), rod and cone photoreceptor outer segments (ROS and COS) and inner segments (RIS and CIS), and the photoreceptor outer nuclear layer (ONL) are avascular. These areas of the retina are supplied by the choriocapillaris: a dense, one-layered network of fenestrated vessels formed by the short posterior ciliary arteries and located next to the RPE. Consistent with their known structure and function, these capillaries have loose endothelial junctions and abundant fenestrae; they are highly permeable to large proteins.

Following systemic exposure to drugs and chemicals by the oral, inhalation, dermal, or parenteral route, these compounds are distributed to all parts of the eye by the blood in the uveal blood vessels and retinal vessels (Figure 17–3). Most chemicals rapidly equilibrate with the extravascular space of the

Cataracts are decreases in the optic transparency of the lens that ultimately can lead to functional visual disturbances. Cataracts can occur at any age; they can also be congenital. Risk factors for the development of cataracts include aging, diabetes, low antioxidant levels, and exposure to a variety of environmental factors, including exposure to UV radiation and visible light, trauma, smoking, and exposure to a large variety of topical and systemic drugs and chemicals.

Several different mechanisms have been hypothesized to account for the development of cataracts. These include the disruption of lens energy metabolism, hydration and/or electrolyte balance, oxidative stress due to the generation of free radicals and ROS, and the occurrence of oxidative stress due to a decrease in antioxidant defense mechanisms such as glutathione, superoxide dismutase, catalase, ascorbic acid, or vitamin E. The generation of ROS leads to oxidation of lens membrane proteins and lipids. A critical pathway is oxidation of protein thiol groups, particularly in methionine or cysteine amino acids, leading to the formation of polypeptide links through disulfide bonds, and in turn, high-molecular-weight protein aggregates. These large aggregations of proteins can attain a size sufficient to scatter light, thus reducing lens transparency. Oxidation of membrane lipids and proteins may also impair membrane transport and permeability.

Corticosteroids

There are two proposed mechanisms by which systemic treatment with corticosteroids may cause cataracts. Corticosteroids alter lens epithelium electrolyte balance, which disrupts the normal lens epithelial cell structure causing gaps to appear between the lateral epithelial cell borders. Another theory is that corticosteroid molecules react with lens crystallin proteins, producing corticosteroid–crystallin adducts that would be light-scattering complexes.

Naphthalene

Accidental exposure to naphthalene results in cortical cataracts and retinal degeneration. The metabolite 1,2-dihydro-1,2-dihydroxynaphthalene (naphthalene dihydrodiol) is the cataract-inducing agent instead of naphthalene itself. Subsequent studies showed that aldose reductase in the rat lens is the enzyme responsible for the formation of naphthalene dihydrodiol, and that treatment with aldose reductase inhibitors prevents naphthalene-induced cataracts.

Phenothiazines

Schizophrenics receiving phenothiazine drugs develop pigmented deposits in their eyes and skin. The phenothiazines combine with melanin to form a photosensitive product that reacts with sunlight, causing formation of the deposits in lens and cornea. The amount of pigmentation is related to the dose of the drug, with the annual yearly dose being the most predictive dose metric. More recent epidemiologic evidence demonstrates a dose-related increase in the risk of cataracts from use of nonantipsychotic phenothiazines.

TARGET SITES AND MECHANISMS OF ACTION: RETINA

The adult mammalian retina is a highly differentiated tissue containing eight distinct layers plus the RPE, 10 major types of neurons, and a Müller glial cell ([MGC] Figure 17–1). The eight layers of the neural retina, which originate from the cells of the inner layer of the embryonic optic cup, are the nerve fiber layer (NFL), ganglion cell layer (GCL), inner plexiform layer (IPL), inner nuclear layer (INL), outer plexiform layer (OPL), outer nuclear layer (ONL), rod and cone photoreceptor inner segment layer (RIS, CIS), and the rod and cone photoreceptor outer segment layer (ROS, COS). The retinal pigment epithelium (RPE) is a single layer of cuboidal epithelial cells that lies on Bruch's membrane adjacent to the vascular choroid. Between the RPE and photoreceptor outer segments lies the subretinal space, which is similar to the brain ventricles. The 10 major types of neurons are the rod and cone photoreceptors, (depolarizing) ON-rod and ON-cone bipolar cells, (hyperpolarizing) OFF-cone bipolar cells, horizontal cells, numerous subtypes of amacrine cells, an interplexiform cell, and ON-RGCs and OFF-RGCs. The MGC is the only glial cell in the retina. The somas of the MGCs are in the INL. The end feet of the MGCs in the proximal or inner retina along with a basal lamina form the internal limiting membrane of the retina, which is similar to the pial surface of the brain. In the distal retina, the MGC end feet join with the photoreceptors and zonula adherens to form the external limiting membrane, which is located between the ONL and RIS/CIS.

The mammalian retina is highly vulnerable to toxicant-induced structural and/or functional damage due to (1) the highly fenestrated choriocapillaris that supplies the distal or outer retina as well as a portion of the inner retina; (2) the very high rate of oxidative mitochondrial metabolism, especially that in the photoreceptors; (3) high daily turnover of rod and cone outer segments; (4) high susceptibility of the rod and cones to degenerate due to inherited retinal dystrophies as well as associated syndromes and metabolic disorders; (5) presence of specialized ribbon synapses and synaptic contact sites; (6) presence of numerous neurotransmitter and neuromodulatory systems, including extensive glutamatergic, GABAergic, and glycinergic systems; (7) presence of numerous and highly specialized gap junctions used in the information signaling process; (8) presence of melanin in the choroid and RPE and also in the iris and pupil; (9) a very high choroidal blood flow rate, as high as 10 times that of the gray matter of the brain; and (10) the additive or synergistic toxic action of certain chemicals with ultraviolet and visible light.

Each of the retinal layers can undergo specific or general toxic effects. These alterations and deficits include, but are not limited to, visual field deficits, scotopic vision deficits such as night blindness and increases in the threshold for dark adaptation, cone-mediated (photopic) deficits such as decreased color perception, decreased visual acuity, macular and general retinal edema, retinal hemorrhages and vasoconstriction, and pigmentary changes.

Retinotoxicity of Systemically Administered Therapeutic Drugs

Cancer Chemotherapeutics—Ocular toxicity is a common side effect of cancer chemotherapy, resulting in blurred vision, diplopia, decreased color vision and visual acuity, optic/retrobular neuritis, transient cortical blindness, and demyelination of the ONs. The retina, due to its high metabolic activity and choroidal circulation (vide infra), appears to be particularly vulnerable to numerous cytotoxic drugs such as the alkylating agents cisplatin, carboplatin, and carmustine; the antimetabolites cytosine arabinoside, 5-fluorouracil, and methotrexate; and the mitotic inhibitors such as docetaxel. The ocular toxicity of different drugs is dependent upon the dose, duration of dosage, and route of administration. If not detected at an early stage of toxicity, the ocular complications are often irreversible even after chemotherapy is discontinued.

Chloroquine and Hydroxychloroquine—Chloroquine (Aralen) and hydroxychloroquine (Plaquenil) are 4-aminoquinoline derivatives used as antimalarial and anti-inflammatory drugs that can cause irreversible loss of retinal function. Chloroquine, its major metabolite desethylchloroquine, and hydroxychloroquine have high affinity for melanin, which results in these drugs accumulating in the choroid and RPE, ciliary body, and iris during and following drug administration. Prolonged exposure of the retina to these drugs, especially chloroquine, may lead to an irreversible retinopathy. Doses of hydroxychloroquine less than 400 mg/day appear to produce little or no retinopathy even after prolonged therapy.

The clinical findings accompanying chloroquine retinopathy can be divided into early and late stages. The early changes include (1) the pathognomonic "bull's-eye retina" visualized as a dark, central pigmented area involving the macula, surrounded by a pale ring of depigmentation, which, in turn, is surrounded by another ring of pigmentation; (2) a diminished EOG; (3) possible granular pigmentation in the peripheral retina; and (4) visual complaints such as blurred vision and problems discerning letters or words. Late-stage findings, which can occur during or even following cessation of drug exposure, include (1) a progressive scotoma, (2) constriction of the peripheral fields commencing in the upper temporal quadrant, (3) narrowing of the retinal artery, (4) color and night blindness, (5) absence of a typical retinal pigment pattern, and (6) very abnormal EOGs and ERGs. These late-stage symptoms are irreversible.

Digoxin and Digitoxin—The cardiac glycosides digoxin and digitoxin are used in the treatment of congestive heart disease and in certain cardiac arrhythmias. Digitalis-induced visual system abnormalities include decreased vision, flickering scotomas, and altered color vision. Digoxin produces more toxicity than digitoxin due to its greater volume of distribution and plasma protein binding. The most frequent visual complaints are color vision impairments and hazy or snowy vision, although complaints of flickering light, colored spots surrounded by bright halos, blurred vision, and glare sensitivity also are reported. Photoreceptors are the primary site of toxicity, with cone photoreceptors being more susceptible to the effects than rod photoreceptors. The retina has the highest number of Na^+,K^+-ATPase sites of any ocular tissue, which are potently inhibited by digoxin and digitoxin.

Indomethacin—Indomethacin is a nonsteroidal anti-inflammatory drug with analgesic and antipyretic properties that is frequently used for the management of arthritis, gout, and musculoskeletal discomfort. Chronic administration of 50 to 200 mg/day of indomethacin for 1 to 2 years has been reported to produce corneal opacities, discrete pigment scattering of the RPE perifoveally, paramacular depigmentation, decreases in visual acuity, altered visual fields, increases in the threshold for dark adaptation, blue–yellow color deficits, and decreases in ERG and EOG amplitudes. Decreases in the ERG a- and b-wave amplitudes, with larger changes observed under scotopic dark-adapted than light-adapted conditions, have been reported. On cessation of drug treatment, the ERG waveforms and color vision changes return to near normal, although the pigmentary changes are irreversible. The mechanism of retinotoxicity is unknown; however, it appears likely that the RPE is a primary target site.

Sildenafil Citrate—Sildenafil citrate (Viagra) is a cGMP-specific phosphodiesterase (PDE) type 5 inhibitor that is utilized in the treatment of erectile dysfunction. Sildenafil is also a weak cGMP PDE type 6 inhibitor, which is present in rod and cone photoreceptors. Transient visual symptoms such as a blue tinge to vision, increased brightness of lights and blurry vision, as well as alterations in scotopic and photopic ERGs have been reported.

Tamoxifen—Tamoxifen (Nolvadex, Tamoplex), a triphenylethylene derivative, is a nonsteroidal antiestrogenic drug that competes with estrogen for its receptor sites. It is a highly effective antitumor agent used for the treatment of metastatic breast carcinoma in postmenopausal women. Chronic high-dose therapy (180–240 mg/day for ~2 years) produces widespread axonal degeneration in the macular and perimacular areas. Clinical symptoms include a permanent decrease in visual acuity and abnormal visual fields, as the axonal degeneration is irreversible. Chronic low-dose tamoxifen (20 mg/day) can result in a small increase in the incidence of keratopathy, with minimal alterations in visual function. Following cessation of low-dose tamoxifen therapy, most of the keratopathy and retinal alterations, except the corneal opacities and retinopathy, are reversible.

Vigabatrin—Vigabatrin, an inhibitor of GABA-transaminase, is used to treat refractory complex partial seizures and infantile spasms. Retinopathy induced by vigabatrin is characterized by irreversible bilateral, concentric peripheral visual constriction, and decreased retinal nerve fiber thickness. Onset of the visual field loss has been observed after six weeks of exposure, but generally requires a couple of years. Rod and cone ERGs as well as flicker responses are altered, indicating that retinal damage also occurs. This drug is now recommended only for epileptic patients with no alternative choices.

Retinotoxicity of Known Neurotoxicants

Inorganic Lead—Lead poisoning (mean blood lead [BPb] ≥ 80 μg/dL) in humans produces amblyopia, blindness, optic neuritis or atrophy, peripheral and central scotomas, paralysis of eye muscles, and decreased visual function. Moderate- to high-level lead exposure produces scotopic and temporal visual system deficits in occupationally exposed factory workers, and developmentally lead-exposed monkeys and rats. This lead exposure dosage produces irreversible retinal deficits in the experimental animals.

Occupational lead exposure produces concentration- and time-dependent alterations in the retina such that higher levels of lead directly and adversely affect both the retina and ON, whereas lower levels of lead appear to primarily affect the rod photoreceptors and the rod pathway. These retinal and oculomotor alterations are, in most cases, correlated with blood lead levels and occurred in the absence of observable ophthalmologic changes, CNS symptoms, and abnormal performance test scores. Thus, these measures of temporal visual function may be among the most sensitive for the early detection of the neurotoxic effects of inorganic lead.

Methanol—Methanol is a low-molecular-weight (32 Da), colorless, and volatile liquid that is readily and rapidly absorbed from all routes of exposure (dermal, inhalation, and oral), easily crosses all membranes, and thus is uniformly distributed to organs and tissues in direct relation to their water content. Following different routes of exposures, the highest concentrations of methanol are found in the blood, aqueous, and vitreous humors, and bile as well as the brain, kidneys, lungs, and spleen. In the liver, methanol is oxidized sequentially to formaldehyde by alcohol dehydrogenase in human and nonhuman primates or by catalase in rodents and then to formic acid. It is excreted as formic acid in the urine or oxidized further to carbon dioxide and then excreted by the lungs. Formic acid is the toxic metabolite of methanol that mediates the metabolic acidosis as well as the retinal and ON toxicity observed in humans, monkeys, and rats with a decreased capacity for folate metabolism.

Human and nonhuman primates are highly sensitive to methanol-induced neurotoxicity due to their limited capacity to oxidize formic acid. The toxicity occurs in several stages. It first occurs as a mild CNS depression, followed by an asymptomatic 12 to 24 h latent period, followed by a syndrome consisting of formic acidemia, uncompensated metabolic acidosis, ocular and visual toxicity, coma, and possibly death. Acute methanol poisoning results in profound and permanent structural alterations in the retina and ON, and visual impairments ranging from blurred vision to decreased visual acuity and light sensitivity to blindness. Formate is directly toxic to Müller glial cell function as well as rod and cone photoreceptors. The mechanism of formate toxicity appears to involve a disruption in oxidative phosphorylation in photoreceptors, Müller glial cells, and ON.

Organic Solvents—Organic solvents produce structural alterations in rods and cones as well as functional alterations such as color vision deficits, decreased contrast sensitivity, and altered visuomotor performance. Dose–response color vision loss and decreases in the contrast sensitivity function occur in workers exposed to organic solvents such as trichlorethylene, alcohols, xylene, toluene, *n*-hexane, styrene, mixtures of these, and others. Adverse effects usually occur only at concentrations above the occupational exposure limits.

TARGET SITES AND MECHANISMS OF ACTION: OPTIC NERVE AND TRACT

The ON consists primarily of RGC axons carrying visual information from the retina to several distinct anatomical destinations in the CNS. Disorders of the ON may be termed *optic neuritis, optic neuropathy,* or *ON atrophy,* referring to inflammation, damage, or degeneration, respectively, of the ON. *Retrobulbar neuritis* refers to inflammation or involvement of the orbital portion of the ON posterior to the globe. Among the symptoms of ON disease are reduced visual acuity, contrast sensitivity, and color vision. Toxic effects observed in the ON may originate from damage to the ON fibers themselves or to the RGC somas that provide axons to the ON. A number of toxic and nutritional disorders can adversely affect the ON. Deficiency of thiamine, vitamin B$_{12}$, or zinc results in degenerative changes in ON fibers. A condition referred to as *alcohol-tobacco amblyopia* or simply as *toxic amblyopia* is observed in habitually heavy users of these substances and is associated with nutritional deficiency.

Acrylamide

Acrylamide monomer is used in a variety of industrial and laboratory applications, where it serves as the basis for the production of polyacrylamide gels and other polyacrylamide products. Exposure to acrylamide produces a distal axonopathy in large-diameter axons of the peripheral nerves and spinal cord that is well documented in humans and laboratory animals. In contrast, middle diameter axons of optic tract are affected, specifically, RGCs that project to the parvocellular layers of the LGN. Why the axons of the optic nerve and tract show a different size-based pattern of vulnerability than do axons of the peripheral nerve and spinal cord is not understood.

Carbon Disulfide

Carbon disulfide (CS_2) is used in industry to manufacture viscose rayon, carbon tetrachloride, and cellophane. CS_2 damages both the PNS and CNS, and has profound effects on vision. In the visual system, workers exposed to CS_2 experience loss of visual function accompanied by observable lesions in the retinal vasculature. Central scotoma, depressed visual sensitivity in the peripheral visual field, optic atrophy, pupillary disturbances, blurred vision, and disorders of color perception have all been reported. The retinal and ON pathologies produced by CS_2 are likely a direct neuropathologic action and not the indirect result of vasculopathy.

Ethambutol

The dextro isomer of ethambutol is widely used as an antimycobacterial drug for the treatment of tuberculosis. Ethambutol produces dose-related alterations in the visual system, such as blue–yellow and red–green dyschromatopsias, decreased contrast sensitivity, reduced visual acuity, and visual field loss. The earliest visual symptoms appear to be a decrease in contrast sensitivity and color vision. Impaired red–green color vision is the most frequently observed and reported complaint. The symptoms are primarily associated with one of the two forms of retrobulbar neuritis (i.e., optic neuropathy). The most common form, seen in almost all cases, involves the central ON fibers and typically results in a central or paracentral scotoma in the visual field and is associated with impaired red–green color vision and decreased visual acuity, whereas the second form involves the peripheral ON fibers and typically results in a peripheral scotoma and visual field loss.

TARGET SITES AND MECHANISMS OF ACTION: THE CENTRAL VISUAL SYSTEM

Many areas of the cerebral cortex are involved in the perception of visual information. The primary visual cortex (V1), Brodmann area 17, or striate cortex receives the primary projections of visual information from the lateral geniculate nucleus (LGN) and also from the superior colliculus. Neurons from the LGN project to the visual cortex maintaining a topographic representation of the receptive field origin in the retina. The receptive fields in the left and right sides of area 17 reflect the contralateral visual world and representations of the upper and lower regions of the visual field are separated below and above, respectively, the calcarine fissure. Cells in the posterior aspects of the calcarine fissure have receptive fields located in the central part of the retina. Cortical cells progressively deeper in the calcarine fissure have retinal receptive fields that are located more and more peripherally in the retina. The central part of the fovea has tightly packed photoreceptors for resolution of fine detailed images, and the cortical representation of the central fovea is proportionately larger than the peripheral retina in order to accommodate a proportionately larger need for neural image processing. The magnocellular and parvocellular pathways project differently to the histologically defined layers of primary striate visual cortex and then to extrastriate visual areas. The receptive fields of neurons in the visual cortex are more complex than the circular center-surround arrangement found in the retina and LGN. Cortical cells respond better to lines of a particular orientation than to simple spots. The receptive fields of cortical cells are thought to represent computational summaries of a number of simpler input signals. As the visual information proceeds from area V1 to extrastriate visual cortical areas, the representation of the visual world reflected in the receptive fields of individual neurons becomes progressively more complex.

Lead

In addition to the retinal effects of lead (see above), lead exposure during adulthood or perinatal development produces structural, biochemical, and functional deficits in the visual cortex of humans, nonhuman primates, and rats. Quantitative morphometric studies in monkeys exposed to high levels of lead from birth or infancy to 6 years of age revealed a decrease in visual cortex (areas V1 and V2), cell volume density, and a decrease in the number of initial arborizations among pyramidal neurons. These alterations could partially contribute to the alterations in the amplitude and latency measures of the flash-evoked and pattern-reversal-evoked potentials in lead-exposed children, workers, monkeys, and rats, and the alterations in tasks assessing visual function in lead-exposed children.

Methyl Mercury

Methyl mercury–poisoned individuals experience a striking and progressive constriction of the visual field (peripheral scotoma). The narrowing of the visual world gives impression of looking through a long tunnel, hence the term *tunnel vision*. The damage is most severe in the regions of primary visual cortex subserving the peripheral visual field, with relative sparing of the cortical areas representing the central vision. Methyl mercury–poisoned individuals also experience poor night vision that is also attributable to peripheral visual field losses.

BIBLIOGRAPHY

Bartlett JD, Jaanus SD: *Clinical Ocular Pharmacology*, 5th ed. Boston, MA: Butterworth-Heinemann, 2008.

Fraunfelder FT, Fraunfelder FW, Chambers WA: *Clinical Ocular Toxicology: Drugs, Chemicals, and Herbs*. Philadelphia, PA: Elsevier Saunders, 2008.

Weir AB, Collins M: *Assessing Ocular Toxicology in Laboratory Animals*. New York: Springer Humana, 2013.

QUESTIONS

1. In which of the following locations would one NOT find melanin?
    a. iris.
    b. ciliary body.
    c. retinal pigment epithelium (RPE).
    d. uveal tract.
    e. sclera.

2. Systemic exposure to drugs and chemicals is most likely to target which of the following retinal sites?
    a. RPE and ganglion cell layer.
    b. optic nerve and inner plexiform layer.
    c. RPE and photoreceptors.
    d. photoreceptors and ganglion cell layer.
    e. inner plexiform layer and RPE.

3. Which of the following structures is NOT part of the ocular fundus?
    a. retina.
    b. lens.
    c. choroid.
    d. sclera.
    e. optic nerve.

4. Drugs and chemicals in systemic blood have better access to which of the following sites because of the presence of loose endothelial junctions at that location?
    a. retinal choroid.
    b. inner retina.
    c. optic nerve.
    d. iris.
    e. ciliary body.

5. All of the following statements regarding ocular irritancy and toxicity are true EXCEPT:
    a. The Draize test involves instillation of a potentially toxic liquid or solid into the eye.
    b. The effect of the irritant in the Draize test is scored on a weighted scale for the cornea, iris, and conjunctiva.
    c. The Draize test usually uses one eye for testing and the other as a control.
    d. The Draize test has strong predictive value in humans.
    e. The cornea is evaluated for opacity and area of involvement in the Draize test.

6. Which of the following statements regarding color vision deficits is FALSE?
    a. Inheritance of a blue–yellow color deficit is common.
    b. Bilateral deficits in the visual cortex can lead to color blindness.
    c. Disorders of the outer retina produce blue–yellow deficits.
    d. Drug and chemical exposure most commonly results in blue–yellow color deficits.
    e. Disorders of the optic nerve produce red–green deficits.

7. A substance with which of the following pH values would be most damaging to the cornea?
    a. 1.0.
    b. 3.0.
    c. 7.0.
    d. 10.0.
    e. 12.0.

8. Which of the following statements concerning the lens is FALSE?
    a. UV radiation exposure is a common environmental risk factor for developing cataracts.
    b. Cataracts are opacities of the lens that can occur at any age.
    c. The lens continues to grow throughout one's life.
    d. Naphthalene and organic solvents both can cause cataracts.
    e. Topical treatment with corticosteroids can cause cataracts.

9. Which of the following is NOT a reason why the retina is highly vulnerable to toxicant-induced damage?
    a. presence of numerous neurotransmitter systems.
    b. presence of melanin in the RPE.
    c. high choroidal blood flow rate.
    d. high rate of oxidative mitochondrial metabolism.
    e. lack of gap junctions.

10. A deficiency in which of the following vitamins can result in degeneration of optic nerve fibers?
    a. vitamin A.
    b. vitamin B_3.
    c. vitamin C.
    d. vitamin B_{12}.
    e. vitamin E.

Psychotropic Agents—Trifluoperazine and chlorpromazine have been shown to cause intracellular cholesterol accumulation in cultured cells of the aortic intima. Aside from the atherogenic effects, postural hypotension has been identified as the most common cardiovascular side effect of tricyclic antidepressants.

Antineoplastic Agents—The vasculotoxic responses elicited by antineoplastic drugs range from asymptomatic arterial lesions to thrombotic microangiopathy. Pulmonary venoocclusive disease has been reported after the administration of various drugs, including 5-fluorouracil, doxorubicin, and mitomycin. Cyclophosphamide causes cerebrovascular and viscerovascular lesions, resulting in hemorrhages.

Analgesics and Nonsteroidal Anti-inflammatory Agents—Aspirin can produce endothelial damage as part of a pattern of gastric erosion. Regular use of analgesics containing phenacetin has been associated with an increased risk of hypertension and cardiovascular morbidity. NSAIDs may induce glomerular and vascular renal lesions.

Oral Contraceptives—Oral contraceptive steroids can produce thromboembolic disorders. Epidemiologic studies have shown that oral contraceptive users have an increased risk of MI relative to nonusers, a correlation that is markedly exacerbated by smoking, and increased risk of cerebral thrombosis, hemorrhage, venous thrombosis, and pulmonary embolism.

Natural Products

Natural products that cause vascular toxicity include those discussed for drugs causing cardiotoxicity. In addition, many other drugs also cause vascular lesions and toxicity such as bacterial endotoxins and homocysteine, which have unique vascular toxic effects.

Bacterial Endotoxins—Bacterial endotoxins are potent toxic agents to the vascular system. These toxins are known to cause thickening of endothelial cells and the formation of fibrin thrombi in small veins. The terminal phase of the effects of endotoxin on the systemic vasculature results in marked hypotension. The action of these agents is somehow related to oxidative stress mechanisms, as evidenced by the ability of vitamin E to prevent some of the toxin-induced damage.

Homocysteine—Moderately elevated levels of homocysteine have been associated with atherosclerosis and venous thrombosis. Toxicity may involve oxidative injury to vascular endothelial and/or smooth muscle cells, leading to deregulation of vascular smooth muscle growth, synthesis and deposition of matrix proteins, and adverse effects on anticoagulant systems.

Hydrazinobenzoic Acid—This nitrogen–nitrogen bonded chemical is present in the cultivated mushroom *Agaricus bisporus*. This hydrazine derivative causes smooth muscle cell

tumors in the aorta and large arteries of mice when administered over the life span of the animals.

T-2 Toxin—Trichothecene mycotoxins, commonly classified as tetracyclic sesquiterpenes, are naturally occurring cytotoxic metabolites of *Fusarium* species. These mycotoxins, including T-2 toxin, are major contaminants of foods and animal feeds and may cause illness in animals and humans. Intravenous infusion of T-2 toxin in rats causes an initial decrease in heart rate and blood pressure, followed by tachycardia and hypertension and finally by bradycardia and hypotension. Acute T-2 toxin exposure causes extensive destruction of myocardial capillaries, while repeated dosing promotes thickening of large coronary arteries.

Vitamin D—The toxic effects of vitamin D may be related to its structural similarity to 25-hydroxycholesterol, a potent vascular toxin. The manifestations of vitamin D hypervitaminosis include medial degeneration, calcification of the coronary arteries, and smooth muscle cell proliferation in laboratory animals.

β-Amyloid—Accumulation of β-amyloid is a major lesion in the brain of Alzheimer's patients. Studies have shown that administration of β-amyloid produces extensive vascular disruption, including endothelial and smooth muscle damage, and adhesion and migration of leukocytes across arteries and venules. Most importantly, the vascular actions of β-amyloid appear to be distinct from the neurotoxic properties of the peptide. It appears that vascular toxicity of β-amyloid makes contributions to Alzheimer's dementia.

Environmental Pollutants and Industrial Chemicals

The environmental pollutants and industrial chemicals discussed in the cardiotoxicity section all have toxic effects on the vascular system. The cardiac effect of some of these agents and pollutants actually may result primarily from the vascular effect. The by-products of vascular tissue damage or the secreted substances, such as cytokines derived from vascular injury, can affect the heart either directly because of the vascular system in the heart or indirectly through blood circulation.

Carbon Monoxide—Carbon monoxide induces focal intimal damage and edema in laboratory animals at a concentration (180 ppm) to which humans may be exposed from environmental sources such as automobile exhaust, tobacco smoke, and fossil fuels. Short-term exposure to carbon monoxide is associated with direct damage to vascular endothelial and smooth muscle cells. The toxic effects of carbon monoxide have been attributed to its reversible interaction with hemoglobin. As a result of this interaction, carboxyhemoglobin decreases the oxygen-carrying capacity of blood, eventually leading to functional anemia. In addition, carbon monoxide interacts with cellular proteins such as myoglobin and cytochrome *c* oxidase and elicits a direct vasodilatory response of the coronary circulation.

Carbon Disulfide—Carbon disulfide (dithiocarbonic anhydride) occurs in coal tar and crude petroleum and is commonly used in the manufacture of rayon and soil disinfectants. This chemical has been identified as an atherogenic agent in laboratory animals. The mechanism for carbon disulfide–atheroma production may involve direct injury to the endothelium coupled with hypothyroidism, because thiocarbamate (thiourea), a potent antithyroid substance, is a principal urinary metabolite of carbon disulfide. Carbon disulfide also modifies low-density lipoprotein in vitro and enhances arterial fatty deposits induced by a high-fat diet in mice.

1,3-Butadiene—Studies have shown that 1,3-butadiene, a chemical used in the production of styrene–butadiene, increases the incidence of cardiac hemangiosarcomas, which are tumors of endothelial origin. Although hemangiosarcomas have also been observed in the liver, lung, and kidney, cardiac tumors are a major cause of death in animals exposed to this chemical. The toxic effects of 1,3-butadiene depend on its metabolic activation by cytochrome P450 to toxic epoxide metabolites.

Metals and Metalloids—The vascular toxicity of food- and water-borne elements (selenium, chromium, copper, zinc, cadmium, lead, and mercury) as well as airborne elements (vanadium and lead) involves reactions of metals with sulfhydryl, carboxyl, or phosphate groups. Metals such as cobalt, magnesium, manganese, nickel, cadmium, and lead also interact with and block calcium channels. Intracellular calcium-binding proteins, such as calmodulin, are biologically relevant targets of heavy metals, including cadmium, mercury, and lead, although the contribution of this mechanism to the toxic effects of metals is not fully understood.

Aromatic Hydrocarbons—Aromatic hydrocarbons, including polycyclic aromatic hydrocarbons and polychlorinated dibenzopdioxins, are persistent toxic environmental contaminants. Aromatic hydrocarbons have been identified as vascular toxins that can initiate and/or promote the atherogenic process in experimental animals. The atherogenic effect is associated with cytochrome P450–mediated conversion of the parent compound to toxic metabolic intermediates, but aromatic hydrocarbons can also initiate the atherogenic process.

Particulate Air Pollution—Recent epidemiologic studies have provided a strong body of evidence that elevated levels of ambient particulate air pollution are associated with increased cardiovascular and respiratory morbidity and mortality. Vascular effects of inhaled ambient particles include endothelial dysfunction and promotion of atherosclerotic lesions. Importantly, these lesions lead to release or secretion of cytokines and chemokines, worsening cardiac complications (discussed previously).

BIBLIOGRAPHY

Acosta D (ed.): *Cardiovascular Toxicology*, 4th ed. New York: Informa Healthcare, 2008.

QUESTIONS

1. In which of the following locations would one NOT find spontaneous depolarization?
   a. SA node.
   b. myocardium.
   c. AV node.
   d. bundle of His.
   e. Purkinje fibers.

2. Which of the following scenarios would increase contractility of the myocardium?
   a. increased activity of the Na^+/K^+-ATPase.
   b. increased activity of sacroplasmic reticulum Ca^{2+} ATPase.
   c. decreased activity of sacroplasmic reticulum Ca^{2+} ATPase.
   d. decreased intracellular calcium levels.
   e. increased intracellular K^+ levels.

3. All of the following statements regarding abnormal cardiac function are true EXCEPT:
   a. Ventricular arrhythmias are generally more severe than atrial arrhythmias.
   b. Ventricular hypertrophy is a common cause of ventricular arrhythmias.
   c. Coronary artery atherosclerosis is a major cause of ischemic heart disease.
   d. Right-sided heart failure results in pulmonary edema.
   e. Tachycardia is classified as a rapid resting heart rate (>100 beats/min).

4. Ion balance is very important in maintaining a normal cardiac rhythm. Which of the following statements is TRUE?
   a. Blockade of K^+ channels decreases the duration of the action potential.
   b. Blockade of Ca^{2+} channels has a positive inotropic effect.
   c. Inhibition of Na^+ channels increases conduction velocity.
   d. Blockage of the Na^+/K^+-ATPase increases contractility.
   e. Calcium is transported into the cell via a Ca^{2+}-ATPase.

5. Which of the following is most likely NOT a cause of myocardial reperfusion injury?
   a. cellular pH fluctuations.
   b. damage to the sarcolemma.
   c. generation of toxic oxygen radicals.
   d. Ca^{2+} overload.
   e. inhibition of the electron transport chain.

6. Which of the following statements regarding the cardio-toxic manifestations of ethanol consumption is FALSE?
   a. Acute ethanol toxicity causes decreased conductivity.
   b. Chronic alcohol consumption is associated with arrhythmias.
   c. Acute ethanol toxicity causes an increased threshold for ventricular fibrillation.
   d. Chronic ethanol toxicity can result in cardiomyopathy.
   e. Acetaldehyde is a mediator of cardiotoxicity.

7. Cardiac glycosides:
   a. increase the activity of the Na^+/K^+-ATPase.
   b. make the resting membrane potential more negative.
   c. can have sympathomimetic and parasympathomimetic effects.
   d. decrease ventricular contractility.
   e. increase AV conduction.

8. Which of the following is NOT a common cardiotoxic manifestation of cocaine abuse?
   a. parasympathomimetic effects.
   b. myocardial infarction.
   c. cardiac myocyte death.
   d. ventricular fibrillation.
   e. ischemia.

9. Using high doses of anabolic–androgenic steroids is NOT likely associated with which of the following?
   a. an increase in LDL.
   b. cardiac hypertrophy.
   c. myocardial infarction.
   d. increased nitric oxide synthase expression.
   e. a decrease in HDL.

10. Which of the following is NOT a common mechanism of vascular toxicity?
    a. membrane disruption.
    b. oxidative stress.
    c. bioactivation of protoxicants.
    d. reduction and accumulation of LDL in endothelium.
    e. accumulation of toxin in vascular cells.

Toxic Responses of the Skin

Robert H. Rice and Theodora M. Mauro

KEY POINTS

- The skin participates directly in thermal, electrolyte, hormonal, metabolic, and immune regulation.
- Percutaneous absorption depends on the xenobiotic's hydrophobicity, which affects its ability to partition into epidermal lipid, and rate of diffusion through this barrier.
- The cells of the epidermis and pilosebaceous units express biotransformation enzymes.
- Irritant dermatitis is a nonimmune-related response caused by the direct action of an agent on the skin.
- Allergic contact dermatitis represents a delayed (type IV) hypersensitivity reaction, whereby minute quantities of material elicit overt reactions.

SKIN AS A BARRIER

The skin protects the body against external insults in order to maintain internal homeostasis. It participates directly in thermal, electrolyte, hormonal, metabolic, and immune regulation. Rather than merely repelling noxious physical agents, the skin may react to them with various defensive mechanisms that serve to prevent internal or widespread cutaneous damage. If an insult is severe or intense enough to overwhelm the protective function of the skin, acute or chronic injury becomes readily manifest. The specific presentation depends on a variety of intrinsic and extrinsic factors including body site, duration of exposure, and other environmental conditions (Table 19–1).

Skin Histology

The skin consists of two major components: the outer epidermis and the underlying dermis, which are separated by a basement membrane (Figure 19–1). The junction ordinarily is not flat but has an undulating appearance (rete ridges). In addition, epidermal appendages (hair follicles, sebaceous glands, and eccrine glands) span the epidermis and are embedded in the dermis. In thickness, the dermis makes up approximately 90% of the skin and has largely a supportive function. Separating the dermis from underlying tissues is a layer of adipocytes, whose accumulation of fat has a cushioning action. The blood supply to the epidermis originates in the capillaries located in the rete ridges at the dermal–epidermal junction. Capillaries also supply the bulbs of the hair follicles and the secretory cells of the eccrine (sweat) glands. The ducts from these glands carry a dilute salt solution to the surface of the skin, where its evaporation provides cooling.

The interfollicular epidermis is a stratified squamous epithelium consisting primarily of keratinocytes, which are tightly attached to each other and to the basement membrane. Melanocytes are distributed sparsely in the dermis, with occasional concentrations beneath the basal lamina and in the papillae of hair follicles. In the epidermis, these cells are stimulated by ultraviolet light to produce melanin granules. The granules are extruded and taken up by the surrounding keratinocytes, which thereby become pigmented. Migrating through the epidermis are numerous Langerhans cells (LCs), which

TABLE 19–1 Factors influencing cutaneous responses.

Variable	Comment
Body site	
Palms/soles	Thick stratum corneum—good physical barrier Common site of contact with chemicals Occlusion with protective clothing
Intertriginous areas (axillae, groin, neck, finger webs, umbilicus, genitalia)	Moist, occluded areas Chemical trapping Enhanced percutaneous absorption
Face	Exposed frequently Surface lipid interacts with hydrophobic substances Chemicals frequently transferred from hands
Eyelids	Poor barrier function—thin epidermis Sensitive to irritants
Postauricular region	Chemical trapping Occlusion
Scalp	Chemical trapping Hair follicles susceptible to metabolic damage
Predisposing cutaneous illnesses—atopic dermatitis	Increased sensitivity to irritants Impaired barrier function
Psoriasis	Impaired barrier function
Genetic factors	Predisposition to skin disorders Variation in sensitivity to irritants Susceptibility to contact sensitization
Temperature	Vasodilation—improved percutaneous absorption Increased sweating—trapping
Humidity	Increased sweating—trapping
Season	Variation in relative humidity Chapping and wind-related skin changes

Known Effects of Plant and Fungal Products in Animals and Humans—Although most naturally occurring environmental estrogens are relatively inactive, the phytoestrogen miroestrol is almost as potent as estradiol in vitro and even more potent than estradiol when administered orally. In addition, many plant estrogens occur in such high concentrations that they induce reproductive alterations in domestic animals. "Clover disease," which is characterized by dystocia, prolapse of the uterus, and infertility, is observed in sheep that graze on highly estrogenic clover pastures. Permanent infertility can be produced in ewes by much lower amounts of estrogen over a longer time period than are needed to produce "clover disease."

Known Effects of Organochlorine Compounds in Humans—Several pesticides and toxic substances have been shown to alter human reproductive function. An accidental high-dose in utero exposure to PCBs and PCDFs has been associated with reproductive alterations in boys, increased stillbirths, low birth weights, malformations, and IQ and behavioral deficits. In addition to the effects associated with this inadvertent exposure, subtle adverse effects were seen in infants and children exposed to relatively low levels of PCBs and PCDFs.

One metabolite of DDT (mitotane, o,p'-DDD) was found to alter adrenal function with sufficient potency to be used as a drug to treat adrenal steroid hypersecretion associated with adrenal tumors. In addition, lower doses of mitotane restored menstruation in women with spanomenorrhea associated with hypertrichosis.

Occupational Exposures—Occupational exposure to pesticides and other toxic substances (i.e., chlordecone and DBCP) in the workplace has been associated with reduced fertility, lowered sperm counts, and/or endocrine alterations in male workers. Workers exposed to high levels of chlordecone, an estrogenic and neurotoxic organochlorine pesticide, displayed intoxication, severe neurotoxicity, and abnormal testicular function. Male workers involved in the manufacture of 4,4′-diaminostilbene-2,2′-disulfonic acid (DAS), a key ingredient in the synthesis of dyes and fluorescent whitening agents, had lower serum testosterone levels and reduced libido as compared with control workers. Thus, it is surprising that occupational exposures to potential EDCs at effective concentrations have not been entirely eliminated from the workplace.

Environmental Androgens

Androgenic activity has been detected in several complex environmental mixtures. Pulp and paper mill effluents (PME) include a chemical mixture that binds androgen receptors (AR) and induces androgen-dependent gene expression in vitro. This mode of action is consistent with the masculinized female mosquitofish (*Gambusia holbrooki*) collected from contaminated sites. Male-biased sex ratios of fish embryos have been reported in broods of eelpout (*Zoarces viviparus*) in the vicinity of a large kraft pulp mill on the Swedish Baltic coast, suggesting that masculinizing compounds in the effluent

were affecting gonadal differentiation and skewing sex ratios. Effluents from beef-cattle concentrated animal feeding operations have been shown to display androgenicity.

Environmental Antiandrogens

Fungicides—Vinclozolin and procymidone are two members of the dicarboximide fungicide class that act as AR antagonists. These pesticides, or their metabolites, competitively inhibit the binding of androgens to AR, leading to an inhibition of androgen-dependent gene expression.

Administration of vinclozolin during sexual differentiation demasculinizes and feminizes the male rat offspring such that treated males display female-like AGD at birth, retained nipples, hypospadias, suprainguinal ectopic testes, a blind vaginal pouch, and small to absent sex accessory glands.

Procymidone induces shortening of the AGD in male pups, and older males display retained nipples, hypospadias, cryptorchidism, cleft phallus, a vaginal pouch, and reduced sex accessory gland size. Fibrosis, cellular infiltration, and epithelial hyperplasia are noted in the dorsolateral and ventral prostatic and seminal vesicular tissues in adult offspring.

Prochloraz is a fungicide that disrupts reproductive development and function by inhibiting the steroidogenic enzymes 17,20-lyase and aromatase and it is an AR antagonist. Prenatal exposure to prochloraz reduces fetal testis testosterone and increases progesterone production without affecting Leydig cell insl3 mRNA levels. Also, prenatal prochloraz treatment delayed parturition and altered reproductive development in the male offspring in a dose-related manner. Treated males displayed reduced AGD and female-like areolas and high-dose males displayed hypospadias, but the epididymides and gubernacular ligaments were relatively unaffected.

Linuron (Herbicide)—This herbicide binds rat and human AR and inhibits DHT–hAR-induced gene expression in vitro. In utero linuron exposure produces male rats displaying epididymal and testicular abnormalities. In contrast to the effects of vinclozolin and procymidone, malformed external genitalia and undescended testes were rarely displayed by linuron-exposed males. Interestingly, the syndrome of effects for linuron is atypical of an AR antagonist and more closely resembles those seen with in utero to phthalates. Also, fetal testosterone production is significantly reduced in linuron-treated fetal males.

***p,p′*-DDE (Pesticide Metabolite)**—p,p'-DDE displays AR antagonism both in vivo and in vitro. In vitro, p,p'-DDE binds to the AR and inhibits androgen-dependent gene expression. In vivo, p,p'-DDE delays pubertal development in male rats by about 5 days at 100 mg/kg/day and inhibits androgen-stimulated tissue growth. p,p'-DDE administered male rats in utero reduces AGD, induces nipples, and permanently reduces androgen-dependent organ weights.

Phthalates (Plasticizers)—In utero, some phthalate esters alter the development of the male rat reproductive tract at relatively low dosages. Prenatal exposures to DBP, benzyl-butyl phthalate (BBP), di-isononyl phthalate (DINP), and diethyl-hexylphthalate (DEHP) cause a syndrome of effects, including underdevelopment and agenesis of the epididymis and other androgen-dependent tissues and testicular abnormalities. The phthalates are unique in their ability to induce agenesis of the gubernacular cords, a tissue whose development is dependent on the peptide hormone insulin-like peptide 3.

Environmental Estrogens

Methoxychlor is an estrogenic pesticide that produces estrogen-like effects. This pesticide requires metabolic activation in order to display full endocrine activity in vitro. The active metabolites of methoxychlor activate estrogen-dependent gene expression in vitro and in vivo in the female rats, thereby stimulating an uterotropic response, accelerating VO and inducing constant estrus, and reducing infertility. In the ovariectomized female rat, methoxychlor also induces estrogen-dependent reproductive and nonreproductive behaviors, including female sex behaviors, running wheel activity, and food consumption.

When given to the dam during pregnancy and lactation, both male and female offspring are affected. Females display irregular estrous cycles and reduced fecundity, whereas male fertility is unaffected at doses up to 200 mg/kg/day.

Ethinylestradiol is a synthetic derivative of estradiol that is in almost all modern formulations of combined oral contraceptive pills. This drug is found in many aquatic systems contaminated by sewage effluents, originating principally from human excretion. Thus, ethinylestradiol plays a major role in causing widespread endocrine disruption in wild populations of fish species and other lower vertebrate species.

EDC Screening Programs

The Endocrine Disruptor Screening and Testing Advisory Committee (EDSTAC) proposed (1) a process to prioritize chemicals for evaluation and recommendations, for (2) screening (Tier 1), and for (3) testing (Tier 2) batteries for EDCs. The recommended screening battery was designed to detect alterations of HPG function; estrogen, androgen, and thyroid hormone synthesis; and AR- and ER-mediated effects in mammals and other taxa.

In Vivo Mammalian Assays—EDSTAC recommended the laboratory rat as the species of choice for the endocrine screening and testing assays. The EDSTAC proposed three short-term in vivo mammalian assays for the tier 1 screening battery: the uterotropic, Hershberger, and pubertal female rat assays.

Uterotropic Assay—Estrogen agonists and antagonists are detected in a 3-day uterotropic assay using subcutaneous administration of the test compound. The selected uterotropic assays for estrogens and antiestrogens use either the intact juvenile or the castrated ovariectomized adult/juvenile female rat.

Hershberger Assay—The second in vivo assay in tier 1, the Hershberger assay, detects antiandrogenic activity simply by weighing androgen-dependent tissues in the castrated male rat. In this assay, weights of the ventral prostate, Cowper's glands, seminal vesicle (with coagulating glands and fluids), glans penis, and levator ani/bulbocavernosus muscles are measured after 10 days of oral treatment with the test compound. This assay is very sensitive for detection of androgens and antiandrogens.

Pubertal Female Rat Assay—The third in vivo mammalian/rat assay in the screening battery is the pubertal female rat assay. Weanling female rats are dosed daily by gavage for 21 days while the age at VO (puberty) is monitored. The females are necropsied at about 42 days of age. This assay detects alterations in thyroid hormone status, HPG function, inhibition of steroidogenesis, estrogens, and antiestrogens, and has been found to be highly reproducible and very sensitive to certain endocrine activities including estrogenicity, inhibition of steroidogenesis, and antithyroid activity.

Alternative Screening Assays—Alternative in vivo assays were also discussed by EDSTAC and are currently being evaluated by the EPA. If they are of sufficient sensitivity, specificity, and relevance, they might replace or augment current tier 1 assays.

Pubertal Male Rat Assay—The pubertal male rat assay detects alterations of thyroid function, HPG maturation, steroidogenesis, and altered steroid hormone function (androgen). Intact weanling males are exposed to the test substance for approximately 30 days. The age at puberty is determined by measuring the age at PPS, and reproductive tissues are evaluated and serum taken for optional hormonal analyses.

In Utero–Lactational Assay—The EDSTAC recommended development of utero-lactational assays due to the unique sensitivity of the fetal reproductive system to certain toxicants. One version of the assay takes about 80 days and uses approximately 10 litters per group (120–150 pups). In this protocol, androgens and antiandrogens can be detected in approximately 2 to 3 weeks, and EDCs with antithyroid activity can be detected in infant or weanling offspring after four to five weeks of maternal treatment.

TESTING FOR REPRODUCTIVE TOXICITY

Screens and Multigeneration Studies

Significant attention has focused on the development of "screens" for reproductive toxicity. The screens currently employed have been developed to prioritize chemicals for more comprehensive testing.

The most comprehensive assessment of reproductive toxicity would be provided by a protocol that exposes the animal model throughout the reproductive cycle (see Figure 20–1)

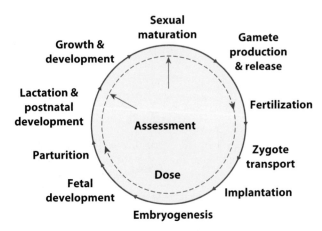

Multigeneration reproduction study

Sexual maturation

Growth & development

Gamete production & release

Lactation & postnatal development

Fertilization

Assessment

Parturition

Zygote transport

Dose

Fetal development

Implantation

Embryogenesis

FIGURE 20–10 **Multigeneration reproduction study.**

and assesses multiple end points at different life stages during this continuous exposure. The protocol and guideline coming closest to this ideal is the multigeneration reproduction study (Figure 20–10) used for the assessment of chemicals, pesticides, and some food additives. Multigeneration studies normally encompass detailed measurements of reproductive performance (number of pregnant females from number of pairs mated, number of females producing a litter, litter size, and number of live pups with their birth weights and sex). Measurement of growth and analysis of the reproductive organs in the F_0 parental generation is conducted. Similar measurements to those undertaken for the F_0 are made on the F_1 parents, and the offspring are examined at birth (and sexually dimorphic end points may be collected such as AGD), at weaning, and at puberty (particularly the assessment of VO and time of first estrus in females and balanopreputial separation in males) in addition to the adult measurements of reproductive performance, organ weights, histology, etc.

Testing for Endocrine-disrupting Chemicals

In the tiered screening and testing approach, only chemicals that display positive reproducible responses in tier 1 screening (T1S) would continue evaluation in full-life cycle or multigenerational tests. In tier 2 testing (T2T), issues of dose–response, relevance of the route of exposure, sensitive life stages, and adversity are resolved.

Data should be summarized in a manner that clearly delineates the proportion of animals that are affected. In teratology studies, data are typically presented and analyzed in this manner, indicating the number of malformed/number observed on an individual and litter basis, whereas multigenerational studies are frequently presented and analyzed differently, even when clear teratogenic and other developmental responses are noted after birth. Multigenerational protocols are used in T2T

because only these protocols expose the animals during all critical stages of development and examine reproductive function of offspring after they mature.

Although the EPA multigenerational test provides for a comprehensive evaluation of the F_0 or parental generation, too few F_1 animals (offspring with developmental exposure) are examined after maturity to detect anything but the most profound reproductive teratogens. F_0 animals within a dose group typically respond in a similar fashion to the chemical exposure; however, the response to toxicants in utero can vary greatly even within a litter with only a few animals displaying severe reproductive malformations in the lower dosage groups.

"Transgenerational" protocols typically use fewer litters (7 to 10 per dose group) but examine all of the animals in each litter. These protocols actually use fewer animals but provide enhanced statistical power to detect reproductive effects in the F_1 generation. The lifelong exposure of both males and females in the F_1 generation, which allows one to detect effects induced in utero, during lactation, or from direct exposure after puberty, can confound the identification of when the effect was induced (i.e., during adulthood versus development) or of which sex was affected.

Some EDCs disrupt pregnancy by altering maternal ovarian hormone production in F_0 dams at dosage levels that appear to be without direct effect on the offspring. In such cases, the standard EPA multigenerational protocol with minor enhancements would be recommended, or a transgenerational protocol with exposure continued after weaning. The transgenerational or in utero lactational protocols fill a gap in the testing program for EDCs that should be used only on a case-by-case basis.

Testing Pharmaceuticals

In the case of pharmaceuticals, it is rare for multigeneration studies to be conducted, because it is not common for all the population to use a specific drug and exposure to the drug is over many different life stages, and not necessarily chronic. Typically three specific studies are undertaken:

1. **A study of fertility and early embryonic development** (see Figure 20–11). Parental adults are exposed to the test chemical for 2 weeks (females) or 4 weeks (males) prior to breeding and then during breeding. Females then continue their exposure through to implantation. Males can be necropsied for the end points noted above for the multigeneration studies after pregnancy has been confirmed, and for the pregnant females, necropsy takes place any time after midgestation. Reproductive and target organs are weighed and examined histologically, sperm parameters are assessed in males, and the uterine implantation sites and ovarian *corpora lutea* are counted in females, as well as live and dead embryos.

2. **A study of effects on pre- and postnatal development including maternal function** (see Figure 20–12). In this study, pregnant females are exposed from the time of implantation until weaning of their offspring (usually PND 21 in the rat). After cessation of exposure, selected offspring

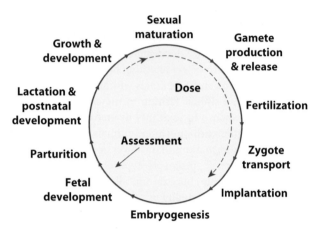

FIGURE 20–11 Fertility and early embryonic study.

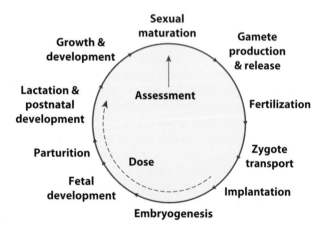

FIGURE 20–12 Pre- and postnatal developmental toxicity study. Dosing is from implantation until the litters are weaned.

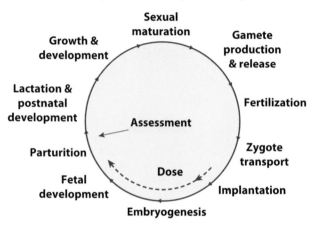

FIGURE 20–13 Embryo–fetal developmental toxicity study as used by FDA guidelines. Dosing starts at implantations and continues to closure of the hard palate with an assessment of fetuses just prior to parturition.

(one male and one female per litter) are raised to adulthood and then mated to assess reproductive competence. These animals are observed for maturation and growth (but are not exposed). Puberty indices, as employed in the multigeneration study, are measured. In addition, sensory function, reflexes, motor activity, learning, and memory are also evaluated.

3. **A study of embryo-fetal development** (see Figure 20–13). This study tests for enhanced toxicity relative to that noted in pregnant females and, unlike the previous two studies, is normally conducted in two species (typically the rat and rabbit). Exposure occurs between implantation and closure of the hard palate and females are killed just prior to parturition. At necropsy, dams are observed for any affected organs and *corpora lutea* are counted. Live and dead fetuses are counted and examined for external, visceral, and skeletal abnormalities.

One of the following three summary risk conclusions would be applied to the drug label: (1) the drug is not anticipated to produce reproductive and/or developmental effects above the background incidence for humans when used in accordance with the dosing information on the product label; (2) the drug may increase the incidence of adverse reproductive and/or developmental events; or (3) the drug is expected to increase the incidence of adverse reproductive and/or developmental effects in humans when used according to the product label.

An examination of the reproductive cycle in a comparison of these three most likely options for FDA studies indicates an obvious gap in the exposure regime for the complete reproductive cycle, namely exposure of weanlings through puberty to adulthood. This exposure period has become of increasing interest to many companies developing drugs for specific administration to infants and juveniles, and "bridging-type" protocols have been developed to specifically address toxicity that may occur after exposure during this specific life stage.

EVALUATION OF TOXICITY TO REPRODUCTION

There are a number of general points that the investigator should note in any estimation of potential reproductive toxicity:

- Adequacy of experimental design and conduct. Was there sufficient statistical power in the evaluation(s)?
- Occurrence of common versus rare reproductive deficits. Biological versus statistical significance.
- Use of historical control data to place concurrent control data into perspective and to estimate population background incidence of various reproductive parameters and deficits.
- Known structure–activity relationships for inducing reproductive toxicity.

- Concordance of reproductive end points. Did a decrease in litter size relate to ovarian histology and changes in vaginal cytology?
- Did the reproductive deficits become more severe with increases in dose? Did histological changes at one dose level become decrements in litter size and then reductions in fertility at higher dose levels in any generation?
- Did the reproductive deficits increase in prevalence (more individuals and/or more litters) with dose level in any generation?
- Special care should be taken for decrements in reproductive parameters noted in the F_1 generation (and potentially later generations) that were not seen in the F_0 generation, which may suggest developmental, as well as reproductive toxicity. Likewise, findings in an F_1 generation animal may (or may not) be reproduced in F_2 offspring. For example, effects in the F_1 generation on reproductive parameters may have resulted in the selection out of sensitive animals in the population, thus not producing F_2 offspring for subsequent evaluation.

BIBLIOGRAPHY

Diamanti-Kandarakis E, Gore AC: *Endocrine Disruptors and Puberty.* New York: Humana Press, 2012.

Gupta RC: *Reproductive and Developmental Toxicology.* Burlington, MA: Academic Press, 2011.

QUESTIONS

1. Which of the following cell types secretes anti-Müllerian hormone (AMH)?
   a. spermatogonium.
   b. Leydig cell.
   c. Sertoli cell.
   d. primary spermatocyte.
   e. spermatid.

2. Penile erections are dependent on:
   a. the CNS.
   b. sympathetic nerve stimulation.
   c. helicine (penile) artery constriction.
   d. corpora cavernosa smooth muscle relaxation.
   e. a spinal reflex arc.

3. The corpus luteum is responsible for the secretion of which of the following hormones during the first part of pregnancy?
   a. estradiol and hCG.
   b. progesterone and estradiol.
   c. progesterone and hCG.
   d. FSH and LH.
   e. FSH and progesterone.

4. All of the following statements regarding the hypothalamo-pituitary–gonadal axis are true EXCEPT:
   a. FSH increases testosterone production by the Leydig cells.
   b. FSH and LH are synthesized in the anterior pituitary.
   c. Estradiol provides negative feedback on the hypothalamus and the anterior pituitary.
   d. GnRH from the hypothalamus increases FSH and LH release from the anterior pituitary.
   e. The LH spike during the menstrual cycle is responsible for ovulation.

5. Which of the following statements is FALSE regarding gametal DNA repair?
   a. DNA repair in spermatogenic cells is dependent on the dose of chemical.
   b. Spermiogenic cells are less able to repair damage from alkylating agents.
   c. Female gametes have base excision repair capacity.
   d. Meiotic maturation of the oocyte decreases its ability to repair DNA damage.
   e. Mature oocytes and mature sperm no longer have the ability to repair DNA damage.

6. Reduction division takes place during the transition between which two cell types during spermatogenesis?
   a. spermatogonium and primary spermatocyte.
   b. primary spermatocyte and secondary spermatocyte.
   c. secondary spermatocyte and spermatid.
   d. spermatid and spermatozoon.
   e. spermatozoon and mature sperm.

7. Which of the following cell types is properly paired with the substance that it secretes?
   a. ovarian granulosa cells—progesterone.
   b. Leydig cells—ABP.
   c. ovarian thecal cells—estrogens.
   d. Sertoli cells—testosterone.
   e. gonadotroph—LH.

8. Which of the following statements regarding male reproductive capacity is FALSE?
   a. Klinefelter's syndrome males are sterile.
   b. FSH levels are often measured in order to determine male reproductive toxicity of a particular toxin.
   c. Divalent metal ions, such as An, Hg, and Cu, act as androgen receptor antagonists and affect male reproduction.
   d. The number of sperms produced per day is approximately the same in all males.
   e. ABP is an important biochemical marker for testicular injury.

9. Reduction of sperm production can be caused by all of the following diseases EXCEPT:
   a. hypothyroidism.
   b. measles.
   c. Crohn's disease.
   d. renal failure.
   e. mumps.

10. Of the following, which is LEAST likely to be affected by estrogen?
    a. nervous system.
    b. musculoskeletal system.
    c. digestive system.
    d. cardiovascular system.
    e. urinary system.

Toxic Responses of the Endocrine System

Patricia B. Hoyer and Jodi A. Flaws

- Endocrine glands are collections of specialized cells that synthesize, store, and release their secretions directly into the bloodstream.
- Each type of endocrine cell in the adenohypophysis is under the control of a specific releasing hormone from the hypothalamus.

- Toxicants can influence the synthesis, storage, and release of hypothalamic-releasing hormones, adenohypophyseal-releasing hormones, and the endocrine gland–specific hormones.

INTRODUCTION

Higher animals have developed the ability to regulate their internal environment, independent of wide external fluctuations via the endocrine system. An endocrine system consists of an endocrine gland that secretes a hormone, the hormone itself, and a target tissue that responds to the hormone. A hormone is a chemical substance produced by a ductless endocrine gland that is secreted into the blood. The hormone-producing glands include the pituitary, the thyroid and parathyroids, the adrenals, the gonads, and the pancreas. There are primarily three chemical classes of hormones: amino acid derivatives (catecholamines and thyroid hormones), peptide hormones (pancreatic), and steroids (derivatives of cholesterol). Endocrine glands are sensing and signaling devices that are capable of responding to changes in the internal and external environments and coordinating multiple activities that maintain homeostasis.

PITUITARY GLAND

Anatomy and Physiology

The pituitary may be divided into two major subdivisions: the pars distalis and the pars nervosa (Figure 21–1). The pars distalis, adenohypophysis or anterior pituitary, is the largest subdivision and it receives peptides from the hypothalamus through a capillary portal system (hypothalamo–hypophyseal vessels). The pars nervosa, neurohypophysis or posterior pituitary, has its cell bodies in the hypothalamus with their axons stretching to the posterior lobe of the pituitary; therefore, functionally and anatomically, the posterior pituitary is an extension of the hypothalamus.

The releasing and release-inhibiting hormones are synthesized by neurons in the hypothalamus, transported by axonal processes, and released into capillary plexus. They are transported to the adenohypophysis by the hypothalamic–hypophyseal portal system, where they interact with specific populations of trophic hormone-secreting cells to govern the rate of release of preformed hormones, such as growth hormone (GH), somatotropic hormone (STH), prolactin (PRL),

luteinizing hormone (LH), follicle-stimulating hormone (FSH), thyrotropic hormone (TTH), adrenocorticotropic hormone (ACTH), and melanocyte-stimulating hormone (MSH). From the pars nervosa, ADH enhances reabsorption of water by the kidney and causes contraction of vascular smooth muscle, whereas oxytocin stimulates contraction of smooth muscle for parturition and milk let-down. These neurohypophyseal hormones are synthetized in the cell body of hypothalamic neurons, packaged in secretory granules, transported along the axon to terminal processes in the pars nervosa for release into the blood.

To maintain appropriate homeostasis, the endocrine organ must constantly monitor systemic hormone concentrations accomplished in the form of negative feedback loops. For example, high circulating levels of cortisol will inhibit corticotrophin-releasing hormone (CRH) release from the hypothalamus, and the adrenocorticotropic hormone (ACTH) release from the pituitary.

Pituitary Toxicity

Studies consistently show that heavy metals may target pituitary gland structure or function. Cadmium inhibits prolactin, LH, and FSH secretion. Cadmium exposure increases ACTH levels in rodents exposed during puberty and decreases ACTH levels in animals exposed during adulthood. Furthermore, studies indicate that acute exposure to cadmium decreases circulating GH levels, while longer period treatment increases circulating GH levels. Lead and mercury also decrease LH and FSH.

Environmental contaminants such as polychlorinated biphenyls (PCBs) and polybrominated diphenylethers inhibit release of LH and FSH as well as TSH. The insecticide dimethoate causes pituitary tumors in rats. Methoxychlor, dieldrin, and endosulfan increase prolactin and LH levels.

Several phytoestrogens affect pituitary cells: coumestrol reduces pulsatile LH and suppresses the pituitary response to exogenous GnRH. Acute exposure to genistein or bisphenol A alter LH secretion as well.

Industrial chemicals alter pituitary structure or function. Flame retardants tetrabromo- and tetrachlorobisphenol A stimulate

THYROID GLAND

General Anatomy

The thyroid gland consists of two lobes of endocrine tissue located just below the larynx on each side of the trachea with an isthmus connecting the two lobes. The thyroid secretes two hormones known as thyroxine (T_4) and triiodothyronine (T_3), which are produced in the thyroid follicle (Figure 21–3).

T_4 and T_3 are important regulators of overall metabolism with their primary target tissues including the liver, kidney, heart, brain, pituitary, gonads, and spleen. Some studies indicate that xenobiotics directly affect the structure of the thyroid gland. For example, heavy metals and red dye #3 are known to decrease the size of the colloid space within the follicle. This leads to an impaired ability of the thyroid gland to synthesize and store thyroid hormones.

Thyroid Hormone Structure and Synthesis

Thyroid hormones are composed of two covalently linked tyrosine amino acids. Both T_4 and T_3 contain iodides that are derived from dietary intake and are required for biological activity. While the thyroid gland synthesizes and secretes both T_4 and T_3, it primarily releases T_4. Figure 21–3 shows the structures required to make T_3 and T_4. At the apical membrane of the follicular cells, I_2 combines with tyrosine residues on thyroglobulin (TGB) to form monoiodotyrosine (MIT) and diiodotyrosine (DIT). Coupling between MIT and DIT occurs such that combined MIT and DIT forms T_3, whereas combined DIT and DIT forms T_4. T_4 from the thyroid gland can be peripherally converted to T_3 (active hormone) or rT_3 (inactive metabolite), then successively diodinated by the monodeiodinases.

Several studies indicate that xenobiotics can interfere with the thyroid gland function by adversely affecting the process of thyroid hormone synthesis. For example, environmental chemicals such as perchlorate, chlorate, and bromate inhibit uptake of iodide and thus decrease thyroid hormone synthesis. Other goitrogenic chemicals are indicated at the bottom of Figure 21–3.

Thyroid Hormone Binding Proteins

Once released into the blood, thyroid hormones are rapidly bound to high-affinity serum binding proteins. Less than

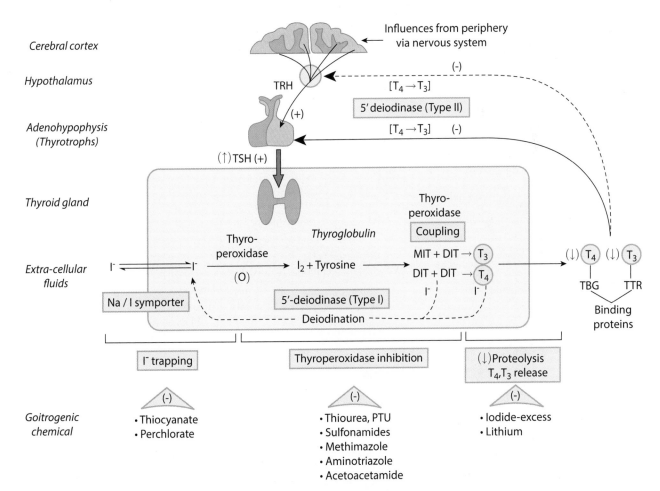

FIGURE 21–3 Mechanism of action of goitrogenic chemicals on thyroid hormone synthesis and secretion. (Reproduced with permission from Dunlop RH, Malbert C, Capen CC, O'Brien TD: *Pathophysiology of Endocrine Homeostasis: Examples IN Veterinary Pathophysiology*, Blackwell Publishing, 2004.)

1% of T_3 is free in circulation. Only this small-unbound fraction has access to receptors in target cells. Environmental chemicals such as PCBs are known to displace thyroid hormones from serum binding proteins and lead to a rapid decline in serum thyroid hormone levels.

Thyroid Hormone Receptors

Thyroid hormones act by binding to the thyroid hormone receptors (TRs). Environmental chemicals can interfere with thyroid hormone binding to TRs and thyroid hormone–related transcription at multiple levels. Some can bind directly to TRs and induce either agonistic or antagonistic effects. Others interfere with the thyroid hormone binding to receptors via indirect mechanisms. There are xenobiotics that can interfere with cross-talk between TRs and other nuclear receptors.

Thyroid Hormone Clearance

The main pathway for clearance of thyroid hormones from the serum is via conjugation to glucuronic acid or sulfate (Figure 21–4). Studies indicate that some xenobiotics including coplanar and noncoplanar congeners of PCBs may increase the clearance of thyroid hormones from the serum by inducing glucuronosyltransferases and sulfotransferases. Others have shown that xenobiotics such as rifampicin and phenobarbital may decrease the transport of thyroid hormones into the brain and liver by inhibiting transporters.

Regulation of Thyroid Hormone Release

Thyroid hormone secretion is regulated by thyroid-stimulating hormone (TSH) from the anterior pituitary gland. The rate of release of TSH is under a hypothalamic–pituitary–thyroid regulatory axis involving negative feedback. The hypothalamus synthesizes and secretes thyroid-releasing hormone (TRH). TRH travels to the anterior pituitary via the portal plexus and stimulates synthesis and secretion of TSH. TSH acts on the thyroid gland to stimulate production and/or release of T_3 and T_4. These can then exert negative feedback control at the level of the anterior pituitary to inhibit further release of TSH. Chemicals such PBDEs may increase TSH levels, leading to increased levels of T_3 and T_4.

Physiological Effects

Thyroid hormones influence nearly every tissue in the body with its primary function being the determination of metabolic rate. In general, thyroid hormone stimulates both anabolic and catabolic biochemical pathways; however, its overriding effect is catabolism. Thyroid hormone also produces significant effects on growth and development of the CNS and skeleton early in life.

Thyroid Toxicity

Given the influence of thyroid hormones on numerous tissues in the body, it is not surprising that xenobiotics that affect

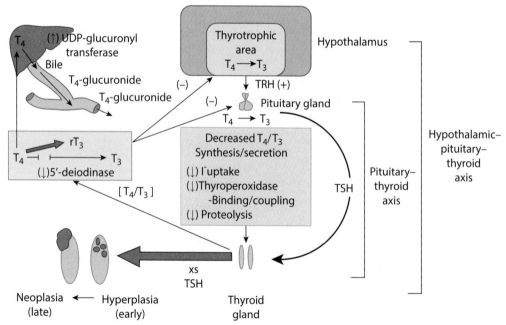

FIGURE 21–4 **Multiple sites of disruption of the hypothalamic–pituitary–thyroid axis by xenobiotic chemicals.** Chemicals can exert direct effects by disrupting thyroid hormone synthesis or secretion and indirectly influence the thyroid through an inhibition of 5'-deiodinase or by inducing hepatic microsomal enzymes (e.g., T_4–UDP-glucuronyltransferase). All of these mechanisms can lower circulating levels of thyroid hormones (T_4 and/or T_3), resulting in a release from negative feedback inhibition and increased secretion of thyroid-stimulating hormone (TSH) by the pituitary gland. The chronic hypersecretion of TSH predisposes the sensitive rodent thyroid gland to develop an increased incidence of focal hyperplastic and neoplastic lesions (adenomas) by a secondary (epigenetic) mechanism.

thyroid hormone levels often cause symptoms of hypothyroidism or hyperthyroidism, or lead to a significant impairment in brain development and function.

PCBs—PCBs are some of the best characterized thyroid disrupting chemicals. PCBs are known to interfere with the thyroid system in a manner that leads to serious neurocognitive defect. Several studies indicate that PCBs decrease the level of thyroid hormone by inhibiting synthesis and/or increasing the metabolism. Further, some studies indicate that they interfere with thyroid hormone action by inhibiting the binding of thyroid hormones to binding proteins or blocking their ability to bind to TRs.

PBDEs—Polybrominated diphenyl ethers (PBDEs) are structurally similar to that of PCBs. Thus, it is not surprising that many of the toxic effects between the two are similar leading to neurocognitive defects.

Perchlorate—A few studies indicate that perchlorate exposure inhibits thyroid hormone levels, possibly leading to hypothyroid-like outcomes.

Pesticides—Pesticide mixtures containing dichlorodiphenyltrichloroethane (DDT) have been shown to increase thyroid volume and to induce antibodies that attack the thyroid gland, resulting in autoimmune thyroid disease.

Perfluorinated Chemicals—Some studies have shown that perfluorooctane sulfonate and perfluorooctanoic acid decrease T_3 and T_4 levels by potentially upregulating phase II enzymes in liver and deiodinases in the thyroid.

Bisphenol A—BPA blocks T_3 action by antagonizing the binding of T_3 to its receptor. Further, some studies have shown that BPA inhibits T_3-mediated gene expression in cell lines. It is suggested that BPA leads to symptoms of hypothyroidism or thyroid resistance syndrome in animal models.

Phthalates—To date, a few small human studies have shown that phthalate exposures may alter the levels of T_3 and T_4 in adult men and pregnant women. They result in low thyroid hormone levels and to symptoms of hypothyroidism.

PARATHYROID GLAND

General Anatomy

Humans have four parathyroid glands that are embedded in the surface of the thyroid gland. They are composed of mainly chief cells that produce parathyroid hormone (PTH). The parathyroid glands are critical for life largely because PTH helps maintain normal plasma calcium levels (Figure 21–5). Calcium is required in optimal concentrations for processes such as fertilization, vision, locomotion-muscle contraction, nerve conduction, blood clotting, exocytosis, cell division, and the activity of a number of enzymes and hormones. When the parathyroids are removed or damaged, PTH levels drop, causing a major drop in circulating calcium levels. In turn, this can lead to tetanic convulsions and death.

Parathyroid Toxicity

Xenobiotic exposures may alter the structure of the parathyroid gland. In some cases, chemicals cause death of the parathyroid cells resulting in a reduced size and limited release of

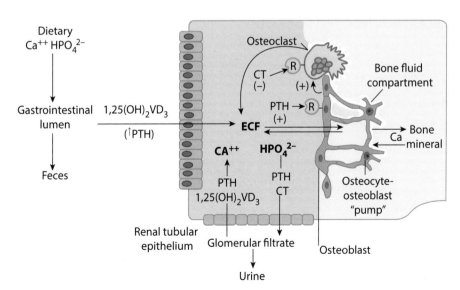

FIGURE 21–5 **Interrelationship of parathyroid hormone (PTH), calcitonin (CT), and 1,25-dihydroxycholecalciferol (1,25(OH)$_2$VD$_3$) in the regulation of calcium (Ca) and phosphorus in extracellular fluids.** Receptors for PTH are on osteoblasts and for CT on osteoclasts in bone. PTH and CT are antagonistic in their action on bone but synergistic in stimulating the renal excretion of phosphorous. Vitamin D exerts its action primarily on the intestine to enhance the absorption of both calcium and phosphorus.

PTH. Other xenobiotic exposures have been shown to increase the size of the parathyroid gland (lead, rotenone, malathion, hexachlorobenzene) often leading to parathyroid cancer.

PTH Structure and Synthesis

PTH is a polypeptide hormone that is derived from a precursor molecule called preproparathyroid hormone (Figure 21–6). Xenobiotics may interfere with the normal synthesis of PTH. Metals such as aluminum and cadmium have been shown to inhibit PTH secretion. Similarly, alcohol consumption has been shown to decrease PTH levels in pregnant rats. Lithium has been associated with a rise in PTH levels as well as abnormally high calcium levels.

PTH Receptors

The PTH receptor is a single G-protein-coupled receptor called PTHR1. A study shows that xenobiotics may alter the expression of PTHR1. Specifically, studies have shown that binge alcohol drinking significantly decreases expression of PTHR1 in male rats.

Physiological Effects

The main physiological role of the parathyroid gland is to control circulating calcium levels (Figure 21–5). PTH works in concert with calcitonin (CT) and vitamin D. PTH serves to increase circulating calcium levels by increasing the release of calcium from bone through demineralization. PTH also serves to increase calcium levels by increasing the tubular reabsorption of calcium by the kidney. Further, it inhibits the renal reabsorption of phosphate, which aids in increasing the solubility of calcium. PTH also enhances magnesium reabsorption, inhibits bicarbonate ion reabsorption, and blocks exchange of sodium ions by the tubules. These actions of PTH result in metabolic acidosis, which favors removal of calcium from plasma proteins and bones. In turn, this increases circulating levels of ionized calcium.

CT reduces circulating calcium levels by reversing the action of PTH on bone resorption. CT serves to prevent hypercalcemia by shutting down efflux of calcium from bone, and it negatively regulates PTH to prevent kidney calcification. Vitamin D also serves to inhibit PTH actions and build bone. Vitamin D_3 is essential for calcium absorption in the GI tract.

Some xenobiotics such as pesticides and fungicides can cause excessive PTH secretion by the parathyroid gland and lead to hyperparathyroidism. Other xenobiotic exposures such as those to heavy metals may cause low PTH secretion and lead to hypoparathyroidism.

Regulation of PTH Release

When the calcium receptors in the parathyroid gland sense low calcium levels, they stimulate the parathyroid gland to release PTH.

ENDOCRINE PANCREAS

Scattered among the pancreatic acini are the endocrine units of the pancreas, the Islets of Langerhans. The major physiological function of the endocrine pancreas is to serve as the primary homeostatic regulator of fuel metabolism, particularly circulating glucose. Islet cells are sensors of glucose homeostasis that respond to changes in their nutrient and hormonal environment.

Role of the Liver in Glucose Production

Energy for cellular metabolism can be derived from fatty acids or glucose in the blood. The liver is the primary contributor to increasing blood glucose levels.

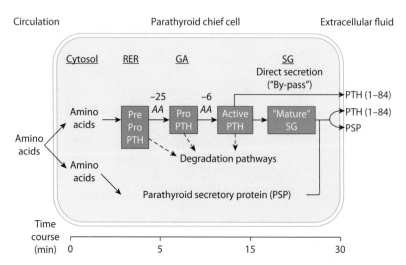

FIGURE 21–6 Biosynthesis of PTH. Active PTH is synthetized as a larger biosynthetic precursor (preproPTH) that undergoes rapid posttranslational processing to proPTH prior to secretion as active PTH (aminoacids 1-84) from chief cells in the parathyroid glands.

Pancreatic Hormones

Insulin—The overall effects of insulin are to stimulate anabolic processes (energy storage). Specifically, insulin functions to lower blood levels of glucose, fatty acids, and amino acids and to promote their conversion to the storage form of each: glycogen, triglycerides, and protein, respectively.

Glucagon—Glucagon is the primary hormone with action counterregulatory to insulin, because it stimulates catabolic processes to prevent hypoglycemia. The release of glucagon is stimulated by epinephrine and norepinephrine, and by the amino acids, arginine, leucine, and alanine. Conversely, glucagon secretion is inhibited by insulin and somatostatin.

Somatostatin—The role of somatostatin is its role in regulation of neuroendocrine function to inhibit secretion of growth hormone in the anterior pituitary. The generalized function of somatostatin appears to be as a hormone release inhibitor.

Interactions of Release

Although glucagon and insulin exert opposing effects on carbohydrate metabolism, they act in concert to preserve normoglycemia in the face of perturbations that might tend to elevate or lower blood glucose. Insulin and glucagon exert opposing effects on various metabolic processes. Therefore, many investigators like to think of the insulin-to-glucagon ratio in blood as an important determinant of the overall metabolic status. When there is a high ratio of insulin to glucagon, a relative anabolic state exists. When the ratio of insulin to glucagon is low, a catabolic state exists.

Metabolic Responses in Diabetes

Two major forms of diabetes mellitus result from either decreased insulin production (type 1) due to autoimmune destruction of pancreatic β cells or reduced insulin function (type 2) owing to end organ insensitivity or resistance to insulin. Insufficient insulin action leads to decreased glycogen, lipid, and protein synthesis (Figure 21–7). Reduced removal of glucose from the blood causes hyperglycemia and various metabolic alterations. Increased action of the counter-regulatory hormone glucagon stimulates glycogenolysis, lipolysis, and protein breakdown. Stimulation of glycogenolysis and gluconeogenesis increases circulating glucose.

Pancreatic Toxicity

The insulin-secreting beta cells are particularly sensitive to chemical attack. The clinical consequences of insulin deficiency are physiologically more severe than those that would result from glucagon deficiency because the other counterregulatory hormones that oppose insulin action can compensate for reduced glucagon regulation. Two chemicals that have been

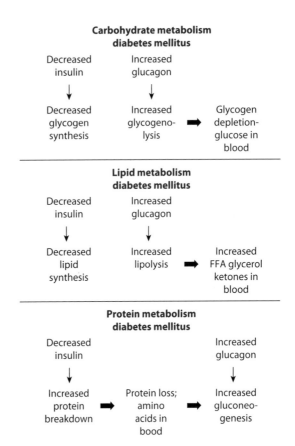

FIGURE 21–7 **Effects of diabetes mellitus on metabolism.** Decreased insulin (type 1) or insulin action (type 2) inhibits glycogen, lipid, and protein synthesis. Increased glucagon stimulates glycogenolysis, lipolysis, and protein breakdown. Glycogenolysis increases circulating glucose. Increased glycerol and amino acids serve as substrates for gluconeogenesis to further increase circulating glucose.

widely used to generate animal models of diabetes are alloxan and streptozotocin. A common target of these in pancreatic beta cells is DNA. There are data to support that DNA damage occurs, poly(ADP-ribose) synthetase is activated, polyadenylation increases, and NAD declines.

Insulin Resistance

Insulin resistance and defective function of pancreatic beta cells usually occur sometime before the development of type 2 diabetes. In a study investigating nondiabetic residents living near a deserted pentachlorophenol and chloralkali factory in Taiwan, insulin resistance was associated with increasing circulating levels of dioxins and mercury. In addition, BPA exposure of pregnant mice resulted in increased insulin, leptin, triglyceride, and glycerol levels.

In Vitro Testing

Several cell lines are available for testing of insulin secretion. Pancreatic beta-cell-derived RINm5F cells were exposed to a combination of the cytokines, IL-1β, TNF-α, and IFN-γ to simulate type 1 diabetes mellitus conditions. This study showed that hydrogen peroxide produced by these cytokines reacted in the presence of trace metal Fe^{++} with nitric oxide to form highly toxic hydroxyl radicals. RINm5F cells were also used to investigate the role of oxidative stress in inorganic arsenic exposure. A number of proapoptotic mitochondrial and cytosolic markers were investigated and found to be elevated during β-cell toxicity.

BIBLIOGRAPHY

Eldridge JC, Stevens JT: *Endocrine Toxicology*, 3rd ed. London: Informa Healthcare, 2010.

Gardner DG, Shoback DM, Greenspan FS: *Greenspan's Basic and Clinical Endocrinology*. New York: McGraw-Hill, 2007.

Jameson JL: *Harrison's Endocrinology*, 11th ed. New York: McGraw-Hill, 2013.

QUESTIONS

1. The inability to release hormones from the anterior pituitary would NOT affect the release of which of the following?
   a. LH.
   b. PRL.
   c. ADH.
   d. TSH.
   e. ACTH.

2. Which of the following statements regarding pituitary hormones is TRUE?
   a. The hypothalamic–hypophyseal portal system transports releasing hormones to the neurohypophysis.
   b. Dopamine enhances prolactin secretion from the anterior pituitary.
   c. Somatostatin inhibits the release of GH.
   d. The function of chromophobes in the anterior pituitary is unknown.
   e. Oxytocin and ADH are synthesized by hypothalamic nuclei.

3. 21-Hydroxylase deficiency causes masculinization of female genitals at birth by increasing androgen secretion from which region of the adrenal gland?
   a. zona glomerulosa.
   b. zona reticularis.
   c. adrenal medulla.
   d. zona fasciculata.
   e. chromaffin cells.

4. Which of the following statements regarding adrenal toxicity is TRUE?
   a. The adrenal cortex and adrenal medulla are equally susceptible to fat-soluble toxins.
   b. Adrenal cortical cells lack the enzymes necessary to metabolize xenobiotic chemicals.
   c. Pheochromocytomas of the adrenal medulla can cause high blood pressure and clammy skin due to increased epinephrine release.
   d. Xenobiotics primarily affect the hydroxylase enzymes in the zona reticularis.
   e. Vitamin D is an important stimulus for adrenal cortex steroid secretion.

5. Chemical blockage of iodine transport in the thyroid gland:
   a. affects export of T_3 and T_4.
   b. prevents reduction to I_2 by thyroid peroxidase.
   c. decreases TRH release from the hypothalamus.
   d. interrupts intracellular thyroid biosynthesis.
   e. mimics goiter.

6. Chromaffin cells of the adrenal gland are responsible for secretion of which of the following?
   a. aldosterone.
   b. epinephrine.
   c. corticosterone.
   d. testosterone.
   e. estradiol.

7. The parafollicular cells of the thyroid gland are responsible for secreting a hormone that:
   a. increases blood glucose levels.
   b. decreases plasma sodium levels.
   c. increases calcium storage.
   d. decreases metabolic rate.
   e. increases bone resorption.

8. Parathyroid adenomas resulting in increased PTH levels would be expected to cause which of the following?
   a. hypocalcemia.
   b. hyperphosphatemia.
   c. increased bone formation.
   d. osteoporosis.
   e. rickets.

9. Which of the following vitamins increases calcium and phosphorus absorption in the gut?
   a. vitamin D.
   b. niacin.
   c. vitamin A.
   d. vitamin B_{12}.
   e. thiamine.

10. All of the following statements regarding glucose control are true EXCEPT:
    a. Glucagon stimulates glycogenolysis, gluconeogenesis, and lipolysis.
    b. Insulin stimulates glycogen synthesis, gluconeogenesis, and lipolysis.
    c. Glucagon stimulates catabolic processes (mobilizes energy) to prevent hypoglycemia.
    d. Insulin promotes storage of glucose, fatty acids, and aminoacids by their conversion to glycogen, triglycerides, and protein, respectively.
    e. Insulin and glucagon exert opposing effects on blood glucose concentrations.

C H A P T E R

22

Toxic Effects of Pesticides

Lucio G. Costa

■ A pesticide may be defined as any substance or mixture of substances intended for preventing, destroying, repelling, or mitigating any pest.

■ Pesticide exposures include (1) accidental and/or suicidal poisonings; (2) occupational exposure (manufacturing, mixing/loading, application, harvesting, and handling of crops); (3) bystander exposure to off-target drift from spraying operations; and (4) the general public who consume food items containing pesticide residues.

■ Chemical insecticides in use today poison the nervous systems of the target organisms.

■ An herbicide is any compound that is capable of either killing or severely injuring plants.

■ A fungicide is any chemical capable of preventing growth and reproduction of fungi.

INTRODUCTION

Pesticides can be defined as any substance or mixture of substances intended for preventing, destroying, repelling, or mitigating pests. Pests can be insects, rodents, weeds, and a host of other unwanted organisms. Pesticides may be more specifically identified as insecticides (insects), herbicides (weeds), fungicides (fungi and molds), rodenticides (rodents), acaricides (mites), molluscides (snails and other mollusks), miticides (mites), larvicides (larvae), and pediculocides (lice). In addition, for regulatory purposes, plant growth regulators, repellants, and attractants (pheromones) often also fall in this broad classification of chemicals.

ECONOMICS AND PUBLIC HEALTH

The use of pesticides must consider the balance of the benefits versus the possible risks of injury to human health or degradation of environmental quality. Pesticides play a major role in the control of vector-borne diseases, which represent a major threat to the health of large human populations. When introduced in 1942, DDT appeared to hold immense promise of benefit to agriculture and public health by controlling vector-borne diseases. However, because of its bioaccumulation in the environment and its detrimental effects on bird reproduction, DDT was eventually banned in most countries by the mid-1970s. When DDT was banned in 1996 in South Africa, less than 10 000 cases of malaria were registered in that country. By 2000, the number of malaria cases had increased to 62 000, but with the reintroduction of DDT at the end of that year, cases were down to 12 500.

Excessive loss of food crops to insects or other pests contributes to economic loss and possible starvation. In developed countries, pesticides allow production of abundant, inexpensive, and attractive fruits and vegetables, as well as grains. Along with insecticides, herbicides and fungicides play a major role in this endeavor.

Use of Pesticides

In the past 20 years, use of pesticides (as amount of active ingredient) has plateaued due to the utilization of more efficacious compounds, which require less active ingredient. Pesticides are often, if not always, used as multiagent formulations, in which the active ingredient is present together with other ingredients to allow mixing, dilution, application, and stability. These other ingredients are lumped under the term "inert" or "other." Though they do not have pesticidal action, such inert ingredients may not always be devoid of toxicity.

Exposure

Exposure to pesticides can occur via the oral or dermal routes or by inhalation. High oral doses, leading to severe poisoning and death, are achieved as a result of pesticide ingestion for suicidal intent, or of accidental ingestion, commonly due to storage of pesticides in improper containers. Chronic low doses, on the other hand, are consumed by the general population as pesticide residues in food or as contaminants in drinking water. Regulations exist to ensure that pesticide residues are maintained at levels below those that would cause any adverse effects. Workers involved in the production, transport, mixing and loading, and application of pesticides, as well as in harvesting of pesticide-sprayed crops, are at the highest risk for pesticide exposure. Dermal exposure during normal handling or application of pesticides, or in case of accidental spillings, occurs in body areas not covered by protective clothing, such as the face or the hands, or by inhalation. Furthermore, pesticides deposited on clothing may penetrate the skin and/or potentially expose others, if clothes are not changed and washed on termination of exposure.

Human Poisoning

Pesticides are not always selective for their intended target species, and adverse health effects can occur in nontarget

TABLE 22–1 WHO-recommended classification of pesticides by hazard.

Class	LD$_{50}$ in Rat (mg/kg Body Weight)			
	Oral		Dermal	
	Solids	Liquids	Solids	Liquids
Ia: Extremely hazardous	5 or less	20 or less	10 or less	40 or less
Ib: Highly hazardous	5–50	20–200	10–100	40–400
II: Moderately hazardous	50–500	200–2000	100–1000	400–4000
III: Slightly hazardous	Over 500	Over 2000	Over 1000	Over 4000
IV+: Unlikely to present hazard in normal use	Over 2000	Over 3000	Over 4000	Over 6000

species, including humans. In the general population and in occupationally exposed workers, concerns range from acute human poisoning to a possible association between pesticide exposure and increased risk of cancer, reproductive and developmental toxicity.

With several million poisonings causing hospital admission and a couple hundred thousand deaths, the World Health Organization (WHO) has recommended a classification of pesticides by hazard, where acute oral or dermal toxicities in rats were considered (Table 22–1). As a class, insecticides are the most acutely toxic followed by herbicides and fungicides.

Regulatory Mandate

In the United States, the Environmental Protection Agency (EPA) regulates pesticide use under the Federal Insecticide, Fungicide and Rodenticide Act and the Federal Food, Drug and Cosmetic Act through registration for use and establishment of maximum allowable levels of pesticide residues (tolerances) in foods and animal feeds.

The Food Quality Protection Act gives EPA the mandate to assess risks of pesticides to infants and children based on dietary consumption patterns of children, possible susceptibility of infants and children to pesticides, and cumulative effects of compounds that share the same mechanism of toxicity. Additional regulations concerning pesticides are present in other laws, such as the Safe Drinking Water Act or the Clean Air Act.

All pesticides sold or distributed in the United States must be registered by the EPA. To register a pesticide or a formulated product, a large number of studies (over 140) are required, a process that takes several years and costs between $50 and $100 million. The database includes information on product and residue chemistry, environmental fate, toxicology, biotransformation/degradation, occupational exposure and reentry protection, spray drift, environmental impact on nontarget species (birds, mammals, aquatic organisms, plants, and soil), environmental persistence and bioaccumulation, as well as product performance and efficacy. Table 22–2 lists basic toxicology data needed for new pesticide registration.

Other nations, such as Canada, Japan, and most European countries, have legislated similar procedures for pesticide registration. The European Union (EU) has created a harmonized Union-wide framework for pesticide regulation. The WHO provides guidance, particularly with the setting of acceptable daily intake (ADI) values for pesticides.

TABLE 22–2 Basic toxicology testing requirements for pesticide registration.

Test	Animal Species*
Acute lethality (oral, dermal, inhalation)	Rat, mouse, guinea pig, rabbit
Dermal irritation	Rabbit, rat, guinea pig
Dermal sensitization	Guinea pig
Eye irritation	Rabbit
Acute delayed neurotoxicity	Hen
Genotoxicity studies (in vitro, in vivo)	Bacteria, mammalian cells, mouse, rat, *Drosophila*
Teratogenicity	Rabbit, rodent (mouse, rat, hamster)
2- to 4-week toxicity study (oral, dermal, inhalation)	Rat, mouse
90-Day toxicity study (oral)	Rat
Chronic toxicity study (oral; 6 months to 2 years)	Rat, dog
Oncogenicity study	Rat, mouse
Reproductive/fertility study	Rat
Developmental neurotoxicity study	Rat

*Substantial efforts are being devoted to develop alternative nonanimal test systems. Only one in vitro test for primary irritation has been validated and accepted by regulatory bodies.

INSECTICIDES

Insecticides play a most relevant role in the control of insect pests, particularly in developing countries. All of the chemical insecticides in use today are neurotoxicants, and act by poisoning the nervous systems of the target organisms (Table 22–3). The central nervous system of insects is highly developed and not unlike that of mammals. As a class, insecticides have high acute toxicity toward nontarget species compared with other pesticides. Some of them, most notably the organophosphates, are involved in a great number of human poisonings and deaths each year.

Organophosphorus Compounds

The general structure of organophosphorus (OP) insecticides can be represented by:

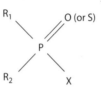

where X is the so-called leaving group that is displaced when the OP phosphorylates acetylcholinesterase (AChE), and is the most sensitive to hydrolysis; R_1 and R_2 are commonly alkoxy groups (i.e., OCH_3 or OC_2H_5) or other chemical substituents; either an oxygen or a sulfur (in this case the compound should be defined as a phosphorothioate) is also attached to

TABLE 22–3 Molecular targets of the major classes of insecticides.

Target	Insecticide	Effect
Acetylcholinesterase	Organophosphates	Inhibition
	Carbamates	Inhibition
Sodium channels	Pyrethroids (types I and II)	Activation
	DDT	Activation
	Dihydropyrazoles	Inhibition
Nicotinic acetylcholine receptors	Nicotine	Activation
	Neonicotinoids	Activation
GABA receptor–gated chloride channels	Cyclodienes	Inhibition
	Phenylpyrazoles	Inhibition
	Pyrethroids (type II)	Inhibition
Glutamate-gated chloride channels*	Avermectins	Activation
Octopamine receptors†	Formamidines	Activation
Mitochondrial complex I	Rotenoids	Inhibition
Ryanodine receptors	Diamides	Activation

*Found only in insects. In mammals, avermectins activate $GABA_A$ receptors.
†In mammals, formamidines activate alpha$_2$-adrenoceptors.

the phosphorus with a double bond. Based on chemical differences, OPs can be divided into several subclasses, which include phosphates, phosphorothioates, phosphoramidates, phosphonates, and others. Figure 22–1 shows the chemical structures of some commonly used OPs.

Biotransformation—For all compounds that contain a sulfur bound to the phosphorus, a metabolic bioactivation is necessary for their biological activity to be manifest, as only compounds with a P=O moiety are effective inhibitors of AChE. Oxidative desulfuration (leads to the formation of an "oxon," or oxygen analog of the parent insecticide) and thioether oxidation (formation of a sulfoxide, S=O, followed by the formation of a sulfone, O=S=O) are catalyzed by cytochrome P450s. Catalytic hydrolysis by phosphotriesterases, known as A-esterases (which are not inhibited by OPs), plays an important role in the detoxication of certain OPs. Noncatalytic hydrolysis of OPs also occurs when these compounds phosphorylate serine esterases classified as B-esterases.

Signs and Symptoms of Toxicity and Mechanism of Action—OP insecticides have high acute toxicity, with oral LD_{50} values in rat often below 50 mg/kg. For several OPs, acute dermal toxicity is also high. Inhibition of AChE by OPs causes accumulation of acetylcholine at cholinergic synapses, with overstimulation of muscarinic and nicotinic cholinergic receptors. As these receptors are localized in most organs of the body, a "cholinergic syndrome" ensues, which includes increased sweating, salivation, bronchial secretion, bronchoconstriction, miosis, increased gastrointestinal motility, diarrhea, tremors, muscular twitching, and various central nervous system effects (Table 22–4). Whereas respiratory failure is a hallmark of severe OP poisoning, mild poisoning and/or early stages of an otherwise severe poisoning may display no clear-cut signs and symptoms.

OPs with a P=O moiety phosphorylate a hydroxyl group on serine in the active (esteratic) site of the enzyme, impeding its action on the physiological substrate. Phosphorylated AChE is hydrolyzed by water slowly, and the rate of "spontaneous reactivation" depends on the chemical nature of the R substituents. Reactivation of phosphorylated AChE does not occur once the enzyme-inhibitor complex has "aged," which occurs when there is loss by nonenzymatic hydrolysis of one of the two alkyl (R) groups. When phosphorylated AChE has aged, the enzyme is considered to be irreversibly inhibited, and the only means of replacing its activity is through synthesis of new enzyme, a process that may take days.

Treatment of Poisoning—Procedures aimed at decontamination and/or at minimizing absorption depend on the route of exposure. In case of dermal exposure, contaminated clothing should be removed, and the skin washed thoroughly with alkaline soap. In case of ingestion, procedures to reduce absorption from the gastrointestinal tract do not appear to be very effective. Atropine, a muscarinic receptor antagonist, prevents the action of accumulating acetylcholine on

filariasis. In insects and nematodes, avermectins exert their toxic effects by binding to, and activating, glutamate-dependent chloride channel. Signs and symptoms of intoxication include hyperexcitability, tremors, and incoordination, followed by ataxia and coma-like sedation.

INSECT REPELLENTS

Insect-transmitted diseases remain a major source of illness and death worldwide, as mosquitoes alone transmit disease to more than 700 million persons annually. DEET (*N*,*N*-diethyl-*m*-toluamide or *N*,*N*-diethyl-3-methylbenzamide) is very effective at repelling insects, flies, fleas, and ticks, and protection time increases with increasing concentrations. Subchronic toxicity studies in various species did not reveal major toxic effects and no significant effects of DEET were seen in mutagenicity, reproductive toxicity, and carcinogenicity studies. Acute and chronic neurotoxicity studies also provided negative results. However, in children DEET is possibly responsible for neurotoxic effects and children should only be exposed to products with up to 10% DEET.

Picaridin

Picaridin was developed as an alternative to DEET. Insect repellent formulations (cream, aerosol, wipe) containing 5% to 20% picaridin are highly effective against a variety of arthropod pests, especially mosquitoes, ticks, and flies. Its action in insects is believed to be due to the interaction with specific olfactory receptors of the arthropod. In humans it is absorbed through the skin to a limited degree, and is metabolized via hydroxylation and glucuronidation, before excretion in the urine. The toxicological profile of picaridin is unremarkable. Acute dermal toxicity is low. There is no evidence of genotoxicity, carcinogenicity, teratogenicity, reproductive toxicity, or neurotoxicity. When used as directed, picaridin-containing formulations are deemed to be safe and effective.

HERBICIDES

Herbicides are chemicals that are capable of either killing or severely injuring plants. Some of the various mechanisms by which herbicides exert their biological effects are shown in Table 22–6, together with examples for each class. Another method of classification pertains to how and when herbicides are applied. Thus, *preplanting* herbicides are applied to the soil before a crop is seeded, *preemergent* herbicides are applied to the soil before the time of appearance of unwanted vegetation, and *postemergent* herbicides are applied to the soil or foliage after the germination of the crop and/or weeds. Herbicides are also divided according to the manner they are applied to plants. *Contact* herbicides are those that affect the plant that was treated, whereas *translocated* herbicides are applied to the soil or to above-ground parts of the plant, and are absorbed and circulated to distant tissues. Nonselective herbicides will

TABLE 22–6 Some mechanisms of action of herbicides.

Mechanism	Chemical Classes (Example)
Inhibition of photosynthesis	Triazines (atrazine), substituted ureas (diuron), uracils (bromacil)
Inhibition of respiration	Dinitrophenols
Auxin growth regulators	Phenoxy acids (2,4-D), benzoic acids (dicamba), pyridine acids (picloram)
Inhibition of protein synthesis	Dinitroanilines
Inhibition of lipid synthesis	Aryloxyphenoxypropionates (diclofop)
Inhibition of specific enzymes • Glutamine synthetase • Enolpyruvylshikimate-3-phosphate synthetase • Acetolactate synthase	 Glufosinate Glyphosate Sulfonylureas
Cell membrane disruptors	Bipyridyl derivatives (paraquat)

kill all vegetation, whereas selective compounds are those used to kill weeds without harming the crops.

A number of herbicides can cause dermal irritation and contact dermatitis, particularly in individuals prone to allergic reactions. Other compounds have generated much debate for their suspected carcinogenicity or neurotoxicity. The principal classes of herbicides associated with reported adverse health effects in humans are discussed below.

Chlorophenoxy Compounds

Chlorophenoxy herbicides are chemical analogs of auxin, a plant growth hormone, that produce uncontrolled and lethal growth in target plants. Because the auxin hormone is critical to the growth of many broad-leaved plants, but is not used by grasses, chlorophenoxy compounds can suppress the growth of weeds (e.g., dandelions) without affecting the grass. The most commonly used compound of this class is 2,4-dichlorophenoxyacetic acid (2,4-D).

Ingestion of 2,4-D has caused acute poisoning in humans, resulting in vomiting, burning of the mouth, abdominal pain, hypotension, myotonia, and CNS involvement including coma. Dermal exposure is the major route of unintentional exposure to 2,4-D in humans.

There are several case reports suggesting an association between exposure to 2,4-D and neurologic effects like peripheral neuropathy, demyelination and ganglion degeneration in the CNS, reduced nerve conduction velocity, myotonia, and behavioral alterations. 2,4-D does not appear to have genotoxic or carcinogenic properties in rats, mice, and dogs. The chlorophenoxy herbicides have attracted much attention because of an association between exposure and non-Hodgkin's lymphoma or soft-tissue sarcoma, found in a few epidemiological studies. Nevertheless, 2,4-D is classified as a group D agent (not classifiable as to human carcinogenicity).

Bipyridil Compounds

Paraquat is a fast-acting, nonselective contact herbicide, used to control broad-leaved weeds and grasses in plantations and fruit orchards, and for general weed control. Paraquat has one of the highest acute toxicities among herbicides. On absorption, independent of the route of exposure, paraquat accumulates in the lung and the kidney. Paraquat is very poorly metabolized, and is excreted almost unchanged in the urine. It has minimal to no genotoxic activity, is not carcinogenic in rodents, has no effect on fertility, is not teratogenic, and only produces fetotoxicity at maternally toxic doses. The major toxicologic concerns for paraquat are related to its acute systemic effects, particularly in the lung, and secondarily, the kidney.

Once paraquat enters a cell, it undergoes alternate reduction followed by reoxidation, a process known as redox cycling. Intracellular redox cycling of paraquat would also result in the oxidation of NADPH, leading to its cellular depletion, which is augmented by the detoxification of hydrogen peroxide formed in the glutathione peroxidase/reductase enzyme system to regenerate GSH (Figure 22–3).

Damage to alveolar epithelial cells occurs within 24h after acute exposure to lethal doses of paraquat. Damage progresses in the following 2 to 4 days with loss of the alveolar epithelium, alveolar edema, extensive infiltration of inflammatory cells into the alveolar interstitium, and finally death due to severe anoxia. Survivors of this destructive first phase show extensive proliferation of fibroblasts in the lung. The second phase is characterized by attempts by the alveolar epithelium to regenerate and restore normal architecture, and presents as an intensive fibrosis. Individuals who survive the first phase may still die from the progressive loss of lung function several weeks after exposure.

The herbicide diquat presents a different toxicologic profile. Acute toxicity is somewhat lower. In contrast to paraquat, diquat does not accumulate in the lung, and no lung toxicity is seen on acute or chronic exposure. On chronic exposure, target organs for toxicity are the gastrointestinal tract, the kidney, and particularly the eye. Like paraquat, diquat can be reduced to form a free radical and then reoxidized in the presence of oxygen, with the concomitant production of superoxide anion. This process of redox cycling occurs in the eye and is believed to be the likely mechanism of cataract formation. Human clinical symptoms include nausea, vomiting, diarrhea, ulceration of mouth and esophagus, decline in renal functions, and neurologic effects, but no pulmonary fibrosis.

Chloroacetanilides

Representative compounds of this class of herbicides are alachlor, acetochlor, and metolachlor, which are used to control herbal grasses and broad-leaved weeds in a number of crops

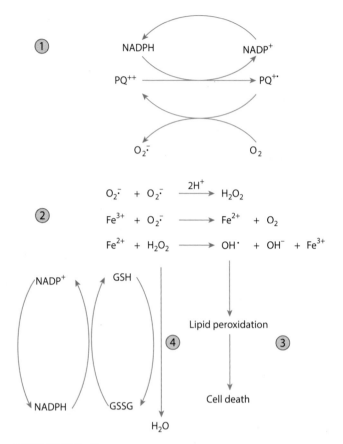

FIGURE 22–3 **Mechanism of toxicity of paraquat.** (1) Redox cycling of paraquat utilizing NADPH; (2) formation of hydroxy radicals leading to lipid peroxidation (3); (4) detoxication of H_2O_2 via glutathione reductase/peroxidase couple, utilizing NADPH. (Modified from Smith LL: Mechanism of paraquat toxicity in the lung and its relevance to treatment, *Hum Toxicol*, 1987 Jan;6(1):31–36).

(corn, soybeans, and peanuts). Alachlor, acetochlor, and butachlor are probable human carcinogens (Group B2). The discovery of alachlor in well water led to cancellation of its registration in some countries, and to its restriction in others. Both are believed to be threshold-sensitive phenomena.

Triazines

The family of triazine herbicides comprises several compounds (atrazine, simazine, and propazine) that are extensively used for the preemergent control of broad-leaved weeds. Triazines have low acute oral and dermal toxicity, and chronic toxicity studies indicate primarily decreased body weight gain. There is no evidence that triazines are teratogenic, genotoxic, or developmental or reproductive toxicants. However, a more recent study has suggested a possible clastogenic effect. Though exposure to atrazine through residues in food commodities is very low, contamination of ground water and drinking water is common. Nevertheless, the known hormonal effects of triazines call for careful evaluation of the endocrine-disrupting effects of these herbicides.

Phosphonomethyl Amino Acids

The two compounds of this class are glyphosate (*N*-phos phonomethyl glycine) and glufosinate (*N*-phosphonomethyl homoalanine). Both are broad-spectrum nonselective systemic herbicides used for postemergent control of annual and perennial plants. Though both compounds contain a P=O moiety, they are organophosphonates and do not inhibit AChE.

Glyphosate—Glyphosate exerts its herbicidal action by inhibiting the enzyme 5-enolpyruvylshikimate-3-phosphate synthase, responsible for the synthesis of an intermediate in the biosynthesis of various amino acids. Although important in plant growth, this metabolic pathway is not present in mammals. It has no teratogenic, developmental, or reproductive effects. Genotoxicity and carcinogenicity studies in animals were negative.

Glyphosate is one of the most widely used herbicides, and the development of transgenic crops that can tolerate glyphosate treatment has expanded its utilization. Given its widespread use, including the home and garden market, accidental or intentional exposure to glyphosate is inevitable. The most widely used glyphosate product is Roundup® which is formulated as a concentrate containing water, 41% glyphosate (as isopropylamine salt), and 15% polyoxethyleneamine (POEA). Mild intoxication results mainly in transient gastrointestinal symptoms. Moderate or severe poisoning presents with gastrointestinal bleeding, hypotension, pulmonary dysfunction, and renal damage.

Glufosinate—Glufosinate is a nonselective contact herbicide that acts by irreversibly inhibiting glutamine synthetase. Plants die as a consequence of the increased levels of ammonia. Mammals have other metabolizing systems that can cope with the effects on glutamine synthetase activity to a certain limit. There is no evidence of genotoxicity or carcinogenicity, or direct effects on reproductive performance and fertility. Developmental toxic effects were found in rabbits (premature deliveries, abortions, and dead fetuses). Humans experience gastrointestinal effects, impaired respiration, neurologic disturbance, and cardiovascular effects.

FUNGICIDES

Fungal diseases are virtually impossible to control without chemical application. Fungicidal chemicals are derived from a variety of structures, ranging from simple inorganic compounds, such as copper sulfate, to complex organic compounds. Most fungicides are surface or plant protectants, and are applied prior to potential infection by fungal spores, either to plants or to postharvest crops. Other fungicides can be used therapeutically, to cure plants when an infestation has already begun. Still others are used as systemic fungicides that are absorbed and distributed throughout the plant. With a few exceptions, fungicides have low acute toxicity in mammals. Some fungicides have been associated with severe epidemics of poisoning.

Captan and Folpet

Captan and folpet are broad-spectrum protectant fungicides; together with captafol, they are called chloroalkylthio fungicides, due to the presence of side chains containing chlorine, carbon, and sulfur. They are potent eye irritants, but only mild skin irritants. Dermal absorption is low. Captan and folpet, as well as thiophosgene, are mutagenic in vitro tests; however, in vivo mutagenicity tests are mostly negative, possibly because of the rapid degradation of these compounds. These fungicides induce the development of duodenal tumors in mice, and on this basis, they are classified by the US EPA as probable human carcinogens. Because of their structural similarity to the potent teratogen thalidomide, chloroalkylthio fungicides have been extensively tested in reproductive/developmental studies in multiple species, but no evidence of teratogenicity has been found.

Dithiocarbamates

The nomenclature of many of these compounds arises from the metal cations with which they are associated; thus, there are, e.g., Maneb (Mn), Ziram and Zineb (Zn), and Mancozeb (Mn and Zn) (Figure 22–4). Thiram is an example of dithiocarbamate without a metal moiety (Figure 22–4). The dithiocarbamates have low acute toxicity by the oral, dermal, and respiratory routes. However, chronic exposure is associated with adverse effects that may be due to the dithiocarbamate

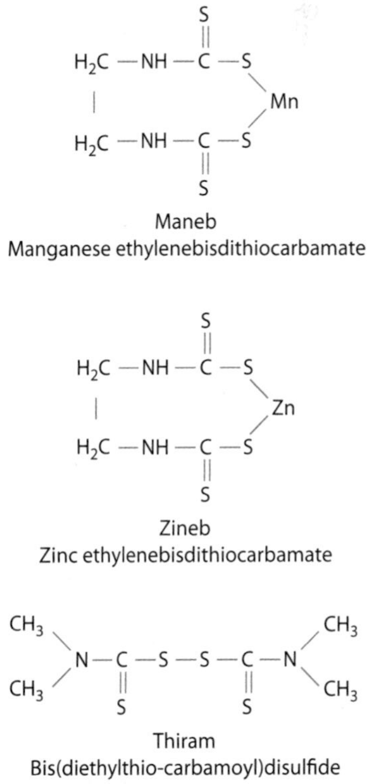

FIGURE 22–4 **Structures of three dithiocarbamate fungicides.**

acid or the metal moiety. These compounds are metabolized to a common metabolite, ethylenethiourea, that is responsible for the effects of dithiocarbamates on the thyroid, which include hypertrophy and hyperplasia of thyroid follicular cells that progress to adenomas and carcinomas. Similarly, dithiocarbamates alter thyroid hormone levels, and cause thyroid hypertrophy. Also, the structure of dithiocarbamate fungicides resembles that of disulfiram, which inhibits aldehyde dehydrogenase and may, after ingestion of ethanol, lead to elevated acetaldehyde levels.

Inorganic and Organometal Fungicides

Copper sulfate has overall low toxicity and remains one of the most widely used fungicides. Triphenyltin acetate is used as a fungicide, whereas tributyltin is utilized as an antifouling agent. Triphenyltin has moderate to high acute toxicity, but may cause reproductive toxicity and endocrine disruption. Organic mercury compounds, such as methylmercury, were used extensively as fungicides in the past for the prevention of seed-borne diseases in grains and cereals.

RODENTICIDES

Rats and mice can cause health and economic damages to humans. Rodents are vectors for several human diseases, including plague, endemic rickettsiosis, spirochetosis, and several others; they can occasionally bite people; they can consume large quantities of postharvest stored foods, and can contaminate foods with urine, feces, and hair. Rodenticides play an important role in rodent control. To be effective, yet safe, rodenticides must satisfy several criteria: (1) the poison must be very effective in the target species once incorporated into bait in small quantity; (2) baits containing the poison must not excite bait shyness, so that the animal will continue to eat it; (3) the manner of death must be such that survivors do not become suspicious of its cause; and (4) it should be species-specific, with considerably lower toxicity to other animals. Toxicologic problems can arise from acute accidental ingestions or from suicidal and homicidal attempts. Every year, thousands of accidental ingestions of rodenticide baits by children occur, most of which resolve without serious consequences.

Fluoroacetic Acid and Its Derivatives

Sodium fluoroacetate (Compound 1080) and fluoroacetamide are white in color and odorless. Their high mammalian toxicity limits use to trained personnel. The main targets of toxicity are the central nervous system and the heart. Initial gastrointestinal symptoms are followed by severe cardiovascular effects (ventricular tachycardia, fibrillation, and hypotension), as well as CNS effects (agitation, convulsions, and coma). Use of Compound 1080 in the United States is severely restricted primarily because of toxicity to nontarget animals, such as dogs.

Anticoagulants

In addition to their use as rodenticides, coumarin derivatives, including warfarin itself, are used as anticoagulant drugs and have become a mainstay for prevention of thromboembolic disease. Coumarins antagonize the action of vitamin K in the synthesis of clotting factors (factors II, VII, IX, and X). Their specific mechanism involves inhibition of vitamin K epoxide reductase, which regenerates the reduced vitamin K necessary for sustained carboxylation and synthesis of relevant clotting factors. Human poisonings by these rodenticides are rare because they are dispersed in grain-based baits. However, there are a significant number of suicide or homicide attempts or of accidental consumption of warfarin.

FUMIGANTS

These agents are active toward insects, mites, nematodes, weed seeds, fungi, or rodents, and have in common the property of being in the gaseous form at the time they exert their pesticidal action. They can be liquids that readily vaporize (e.g., ethylene dibromide), solids that can release a toxic gas on reaction with water (e.g., phosphine released by aluminum phosphide), or gases (e.g., methyl bromide). For soil fumigation, the compound is injected directly into the soil, which is then covered with plastic sheeting, which is sealed. Compounds used as fumigants are usually nonselective, highly reactive, and cytotoxic. They provide a potential hazard from the standpoint of inhalation exposure, and to a minor degree for dermal exposure or ingestion, in case of solids or liquids.

Methyl Bromide

Methyl bromide is a broad-spectrum pesticide, used for soil fumigation, commodity treatment, and structural fumigation. Acute exposure results in respiratory, gastrointestinal, and neurologic symptoms; the latter include lethargy, headache, seizures, paresthesias, peripheral neuropathy, and ataxia, and are considered to be more relevant than other toxic effects for human risk assessment. Acute and chronic neurotoxicity studies in rats have demonstrated behavioral effects and morphological lesions, which were concentration- and time-dependent. Methyl bromide is positive in some genotoxicity tests, but it is listed in Group 3 as not classifiable as a human carcinogen. Methyl bromide is an odorless and colorless gas, but chloropicrin, with a pungent odor and eye irritation, is often used in conjunction with methyl bromide and other fumigant mixtures, to warn against potentially harmful exposures.

1,3-Dichloropropene

1,3-Dichloropropene is a soil fumigant, extensively utilized for its ability to control soil nematodes. It is an irritant, and can cause redness and necrosis of the skin. It is extensively metabolized, with the mercapturic acid conjugate being the major urinary metabolite. Data on genotoxicity are contradictory, and carcinogenicity studies in rodents have found an increase in benign liver tumors in rats but not in mice, after oral administration.

Sulfur

Elemental sulfur is an effective fumigant for the control of many plant diseases, particularly fungal diseases, and represents the most heavily used crop protection chemical in the United States. Sulfur finds its major uses in grapes and tomatoes, and can be used in organic farming. The primary health effect in humans associated with the agricultural use of elemental sulfur is dermatitis. In ruminants, excessive sulfur ingestion can cause cerebrocortical necrosis (polioencephalomalacia), possibly due to its conversion by microorganisms in the rumen to hydrogen sulfide.

BIBLIOGRAPHY

Davis FR: *Banned: A History of Pesticides and the Science of Toxicology*. New Haven, CO: Yale University Press, 2014.

Marrs TT, Ballantyne B: *Pesticide Toxicology and International Regulation*. Hoboken NJ: John Wiley & Sons, 2004.

Yu SJ: *The Toxicology and Biochemistry of Insecticides*, 2nd ed. Boca Raton, FL: CRC Press/Taylor & Francis, 2014.

QUESTIONS

1. Which of the following does NOT contribute to the environmental presence of organochlorine insecticides?
   a. high water solubility.
   b. low volatility.
   c. chemical stability.
   d. low cost.
   e. slow rate of degradation.

2. All of the following are characteristic of DDT poisoning EXCEPT:
   a. paresthesia.
   b. hypertrophy of hepatocytes.
   c. increased potassium transport across the membrane.
   d. slow closing of sodium ion channels.
   e. dizziness.

3. Anticholinesterase agents:
   a. enhance the activity of AChE.
   b. increase ACh concentration in the synaptic cleft.
   c. only target the neuromuscular junction.
   d. antagonize ACh receptors.
   e. cause decreased autonomic nervous system stimulation.

4. All of the following symptoms would be expected following anticholinesterase insecticide poisoning EXCEPT:
   a. bronchodilation.
   b. tachycardia.
   c. diarrhea.
   d. increased blood pressure.
   e. dyspnea.

5. Which of the following insecticides blocks the electron transport chain at NADH–ubiquinone reductase?
   a. nicotine.
   b. carbamate esters.
   c. nitromethylenes.
   d. pyrethroid esters.
   e. rotenoids.

6. What is the main mechanism of pyrethroid ester toxicity?
   a. blockage of neurotransmitter release.
   b. inhibition of neurotransmitter reuptake.
   c. acting as a receptor agonist.
   d. causing hyperexcitability of the membrane by interfering with sodium transport.
   e. interfering with Cl^- transport across the axonal membrane.

7. Which of the following herbicides is NOT correctly paired with its mechanism of action?
   a. glufosinate—inhibition of glutamine synthetase.
   b. paraquat—interference with protein synthesis.
   c. glyphosate—inhibition of amino acid synthesis.
   d. chlorophenoxy compounds—growth stimulants.
   e. diquat—production of superoxide anion through redox cycling.

8. Captan:
   a. is a herbicide that inhibits root growth.
   b. is an insecticide that targets the reproductive organs.
   c. is a fungicide that could cause duodenal tumors.
   d. is a herbicide that stimulates growth.
   e. is a fungicide that is a known teratogen.

9. What is a mechanism of action of nicotine?
   a. Nicotine antagonizes ACh at the neuromuscular junction.
   b. Nicotine decreases the rate of repolarization of the axonal membrane.
   c. Nicotine interferes with sodium permeability.
   d. Nicotine acts as an ACh agonist in the synapse.
   e. Nicotine inhibits the release of neurotransmitter.

10. Which of the following is the most characteristic of warfarin poisoning?
    a. diarrhea.
    b. cyanosis.
    c. decreased glucose metabolism.
    d. hematomas.
    e. seizures.

Toxic Effects of Metals

Erik J. Tokar, Windy A. Boyd, Jonathan H. Freedman, and Michael P. Waalkes

KEY POINTS

- Persons at either end of the life span, young children or elderly people, are more susceptible to toxicity from exposure to a particular level of metal than most adults.
- Metals that provoke immune reactions include mercury, gold, platinum, beryllium, chromium, and nickel.
- *Complexation* is the formation of a metal ion complex in which the metal ion is associated with a charged or uncharged electron donor, referred to as a *ligand*.

- *Chelation* occurs when bidentate ligands form ring structures that include the metal ion and the two ligand atoms attached to the metal.
- Metal–protein interactions include binding to numerous enzymes, the metallothioneins, nonspecific binding to proteins such as serum albumin or hemoglobin, and specific metal carrier proteins involved in the membrane transport of metals.

INTRODUCTION

What Is a Metal?

Metals are typically defined by physical properties of the element in the solid state. General metal properties include high reflectivity (luster), high electrical conductivity, high thermal conductivity, and mechanical ductility and strength. A toxicologically important characteristic of metals is that they may react in biological systems by losing one or more electrons to form cations.

Many metals have been reported to produce significant toxicity in humans. These include major toxic metals (e.g., lead and cadmium), essential metals (e.g., zinc and copper), medicinal metals (e.g., platinum and bismuth), minor toxic metals including metals in emerging technology (e.g., indium and uranium), toxic metalloids (e.g., arsenic and antimony), and certain nonmetallic elemental toxicants (e.g., selenium and fluoride). An overview of metal toxicology is shown in Figure 23–1.

Metals as Toxicants

Metals are unique among pollutant toxicants in that they are all naturally occurring and are already ubiquitous to some level within the human environment. Regardless of how safely metals are used in industrial processes or consumer products, some level of human exposure is inevitable. Metals differ from other toxic substances because, as elements, they are neither created nor destroyed by human endeavors. Human use of metals has influenced environmental levels of metals in air, water, soil, and food. Human use of metals can also alter the chemical form or speciation of an element and thereby impact toxic potential. As elemental species, metals are nonbiodegradable. This indestructibility combined with bioaccumulation contributes to the high concern for metals as toxicants.

Movement of Metals in the Environment

Metals are redistributed naturally in the environment by both geological and biological cycles. Rainwater dissolves rocks and ores and transports materials, including metals, to rivers and underground water (e.g., arsenic), depositing and stripping materials from adjacent soil and eventually transporting these substances to the ocean to be precipitated as sediment or taken up into forming rainwater to be relocated elsewhere. Biological cycles moving metals include biomagnification by plants and animals resulting in incorporation into food cycles. Human industry greatly enhances metal distribution in the global environment by discharge to soil, water, and air. Reports of metal intoxication are common in plants, aquatic organisms, invertebrates, fish, sea mammals, birds, and domestic animals. Not all human toxicity occurs from metals deposited in the biosphere by human activity. For example, chronic arsenic poisoning from high levels of naturally occurring inorganic arsenic in drinking water is a major health issue in many parts of the world. Endemic intoxication from excess fluoride, selenium, or thallium can all occur from natural high environmental levels.

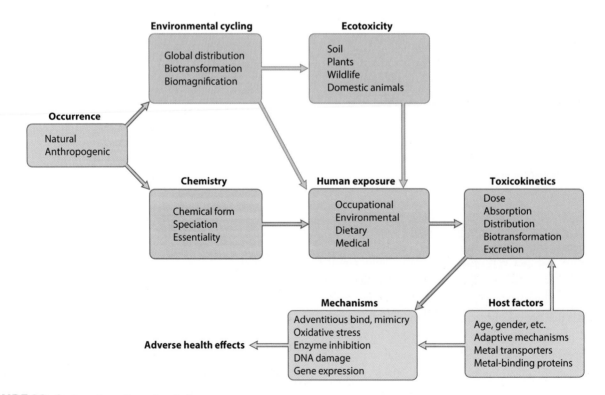

FIGURE 23-1 Overview of metal toxicology.

activity. Single cell necrosis, evident 5 to 6 h postdosing, progresses to maximal centrilobular necrosis within 24 to 48 h. Cellular regeneration is maximal 36 to 48 h postdosing. The rate and extent of tissue repair are important determinants of the ultimate outcome of liver injury.

Perturbation of intracellular calcium (Ca^{2+}) homeostasis appears to be part of CCl_4 cytotoxicity. Increased cytosolic Ca^{2+} levels may result from influx of extracellular Ca^{2+} due to plasma membrane damage and from decreased intracellular Ca^{2+} sequestration. Elevation of intracellular Ca^{2+} in hepatocytes can activate phospholipase A_2 and exacerbate membrane damage. Elevated Ca^{2+} may also be involved in alterations in calmodulin and phosphorylase activity as well as changes in nuclear protein kinase C activity. High intracellular Ca^{2+} levels activate a number of catabolic enzymes including proteases, endonucleases, and phospholipases, which kill cells via apoptosis or necrosis. Increased Ca^{2+} may stimulate the release of cytokines and eicosanoids from Kupffer cells, inducing neutrophil infiltration and hepatocellular injury. CCl_4 hepatotoxicity is obviously a complex, multifactorial process.

Chloroform

Chloroform ($CHCl_3$, trichloromethane) is used primarily in the production of the refrigerant chlorodifluoromethane (Freon 22). Measurable concentrations of $CHCl_3$ are found in municipal drinking water supplies. $CHCl_3$ is hepatotoxic and nephrotoxic. It can invoke CNS symptoms at subanesthetic concentrations similar to those of alcohol intoxication and can sensitize the myocardium to catecholamines, possibly resulting in cardiac arrhythmias.

The metabolite phosgene covalently binds hepatic and renal proteins and lipids, which damages membranes and other intracellular structures, leading to necrosis and subsequent reparative cellular proliferation that promotes tumor formation in rodents by irreversibly "fixing" spontaneously altered DNA and clonally expanding initiated cells. The expression of certain genes, including *myc* and *fos,* is altered during regenerative cell proliferation in response to $CHCl_3$-induced cytotoxicity.

Although a rodent carcinogen, ingestion of $CHCl_3$ in small increments, similar to drinking water patterns of humans, fails to produce sufficient cytotoxic metabolite(s) per unit time to overwhelm detoxification mechanisms. Currently, $CHCl_3$ is classified as a probable human carcinogen (group B2).

AROMATIC HYDROCARBONS

Benzene

Benzene is derived primarily from petroleum and is used in the synthesis of other chemicals and as an antiknock agent in unleaded gasoline. Inhalation is the primary route of exposure in industrial and in everyday settings. Cigarette smoke is the major source of benzene in the home. Smokers have benzene body burdens which are 6 to 10 times greater than those of nonsmokers. Passive smoke can be a significant source of benzene exposure to nonsmokers. Gasoline vapor emissions and auto exhaust are the other key contributors to exposures of the general populace.

The hematopoietic toxicity of chronic exposure to benzene may manifest initially as anemia, leukopenia, thrombocytopenia, or a combination of these. Bone marrow depression appears to be dose-dependent in both laboratory animals and humans. Continued exposure may result in marrow aplasia and pancytopenia, an often fatal outcome. Survivors of aplastic anemia frequently exhibit a preneoplastic state, termed *myelodysplasia,* which may progress to myelogenous leukemia.

There is strong evidence from epidemiologic studies that high-level benzene exposures result in an increased risk of acute myelogenous leukemia (AML) in humans. Evidence of increased risks of other cancers in such populations is less compelling.

Various potential mechanisms require the complementary actions of benzene and several of its metabolites for toxicity. (1) A number of benzene metabolites bind covalently to GSH, proteins, DNA, and RNA. This can result in disruption of the functional hematopoietic microenvironment by inhibition of enzymes, destruction of certain cell populations, and alteration of the growth of other cell types. Covalent binding of hydroquinones to spindle-fiber proteins will inhibit cell replication. (2) Oxidative stress contributes to benzene toxicity. As the bone marrow is rich in peroxidase activity, phenolic metabolites of benzene can be activated there to reactive quinone derivatives, which can cause DNA damage, leading to cell mutation or apoptosis. Modulation of apoptosis may lead to aberrant hematopoiesis and neoplastic progression.

Toluene

Toluene is present in paints, lacquers, thinners, cleaning agents, glues, and many other products. It is also used in the production of other chemicals. Gasoline, which contains 5% to 7% toluene (w/w), is the largest source of atmospheric emissions and exposure of the general populace. Inhalation is the primary route of exposure, though skin contact occurs frequently. Toluene is a favorite of solvent abusers, who intentionally inhale high concentrations of the VOC.

Toluene is well absorbed from the lungs and GI tract. It rapidly accumulates in the brain, and subsequently, is deposited in other tissues according to their lipid content, with adipose tissue attaining the highest levels. Toluene is well metabolized, but a portion is exhaled unchanged.

The CNS is the primary target organ of toluene and other alkylbenzenes. Manifestations of exposure range from slight dizziness and headache to unconsciousness, respiratory depression, and death. Occupational inhalation exposure guidelines are established to prevent significant decrements in psychomotor functions. Acute encephalopathic effects are rapidly reversible on cessation of exposure. Subtle neurologic effects have been reported in some groups of occupationally exposed individuals. Severe neurotoxicity is sometimes diagnosed in persons who have abused toluene for a prolonged period. Clinical signs include abnormal electroencephalographic (EEG) activity, tremors, and nystagmus, as well as impaired hearing, vision, and speech. Magnetic resonance imaging has revealed permanent changes in brain structure, which correspond to the degree of brain dysfunction. These changes include ventricular enlargement, cerebral atrophy, and white matter hyperintensity, a characteristic profile termed *toluene leukoencephalopathy*.

Xylenes and Ethylbenzene

Large numbers of people are exposed to xylenes and ethylbenzene occupationally and environmentally. Xylenes and ethylbenzene, like benzene and toluene, are major components of gasoline and fuel oil. The primary uses of xylenes industrially are as solvents and synthetic intermediates. Most of the aromatics released into the environment evaporate into the atmosphere.

Similar to toluene, xylenes and other aromatic solvents are well absorbed from the lungs and GI tract, distributed to tissues according to tissue blood flow and lipophilicity, exhaled to some extent, well metabolized by hepatic P450s, and largely excreted as urinary metabolites. Acute lethality of hydrocarbons (i.e., CNS depression) varies directly with lipophilicity. There is limited evidence that chronic occupational exposure to xylenes is associated with residual neurologic effects.

Xylenes and ethylbenzene have limited capacity to adversely affect organs other than the CNS. Mild, transient liver and/or kidney toxicity has been reported occasionally in humans exposed to high vapor concentrations of xylenes. The majority of alkylbenzenes do not appear to be genotoxic or carcinogenic. Ethylbenzene and styrene are known animal carcinogens, but there are limited human data.

ALCOHOLS

Ethanol

Many humans experience greater exposure to ethanol (ethyl alcohol and alcohol) than to any other solvent. Ethyl alcohol is used as an additive in gasoline, as a solvent in industry, in many household products and pharmaceuticals including hand sanitizers, and in intoxicating beverages. Frank toxic effects are less important occupationally than injuries resulting from psychomotor impairment. Driving under the influence of alcohol is the major cause of fatal auto accidents. Blood alcohol level and the time necessary to achieve it are controlled largely by the rapidity and extent of ethanol consumption. Ethanol is distributed in body water and to some degree in adipose tissue. The alcohol is eliminated by urinary excretion, exhalation, and metabolism. The blood level in an average adult decreases by ~15 to 20 mg/dL per hour. Thus, a person with a blood alcohol level of 120 mg/dL would require 6 to 8 h to reach negligible levels.

Ethanol is metabolized to acetaldehyde by three enzymes: (1) alcohol dehydrogenase (ADH) catalyzes oxidation of most of the ethanol to acetaldehyde, which is rapidly oxidized by acetaldehyde dehydrogenase (ALDH) to acetate; (2) catalase,

utilizing H_2O_2 supplied by the actions of NADPH oxidase and xanthine oxidase, will normally account for more than 10% of ethanol metabolism; (3) CYP2E1, which is the principal isoform of the hepatic microsomal ethanol oxidizing system (MEOS).

ALDH activity is usually sufficiently high to metabolize large amounts of acetaldehyde to acetate. Caucasians, blacks, and Asians have varying percentages of different ALDH isozymes, which impact the efficiency of acetaldehyde metabolism. Some 50% of Asians have inactive ALDH, and these persons may experience flushing, headache, nausea, vomiting, tachycardia, and hyperventilation on ingestion of ethanol. Whereas this syndrome offers protection against developing alcoholism, it increases the risk of acetaldehyde-related cancers of the esophagus, stomach, colon, lung, head, and neck.

Gender differences in responses to ethanol are well recognized. Females exhibit slightly higher blood ethanol levels than men following ingestion of equivalent doses. This phenomenon is due in part to more extensive ADH-catalyzed metabolism of ethanol by the gastric mucosa of males and to the smaller volume of distribution in women for relatively polar solvents such as alcohols. Also, women are more susceptible to alcohol-induced hepatitis and cirrhosis.

Fetal alcohol syndrome (FAS) is the most common preventable cause of mental retardation. Diagnostic criteria for FAS include (1) heavy maternal alcohol consumption during gestation; (2) pre and postnatal growth retardation; (3) craniofacial malformations including microcephaly; and (4) mental retardation. Less complete manifestations of gestational ethanol exposure are referred to as fetal alcohol spectrum disorder (FASD). Potential mechanisms causing FASD include (1) simple oxidative stress in fetal tissues, (2) alteration of neurotransmitter-gated ion channels such as the NMDA receptor, (3) alterations in the regulation of gene expression with reduced retinoic acid signaling or variant DNA methylation, (4) interference with mitogenic and growth factor responses involved in neural stem cell proliferation, (5) disturbances in molecules that mediate cell–cell interactions, and (6) derangements of glial proliferation, differentiation, and function. Overconsumption during all three trimesters of pregnancy can result in particular manifestations depending on the period of gestation during which insult occurs.

Human CYP2E1 is effective in production of reactive oxygen intermediates from ethanol that cause lipid peroxidation. Also, ethanol induces the release of endotoxin from gram-negative bacteria in the gut. The endotoxin is taken up by Kupffer cells, causing the release of inflammatory mediators, which are cytotoxic to hepatocytes and chemoattractants for neutrophils.

Alcohol-induced tissue damage results from both nutritional disturbances and direct toxic effects. Malabsorption of thiamine, diminished enterohepatic circulation of folate, degradation of pyridoxal phosphate, and disturbances in the metabolism of vitamins A and D can occur. Prostaglandins released from endotoxin-activated Kupffer cells may be responsible for a hypermetabolic state in the liver. With the increase in oxygen demand, the viability of centrilobular hepatocytes would be most compromised due to their relatively poor oxygen supply. Metabolism of ethanol via ADH and ALDH results in a shift in the redox state of the cell. The resulting hyperlacticacidemia, hyperlipidemia, hyperuricemia, and hyperglycemia lead to increased steatosis and collagen synthesis.

Alcoholism can result in damage of extrahepatic tissues. Alcoholic cardiomyopathy is a complex process that may result from decreased synthesis of cardiac contractile proteins, attack of oxygen radicals, increases in endoplasmic reticulum Ca^{2+}-ATPase, and antibody response to acetaldehyde–protein adducts. Heavy drinking appears to deplete antioxidants and increases the risk of both hemorrhagic and ischemic strokes. The brain and pancreas may be adversely affected in alcoholics.

The associations between alcohol and cancers came primarily from epidemiologic case–control and cohort studies. Ethanol and smoking act synergistically to cause oral, pharyngeal, and laryngeal cancers. It is generally believed that alcohol induces liver cancer by causing cirrhosis or other liver damage and/or by enhancing the bioactivation of carcinogens.

Chronic ethanol consumption may promote carcinogenesis by (1) production of acetaldehyde, a weak mutagen and carcinogen; (2) induction of CYP2E1 with conversion of procarcinogens to carcinogens; (3) depletion of SAM and, consequently, global DNA hypomethylation; (4) increased production of inhibitory guanine nucleotide regulatory proteins and components of extracellular signal-regulated kinase-mitogen-activated protein kinase signaling; (5) accumulation of iron and associated oxidative stress; (6) inactivation of the tumor suppressor gene *BRCA1* and increased estrogen responsiveness (primarily in the breast); and (7) impairment of retinoic acid metabolism.

Methanol

Methanol (methyl alcohol and wood alcohol) is found in a host of consumer products including windshield washer fluid, carburetor cleaners, and copy machine toner, and is used in the manufacture of formaldehyde and methyl *tert*-butyl ether. Serious methanol toxicity is most commonly associated with ingestion. Acute methanol poisoning in humans is characterized by an asymptomatic period of 12 to 24 h followed by formic acidemia, ocular toxicity, coma, and in extreme cases death. Visual disturbances develop between 18 and 48 h after ingestion and range from mild photophobia and blurred vision to markedly reduced visual acuity and complete blindness.

The target of methanol within the eye is the retina, specifically the optic disk and optic nerve. Müller cells, rod, and cone cells are altered functionally and structurally, because cytochrome *c* oxidase activity in mitochondria is inhibited, resulting in a reduction in ATP.

Though metabolized in liver, intraretinal conversion of methanol to formaldehyde and formate is critical. Metabolism of formate to CO_2 then occurs via a two-step, tetrahydrofolate (THF)-dependent pathway. Susceptibility to methanol toxicity is dependent on the relative rate of formate clearance. Conversion of formate to CO_2 is slower in primates than in rodents. In fact, formate acts as a direct ocular toxin and the acidotic state potentiates formate toxicity because the inhibition of cytochrome oxidase increases as pH decreases.

GLYCOLS

Ethylene Glycol

Ethylene glycol (EG) (1,2-dihydroxyethane) is a major constituent of antifreeze, deicers, hydraulic fluids, drying agents, and inks, and is used to make plastics and polyester fibers. The most important routes of exposure are dermal and accidental or intentional ingestion. EG is rapidly degraded in environmental media.

Three clinical stages of acute poisoning entail (1) a period of inebriation, the duration and degree depending on dose; (2) the cardiopulmonary stage 12 to 24 h after exposure, characterized by tachycardia and tachypnea, which may progress to cardiac failure and pulmonary edema; and (3) the renal toxicity stage 24 to 72 h postexposure. Metabolic acidosis can progress in severity during stages 2 and 3.

Absorption from the GI tract of rodents is very rapid and virtually complete. Dermal absorption in humans appears to be less extensive. EG is distributed throughout the total body water. As illustrated in Figure 24–2, EG is metabolized by NAD^+-dependent ADH to glycolaldehyde and on to glycolic acid. Glycolic acid is oxidized to glyoxylic acid by glycolic acid oxidase and lactic dehydrogenase. Glyoxylic acid may be converted to formate and CO_2, or oxidized by glyoxylic acid oxidase to oxalic acid. Metabolic acidosis in humans appears to be due to accumulation of glycolic acid. Hypocalcemia can result from calcium chelation by oxalic acid to form calcium oxalate crystals. Deposition of these crystals in tubules of the kidney and small blood vessels in the brain is associated with damage of these organs. Acute renal failure may follow. Additionally, hippuric acid crystals and direct cytotoxicity by other metabolites may act as damaging agents to the kidney in EG exposure. EG appears to have limited chronic toxicity potential, exhibits no evidence of carcinogenicity, and does not appear to be a reproductive toxicant.

Propylene Glycol

Propylene glycol (PG) is used as an intermediate in the synthesis of polyester fibers and resins, as a component of automotive antifreeze/coolants, and as a deicing fluid for aircraft. As PG is "generally recognized as safe" by the FDA, it is a constituent of many cosmetics and processed foods. Furthermore, it serves as a solvent/diluent for a substantial number of oral, dermal, and intravenous drug preparations. The most important routes of exposure are ingesting and dermal contact. PG is readily metabolized by ADH to lactaldehyde, which is then oxidized by aldehyde dehydrogenase to lactate. Excessive lactate is

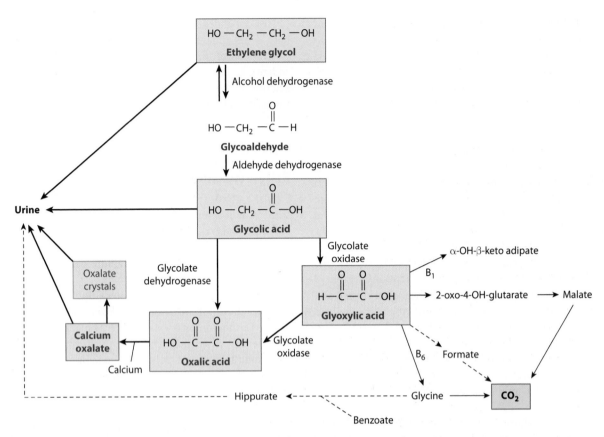

FIGURE 24-2 Metabolic scheme for ethylene glycol in animals. Key metabolites that have been observed in vivo are highlighted in boxes. Dashed lines are theoretical pathways that have not been verified in vivo or in vitro. (Adapted with permission from Corley RA, Bartels MJ, Carney EW, et al.: Development of a physiologically based pharmacokinetic model for ethylene glycol and its metabolite, glycolic acid, in rats and humans. *Toxicol Sci*, 2005 May;85(1):476–490.)

primarily responsible for the acidosis. PG has a very low order of acute and chronic toxicity.

GLYCOL ETHERS

The glycol ethers include EG monomethyl ether, also called 2-methoxyethanol (2-ME; **CH3—O**—CH_2—CH_2—**OH**), EG dimethyl ether (**CH3—O**—CH_2—CH_2—**O—CH3**), 2-butoxyethanol (2-BE; **CH3—CH2—CH2—CH2—O**—CH_2—CH_2—**OH**), and 2-ME acetate (**CH3—CO—O**—CH_2—CH_2—**O—CH3**). These solvents undergo rapid ester hydrolysis in vivo, and exhibit the same toxicity profile as unesterified glycols. The glycol ethers are metabolized to alkoxyacetic acids, which are regarded as the ultimate toxicants. Their acetaldehyde precursors have also been implicated.

Like glycol ether metabolism, glycol ether toxicity varies with chemical structure. With increasing alkyl chain length, reproductive and developmental toxicity decrease, whereas hematotoxicity increases.

Reproductive Toxicity

Epidemiologic studies have reported associations between glycol ether exposure and increased risk for spontaneous abortion, menstrual disturbances, and subfertility among women employed in the semiconductor industry. Reversible spermatotoxicity in males has been described for those exposed to glycol ethers. Typical responses include testicular and seminiferous tubule atrophy, abnormal sperm head morphology, necrotic spermatocytes, decreased sperm motility and count, and infertility.

Developmental Toxicity

Developmental toxicity in rodents includes a variety of minor skeletal variations, hydrocephalus, exencephaly, cardiovascular malformations, dilatation of the renal pelvis, craniofacial malformations, and digit malformations. There are significant associations for glycol ether exposure inducing cleft lip.

Hematotoxicity

Some glycol ethers are hemolytic to red blood cells. Typically, the osmotic balance of the cells is disrupted, they imbibe water and swell, their ATP concentration decreases, and hemolysis occurs. Humans are less susceptible than rodents to glycol ether–induced erythrocyte deformity and hemolysis.

AUTOMOTIVE GASOLINE AND ADDITIVES

Gasoline is a mixture of hundreds of hydrocarbons predominantly in the range of C_4 to C_{12}. Because its composition varies with the crude oil from which it is refined, the refining process, and the use of specific additives, generalizations regarding the toxicity of gasoline must be made carefully. Experiments conducted with fully vaporized gasoline may not be predictive of actual risk, because humans are exposed primarily to the more volatile components in the range of C_4 to C_5, which are generally less toxic than higher molecular-weight fractions.

The most extreme exposures occur to those intentionally sniffing gasoline for its euphoric effects. This dangerous habit can cause acute and chronic encephalopathies that are expressed as both motor and cognitive impairment. Ingestion of gasoline during siphoning events is typically followed by a burning sensation in the mouth and pharynx, as well as nausea, vomiting, and diarrhea resulting from GI irritation. Gasoline aspirated into the lungs may produce pulmonary epithelial damage, edema, and pneumonitis.

Oxygenated gasoline contains additives that boost its octane quality, enhance combustion, and reduce exhaust emissions. Benzene and 1,3-butadiene are classified as known or probable human carcinogens. The co-exposure of ethanol and gasoline shows additive and possibly synergistic toxic effects on growth, neurochemistry, and histopathology of the adrenal gland and respiratory tract. No significant epidemiologic association exists between methyl *tertiary*-butyl ether (MTBE) exposure and the acute symptoms commonly attributed to MTBE, including headache; eye, nose, and throat irritation; cough; nausea; dizziness; and disorientation. Because three MTBE animal cancer bioassays indicate kidney and testicular tumors in male rats and liver adenomas, leukemia, and lymphoma in female rats, MTBE is classified as a possible human carcinogen (group C).

CARBON DISULFIDE

The major uses of CS_2 are in the production of rayon fiber, cellophane, and CCl_4, and as a solubilizer for waxes and oils. Human exposure is predominantly occupational. Two distinct metabolic pathways for CS_2 exist: (1) the direct interaction of CS_2 with free amine and sulfhydryl groups of amino acids and polypeptides to form dithiocarbamates and trithiocarbonates; and (2) microsomal metabolism of CS_2 to reactive sulfur intermediates capable of covalently binding tissue macromolecules. The conjugation of CS_2 with sulfhydryls of cysteine or GSH results in the formation of 2-thiothiazolidine-4-carboxylic acid (TTCA), which is excreted in urine and has been frequently used as a biomarker of CS_2 exposure.

CS_2 is capable of targeting multiple organ systems including the cardiovascular system, CNS and PNS, male and female fertility, and eyes (retinal angiopathy and impairment of color vision). CS_2 toxicity requires frequent and prolonged exposures in occupational settings. The most common neurotoxic effect is a distal sensorimotor neuropathy that preferentially affects long axons in the PNS and CNS (particularly the ascending and descending tracks of the spinal cord and the visual pathways). Encephalopathy with motor and cognitive impairment has also been reported following chronic, low-level exposure to CS_2. The following clinical syndromes have been associated with CS_2: (1) acute and chronic encephalopathy (often with prominent psychiatric manifestations), (2) polyneuropathy (both peripheral and cranial), (3) Parkinsonism, and (4) asymptomatic CNS and PNS dysfunction. Pathological changes occur in both the CNS and PNS. CNS pathology consists of neuronal degeneration throughout the cerebral hemispheres, with maximal diffuse involvement in the frontal regions. Cell loss is also noted in the globus pallidus, putamen, and cerebellar cortex, with loss of Purkinje cells. Vascular abnormalities with endothelial proliferation of arterioles may be seen, sometimes associated with focal necrosis or demyelination. PNS changes consist primarily of myelin swelling and fragmentation and large focal axonal swellings, characteristic of distal axonopathy.

BIBLIOGRAPHY

Karch SB, Drummer O: *Karch's Pathology of Drug Abuse*. 4th ed. Boca Raton, FL: CRC Press, 2009.

Patnaik P: *A Comprehensive Guide to the Hazardous Properties of Chemical Substances*. 3rd ed. Hoboken, NJ: John Wiley & Sons, 2007.

QUESTIONS

1. Which of the following statements regarding solvents is FALSE?
   a. Solvents can be absorbed from the GI tract and through the skin.
   b. Equilibration of absorbed solvents/vapors occurs most quickly in the lungs.
   c. Solvents are small molecules that lack charge.
   d. Volatility of solvents increases with molecular weight.
   e. Most solvents are refined from petroleum.

2. What is the route in which most solvents enter the environment?
   a. chemical spills.
   b. contamination of drinking water.
   c. evaporation.
   d. improper waste disposal.
   e. wind.

3. All of the following statements are true EXCEPT:
   a. Most solvents can pass freely through membranes by diffusion.
   b. A solvent's lipophilicity is important in determining its rate of dermal absorption.
   c. Hydrophilic solvents have a relatively low blood:air partition coefficient.
   d. Biotransformation of a lipophilic solvent can result in the production of a mutagenic compound.
   e. Hepatic first-pass metabolism determines the amount of solvent absorbed in the GI tract.

4. Which of the following statements regarding age solvent toxicity is TRUE?
   a. GI absorption is greater in adults than it is in children.
   b. Polar solvents reach higher blood levels in the elderly than they do in children.
   c. Children are always more susceptible to solvent toxicity than are adults.
   d. Increased alveolar ventilation increases uptake of lipid-soluble solvents to a greater extent than water-soluble solvents.
   e. Increased body fat percentage increases clearance of solvent chemicals.

5. Huffing gasoline can result in which of the following serious health problems?
   a. renal failure.
   b. pneumothorax.
   c. Hodgkin's disease.
   d. encephalopathy.
   e. thrombocytopenia.

6. Which of the following statements regarding benzene is FALSE?
   a. High-level exposure to benzene could result in acute myelogenous leukemia (AML).
   b. Gasoline vapor emissions and auto exhaust are the two main contributors to benzene inhalation.
   c. Benzene is used as an ingredient in unleaded gasoline.
   d. Benzene metabolites covalently bind DNA, RNA, and proteins and interfere with their normal functioning within the cell.
   e. Reactive oxygen species can be derived from benzene.

7. Which of the following is NOT a criterion for fetal alcohol syndrome diagnosis?
   a. maternal alcohol consumption during gestation.
   b. pre and postnatal growth retardation.
   c. microcephaly.
   d. ocular toxicity.
   e. mental retardation.

8. Which of the following is NOT an important enzyme in ethanol metabolism?
   a. alcohol dehydrogenase.
   b. formaldehyde dehydrogenase.
   c. CYP2E1.
   d. catalase.
   e. acetaldehyde dehydrogenase.

9. Which of the following is NOT associated with glycol ether toxicity?
   a. irreversible spermatotoxicity.
   b. craniofacial malformations.
   c. hematotoxicity.
   d. seminiferous tubule atrophy.
   e. cleft lip.

10. Which of the following statements regarding chlorinated hydrocarbons is FALSE?
    a. Toxicities of trichloroethylene (TCE) are mediated mostly by reactive metabolites, not the parent compound.
    b. Glutathione conjugation is an important metabolic step of both trichloroethylene (TCE) and perchloroethylene (PERC).
    c. Many chlorinated hydrocarbons are used as degreasing agents.
    d. Chloroform interferes with intracellular calcium homeostasis.
    e. Carbon tetrachloride causes hepatocellular and kidney toxicity.

Toxic Effects of Radiation and Radioactive Materials

David G. Hoel

KEY POINTS

- The four main types of radiation are due to alpha particles, electrons (negatively charged beta particles or positively charged positrons), gamma-rays, and X-rays.

- Alpha particles are helium nuclei (consisting of two protons and two neutrons), with a charge of +2, that are ejected from the nucleus of an atom.

- Beta particle decay occurs when a neutron in the nucleus of an element is effectively transformed into a proton and an electron, which is ejected.

- Gamma-ray emission occurs in combination with alpha, beta, or positron emission or electron capture. Whenever the ejected particle does not utilize all the available energy for decay, the excess energy is released by the nucleus as photon or gamma-ray emission coincident with the ejection of the particle.

- The Compton Effect occurs when a photon scatters at a small angle from its original path with reduced energy because part of the photon energy is transferred to an electron.

- Ionizing radiation loses energy when passing through matter by producing ion pairs (an electron and a positively charged atom residue).

- Radiation may deposit energy directly in DNA (direct effect) or may ionize other molecules closely associated with DNA, hydrogen, or oxygen, to form free radicals that can damage DNA (indirect effect).

INTRODUCTION

Ionizing radiations such as γ-rays and X-rays are radiations that have sufficient energy to displace electrons from molecules. These freed electrons then have the capability of damaging other molecules and, in particular, DNA. Atoms of the DNA target may be directly ionized or indirectly affected by the creation of a free radical that can interact with the DNA molecule. In particular, the hydroxyl radical is predominant in DNA damage. Thus, the potential health effects of low levels of radiation are important to understand in order to be able to quantify their effects. Cancer has been the major adverse health effect of ionizing radiation. National Council on Radiation Protection (NCRP) Report 160 gives a summary breakdown of exposure sources in Figure 25–1.

RADIATION BACKGROUND

Types of Ionizing Radiation

When ionizing radiation passes through matter, it has the energy to ionize atoms so that one or more of its electrons can be dislodged and chemical bonds broken. Ionizing radiation is of two types: particulate and electromagnetic waves. Particulate

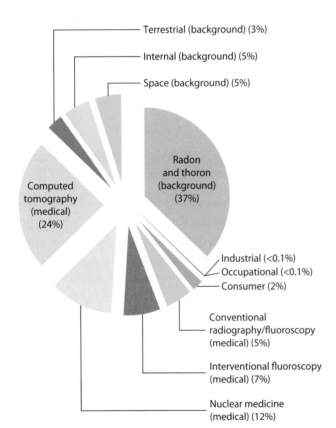

FIGURE 25–1 **Percent contribution of total effective dose to individuals** (Reproduced with permission from NCRP Report No. 160. *Ionizing Radiation Exposure of the Population of the United States.* Bethesda, MD: National Council on Radiation Protection and Measurements; 2009. http://NCRPpublications.org).

radiation may either be electrically charged (α, β, proton) or have no charge (neutron). Ionizing electromagnetic radiation (photons) in the form of X-rays or γ-rays has considerably more energy than nonionizing radiation, such as ultraviolet and visible light. Radionuclides (i.e., radioactive atoms), being unstable, release both electromagnetic and particulate radiation during their radioactive decay. The radionuclides decay into either stable elements or through a decay chain of successive radionuclides called decay daughters. The types of radiation emitted, its rate of decay, and the energies of the released radiation are unique to each type of radionuclide. For example, the uranium decay series is illustrated in Figure 25–2, with specific details provided in Table 25–1.

The rate of energy dissipation by a single event is referred to as linear energy transfer (LET). The LET of a charged particle is the average energy lost due to interactions per unit length of its trajectory given as kiloelectron volts per micrometer (keV/μm).

X-rays, γ-rays, and β particles of similar energies produce sparse ionization tracks and are classified as low-LET radiation. Particulate radiation (e.g., neutrons and α particles) causes interactions with large amounts of energy being dissipated within short distances. α-Particles (helium nucleus), which are released from the nucleus of some radionuclides, are slow-moving with a positive charge. Although they cannot penetrate a piece of paper or skin, they are of concern if ingested or inhaled. The most recognized example is the lung cancer risk from the inhalation of radon (Rn 222) and its daughter products.

Relative Biologic Effectiveness and Quality Factors

The various types of ionizing radiation have similar biologic effects that occur because of the ionization of molecules. However, without knowing the type of radiation, one cannot specify how much radiation is needed to produce a specific biologic effect. This is because a given absorbed dose (energy per unit mass) of X-rays does not have the same biologic effect as an identical dose of neutrons. The relative effectiveness of different types of radiation in producing biologic changes depends on deposition of energy. The relative biologic effectiveness is numerically equal to the inverse of the ratio of absorbed doses of the two radiations required to produce equal biologic effects. The difficulty is that the relative biologic effectiveness may differ depending on the biologic end point and it may also be dose-dependent.

Units of Radiation Activity and Dose

The basic unit of radiation activity is the Becquerel (Bq), which is nuclear disintegrations per second. The older unit of activity is the Curie (Ci), which corresponds to the number of disintegrations in 1 s from 1 g of radium 226 or 1 Ci = 3.7×10^{10} decays per second; thus, 1 Bq = 2.7×10^{-11} Ci. The EPA continues to use the old unit of activity with regard to radon.

The basic unit of dose is the Gray (Gy), which is the amount of energy released in a given mass of tissue. One Gray is defined as 1 joule of energy released in 1 kg of tissue. The other common

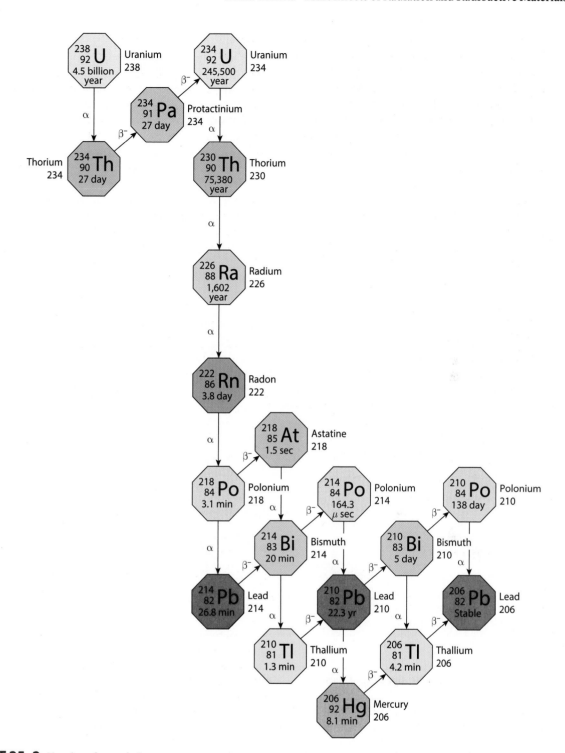

FIGURE 25–2 Uranium decay chain.

measure is the Sievert (Sv), which is a dose equivalent; that is, the dose in Gray multiplied by the appropriate quality factor.

RADIOBIOLOGY

Radiation biology has made significant progress in our understanding of radiation effects at low doses. Currently radiation cancer risk extrapolations make two assumptions: namely that the basic mode of action is linearly related to dose and that the individual cell is the unit of risk. However, effects occurring in nontargeted cells such as with induced genomic instability and bystander effects suggest that responses can occur nonuniformly over time at the tissue level. Following irradiation, various protective cellular processes occur that depend on the degree of damage and the tissue type. These mechanisms include DNA repair, intracellular metabolic oxidation/reduction reactions,

TABLE 25–1 Radioisotopes in the uranium decay series.

Nuclide	Decay Mode	Half-Life (a = Year)	Energy Released, MₑV	Product of Decay
^{238}U	α	4.468×10^9 a	4.270	^{234}Th
^{234}Th	β⁻	24.10 days	0.273	^{234m}Pa
^{234m}Pa	β− 99.84% IT 0.16%	1.16 min	2.271 0.074	^{234}U ^{234}Pa
^{234}Pa	β⁻	6.70 h	2.197	^{234}U
^{234}U	α	245 500 a	4.859	^{230}Th
^{230}Th	α	75 380 a	4.770	^{226}Ra
^{226}Ra	α	1602 a	4.871	^{222}Rn
^{222}Rn	α	3.8235 days	5.590	^{218}Po
^{218}Po	α 99.98% β⁻ 0.02%	3.10 min	6.115 0.265	^{214}Pb ^{218}At
^{218}At	α 99.90% β⁻ 0.10%	1.5 s	6.874 2.883	^{214}Bi ^{218}Rn
^{218}Rn	α	35 ms	7.263	^{214}Po
^{214}Pb	β⁻	26.8 min	1.024	^{214}Bi
^{214}Bi	β⁻ 99.98% α 0.02%	19.9 min	3.272 5.617	^{214}Po ^{210}Tl
^{214}Po	α	0.1643 ms	7.883	^{210}Pb
^{210}Tl	β⁻	1.30 min	5.484	^{210}Pb
^{210}Pb	β⁻	22.3 a	0.064	^{210}Bi
^{210}Bi	β⁻ 99.99987% α 0.00013%	5.013 days	1.426 5.982	^{210}Po ^{206}Tl
^{210}Po	α	138.376 days	5.407	^{206}Pb
^{206}Tl	β⁻	4.199 min	1.533	^{206}Pb
^{206}Pb	—	Stable	—	—

cell cycle checkpoint controls, cellular signaling, senescence, and apoptosis.

A study reviewed in detail the effects of DNA damage after exposure to low doses of ionizing radiation. After an exposure to 5 mGy of low-LET radiation (average background per year), each cell nucleus is on average hit by one electron, resulting in 5 to 10 damaged bases, 2.5 to 5 single-strand breaks and 0.25 double-strand breaks.

Nontargeted Radiation Effects

Exposure to ionizing radiation can result in direct damage to the irradiated cells as well as producing effects in cells that were not irradiated (bystander effects). These nontargeted effects can occur in the nonirradiated neighbors of irradiated cells and at sites distant from the irradiated cells. Effects can also be observed in the progeny of an irradiated cell (genomic instability). Both targeted and nontargeted effects can result in DNA mutations, gene amplifications, chromosomal rearrangements, carcinogenesis, and cell death.

Bystander Effects—Radiation-induced bystander effects are those in which cells that have not been directly exposed to ionizing radiation react as though they have been exposed by receiving a biochemical signal from a radiation-exposed cell. That is, they show chromosomal instability and other abnormalities, or die. For high-LET radiation a bystander effect has been shown for inducing cell lethality, chromosome aberrations, sister-chromatid exchanges, mutations, genomic instability, signal transduction pathways, and in vitro transformation. For low-LET radiation, the bystander effect has been limited to cell lethality and lethal mutations.

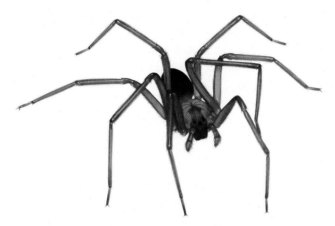

FIGURE 26–9 *Loxosceles reclusa* (male brown recluse spider) with the violin pattern on the dorsal cephalothorax.

The bite of this spider produces about the same degree of pain as does the sting of an ant, but sometimes the patient may be unaware of the bite. Pruritis over the area often occurs with reddening and elevated skin temperature at the lesion. With significant envenomations, hemorrhages may develop throughout the area, lymphadenopathy is common, and necrosis of the surrounding tissue may be visualized. Systemic symptoms and signs include fever, malaise, stomach cramps, nausea and vomiting, jaundice, spleen enlargement, hemolysis, hematuria, and thrombocytopenia. Fatal cases, while rare, usually are preceded by intravascular hemolysis, hemolytic anemia, thrombocytopenia, hemoglobinuria, and renal failure.

***Steatoda* Species—**These spiders are variously known as the false black widow, combfooted, cobweb, or cupboard spiders. The venom of *Steatoda paykulliana* stimulates the release of transmitter substances similar to *Latrodectus*. The venom is said to form ionic channels that are permeable for bivalent and monovalent cations, and the duration of time in the open state depends on the membrane potential. *S. paykulliana* venom induces strong motor unrest, clonic cramps, exhaustion, ataxia, and then paralysis.

***Cheiracanthium* Species (Running Spiders)—** *Cheiracanthium punctorium, C. inclusum, C. mildei, C. diversum,* and *C. japonicum* are often implicated in envenomations. *Cheiracanthium* tends to be tenacious and sometimes must be removed from the bite area. For that reason there is a high degree of identification following the bite of these spiders. The most toxic venom fraction is said to be a protein of 60 kDa, and the venom is high in norepinephrine and serotonin.

The patient usually describes the bite as sharp and painful. A reddened wheal with a hyperemic border develops. Small petechiae may appear near the center of the wheal. Skin temperature over the lesion is often elevated, but body temperature is usually normal. Lymphadenitis and lymphadenopathy may develop. *C. japonicum* produces more severe manifestations,

including severe local pain, nausea and vomiting, headache, chest discomfort, severe pruritus, and shock.

Theraphosidae Species (Tarantulas)—True tarantulas are members of the family Theraphosidae. Tarantulas are predators and they feed on various vertebrate and invertebrate preys that are captured after envenomation with venoms that act rapidly and irreversibly on the central and peripheral nervous systems. In humans, reported bites elicit mild to severe local pain, strong itching, and tenderness that may last for several hours. Edema, erythema, joint stiffness, swollen limbs, burning feelings, and cramps are common.

Theraphosid spiders contain several toxins that are being evaluated for development as antiarrhythmic or as antinociceptive drugs. In particular, *Grammostola* mechanotoxin 4 from *Grammostola spatulata* has considerable promise as an antiarrhythmic. Protoxin I and II from *Thrixopelma pruriens* have promise as analgesics because they inhibit the tetrodotoxin-resistant sodium channels.

Ticks

Tick paralysis is caused by the saliva of certain ticks of the families Ixodidae, Argasidae, and Nuttalliellidae. Ticks are known to transmit the organisms causing Lyme disease, Rocky Mountain spotted fever, babesiosis, leptospirosis, Q fever, ehrlichiosis, typhus, tick-borne encephalitis, and others.

Tick saliva contains a number of active constituents. For example, saliva from *Ixodes scapularis* contains apyrase (ATP-diphosphohydrolase), which hydrolyzes ADP that is released at the bite site thereby inhibiting ADP-induced platelet aggregation; kininase (ACE-like protein or angiotensin-converting enzyme-like protein), which hydrolyzes circulating kinins and reduces the host inflammatory response; glutathione peroxidase; serine protease inhibitors, which inhibit coagulation enzymes; an anti-complement protein that inhibits an enzyme in the alternative pathway for complement; an amine-binding protein that binds serotonin, histamine, and other biogenic amines.

As tick bites are often not felt, the first evidence of envenomation may not appear until several days later, when small macules 3 to 4 mm in diameter develop that are surrounded by erythema and swelling. The patient often complains of difficulty with gait, followed by paresis and eventually locomotor paresis and paralysis. Problems in speech and respiration may ensue and lead to respiratory paralysis if the tick is not removed. The saliva of *Ixodes holocyclus* has yielded a peptide holocyclotoxin-1 that may cause paralysis.

CHILOPODA (CENTIPEDES)

In the United States, the prevalent biting genus is a *Scolopendra* species. The venom is concentrated within the intracellular granules, discharged into vacuoles of the cytoplasm of the secretory cells, and moved by exocytosis into the lumen of the gland; from thence ducts carry the venom to the jaws.

Centipede venoms contain high-molecular-weight proteins, proteinases, esterases, 5-hydroxytryptamine, histamine, lipids, and polysaccharides. The bite produces sharp pain, immediate bleeding, redness, and swelling. Localized tissue changes and necrosis have been reported, and severe envenomations may cause nausea and vomiting, changes in heart rate, vertigo, and headache.

DIPLOPODA (MILLIPEDES)

The repellent secretions expelled from the sides of their bodies contain a toxin of benzoquinone derivatives plus a variety of complex substances such as iodine and hydrocyanic acid, which the animal makes use of to produce hydrogen cyanide. Some species can spray these defensive secretions. The lesions produced by millipedes consist of a burning or prickling sensation and development of a yellowish or brown-purple lesion; subsequently, a blister containing serosanguinous fluid forms, which may rupture. Eye contact can cause acute conjunctivitis, periorbital edema, keratosis, and much pain; such an injury must be treated immediately.

INSECTA

Heteroptera (True Bugs)

The clinically most important of the true bugs are the Reduviidae (the reduviids): the kissing bug, assassin bug, wheel bug, or cone-nose bug of the genus *Triatoma*. The venom of these bugs appears to have apyrase activity and to lack 5-nucleotidase, inorganic pyrophosphatase, phosphatase, and adenylate kinase activities, but it is fairly rich in protease properties. It inhibits collagen-induced platelet aggregation. Three peptides isolated from the saliva are calcium channel inhibitors. The bites of *Triatoma* species are painful and give rise to erythema, pruritus, increased temperature in the bitten part, localized swelling, and—in those allergic to the saliva—systemic reactions such as nausea and vomiting and angioedema.

Hymenoptera (Ants, Bees, Wasps, and Hornets)

Formicidae (Ants)—Most ants have stings, but those that lack them can spray a defensive secretion from the tip of the gaster, which is often placed in the wound of the bite. Clinically important stinging ants are the harvesting ants (*Pagonomyrmex*), fire ants (*Solenopsis*), and little fire ants (*Ochetomyrmex*).

The venoms of the ants vary considerably. Formicinae ant venom contains about 60% formic acid. Fire ant venoms are rich in alkaloids. The sting of the fire ant gives rise to a painful burning sensation, after which a wheal and localized erythema develop, forming a vesicle that becomes purulent and turns into a pustle. The pustule may then break down, become a crust, or become a fibrotic nodule. In multiple stings there may be nausea, vomiting, vertigo, increased perspiration, respiratory difficulties, cyanosis, coma, and even death.

Apidae (Bees)—This family includes the bumble bees, honeybees, carpenter bees, and yellow jackets. The commonest stinging bees are *Apis mellifera* and the Africanized bee, *Apis mellifera adansonii*, and the incidence of Hymenoptera poisonings is increasing.

The venom contains biologically active peptides, such as melittin, apamine, mast cell–degranulating peptide, and others, as well as phospholipases A_2 and B, hyaluronidase, histamine, dopamine, monosaccharides, and lipids. Melittin tetramers cause a breakdown of the resting potential and rapid depolarization of nociceptors, which induces pain. Apamine is a blocker of calcium-dependent potassium channels and is thought to be the "lethal factor".

Bee stings typically produce immediate, sharp or burning pain, slight local erythema, and edema followed by itching. It is said that 50 stings can be serious and lead to respiratory dysfunction, intravascular hemolysis, hypertension, myocardial damage, hepatic changes, shock, and renal failure. With 100 or more stings, death can occur.

Vespidae (Wasps)—This family includes wasps and hornets. These venoms contain a high content of peptides, which include mastoparan in wasps and hornets and crabolin from hornet venom. These peptides release histamine from mast cells. Wasp kinins cause immediate pain, vasodilation, and increased vascular permeability leading to edema. These venoms also contain phospholipases and hyaluronidases, which contribute to the breakdown of membranes and connective tissue to facilitate diffusion of the venom.

Lepidoptera (Caterpillars, Moths, and Butterflies)

The urticating hairs, or setae, of caterpillars are effective defensive weapons that protect some species from predators. The toxic material found in the venom glands contains aristolochic acids, cardenolides, kallikrein, histamine and a fibrinolytic peptide. The spicules of *Thaumetopoea pityocampa* contain a toxin that is a strong dermal irritant and highly allergenic peptide. In some parts of the world the stings of several species of Lepidoptera give rise to a bleeding diathesis, often severe and sometimes fatal.

MOLLUSCA (CONE SNAILS)

Human interest in this group of mollusks has been due to the beautiful patterns on their shells. Cone snails have a venom duct for synthesis and storage of venom and hollow harpoon-like teeth for injection of the venom. There are probably over 100 different venom components per species known as conotoxins. Molecular targets include G-protein-coupled receptors, neuromuscular transporters, and ligand- or voltage-gated ion channels. Some components have enzymatic activity. Figure 26–10 provides an overview of peptidic *Conus* venom components, indicating gene superfamilies, disulfide bond characteristics, and general targets.

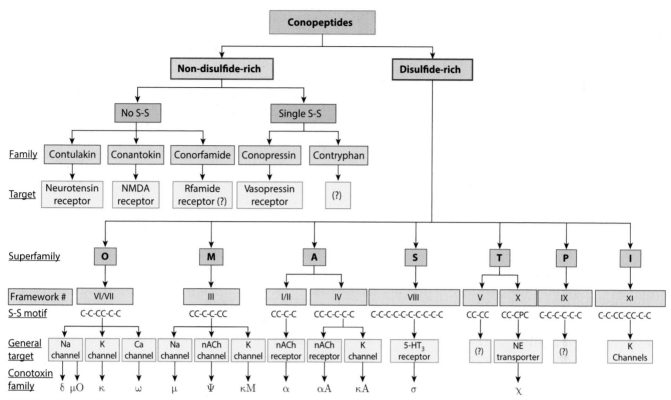

FIGURE 26–10 **Organizational diagram for *Conus* peptides, indicating gene superfamilies, disulfide patterns, and known pharmacologic targets.** Only the superfamilies of the disulfide-rich peptides are shown. (Reproduced with permission from Terlau H, Olivera BM: *Conus* venoms: A rich source of novel ion channel-targeted peptides. *Physiol Rev*, 2004 Jan;84(1):41–68.)

Cone snails could be called sophisticated practitioners of combination drug therapy. After injection, multiple conopeptides act synergistically to affect the targeted prey. The term toxin cabal has been applied to this coordinated action of the conopeptide mixture. The fish-hunting species *Conus purpurascens* apparently has two distinct cabals whose effects differ in time and space. The "lightning-strike cabal" causes immediate immobilization of the injected prey because various venom components inhibit voltage-gated sodium channel inactivation and block potassium channels, resulting in massive depolarization of axons in the vicinity of the injection site and a tetanic state. The second physiologic cabal, the "motor cabal," acts more slowly as conotoxins must be distributed throughout the body of the prey. The overall result is total inhibition of neuromuscular transmission. Various conopeptides inhibit presynaptic calcium channels that control neurotransmitter release, the postsynaptic neuromuscular nicotinic receptors, and the sodium channels involved in the muscle action potential.

REPTILES

Lizards

The Gila monster (*Heloderma suspectum*) and the beaded lizards (*Heloderma horridum*) are far less dangerous than is generally believed. Their venom is transferred from venom glands in the lower jaw through ducts that discharge their contents near the base of the larger teeth of the lower jaw. The venom is then drawn up along grooves in the teeth by capillary action. The venom of this lizard has serotonin, amine oxidase, phospholipase A, a bradykinin-releasing substance, helodermin, gilatoxin, and low-proteolytic as well as high-hyaluronidase activities. The clinical presentation of a helodermatid bite can include pain, edema, hypotension, nausea, vomiting, weakness, and diaphoresis. No antivenin is commercially available.

Snakes

General Information and Classification—Venomous snakes primarily belong to the following families: Viperidae (vipers), Elapidae, Atractaspididae, and Colubridae. Overall the Colubridae are considered the largest venomous family, and are composed of nearly 60% of all snakes.

Snake Venoms—These venoms are complex mixtures: proteins and peptides, consisting of both enzymatic and nonenzymatic compounds. Snake venoms also contain inorganic cations such as sodium, calcium, potassium, magnesium, and small amounts of zinc, iron, cobalt, manganese, and nickel. The metals in snake venoms are likely catalysts for metal-based enzymatic reactions. For example, in the case of some elapid venoms, zinc ions appear to be necessary for anticholinesterase activity, and calcium may play a role in the activation of phospholipase A and the direct lytic factor. Some proteases appear to be metalloproteins. Some snake venoms also contain carbohydrates (glycoproteins), lipids, and biogenic amines, such as histamine, serotonin, and neurotransmitters (catecholamines and acetylcholine) in addition to positively charged metal ions. The complexity of snake venom components is illustrated nicely in Figure 26–11.

Actions of snake venoms can be said to be broad ranging in several areas. A simplistic approach would group toxin components as neurotoxins, coagulants, hemorrhagins, hemolytics, myotoxins, cytotoxins, and nephrotoxins. Neurotoxins produce neuromuscular paralysis ranging from dizziness to ptosis; to ophthalmoplegia, flaccid facial muscle paralysis, and inability to swallow; to paralysis of larger muscle groups; and finally to paralysis of respiratory muscles and death by asphyxiation. Coagulants may have an initial procoagulant action that uses up clotting factors leading to bleeding. Coagulants may directly inhibit normal clotting at several places in the clotting cascade or via inhibition of platelet aggregation. In addition, some venom components may damage the endothelial lining of blood vessels leading to hemorrhage. Bite victims may show bleeding from nose or gums, from the bite site, and in saliva, urine, and stools. Myotoxins can directly impact muscle

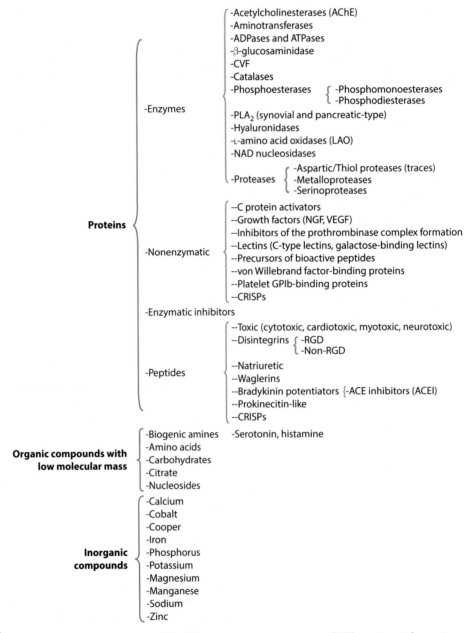

FIGURE 26–11 **Components of snake venoms.** ACE, angiotensin-converting enzyme; CRISP, cysteine-rich secretory protein; CVF, cobra venom factor–like proteins; LAO, L-amino acid oxidase; PLA$_2$, phospholipase A2; RGD, arginine–glycine–aspartate. (Reproduced with permission from Ramos OHP, Selistre-de-Araujo HS: Snake venom metalloproteases—structure and function of catalytic and disintegrin domains. *Comp Biochem Physiol C Toxicol Pharmacol.* 2006 Mar-Apr;142(3-4):328–346.)

contraction leading to paralysis or cause rhabdomyolysis or the breakdown of skeletal muscle. Myoglobinuria, or a dark brown urine, and hyperkalemia may be noted. Cytotoxic agents have proteolytic or necrotic properties leading to the breakdown of tissue. Typical signs include massive swelling, pain, discoloration, blistering, bruising, and wound weeping. Finally, nephrotoxins can cause direct damage to kidney structures leading to bleeding, damage to several parts of the nephron, tissue oxygen deprivation, and renal failure.

Enzymes—At least 26 different enzymes have been isolated from snake venoms. No single snake venom contains all 26 enzymes and some important snake venom enzymes are shown in Figure 26–11. Proteolytic enzymes that catalyze the breakdown of tissue proteins and peptides include peptide hydrolases, proteases, endopeptidases, peptidases, and proteinases. Collagenase is a specific kind of proteinase that digests collagen. This activity has been demonstrated in the venoms of a number of species of crotalids and viperids. Hyaluronidase cleaves internal glycoside bonds in certain acid mucopolysaccharides resulting in a decrease in the viscosity of connective tissues. The breakdown in the hyaluronic barrier allows other fractions of venom to penetrate the tissues, causing hyaluronidase to be called "spreading factor." Fibrin(ogen)olytic enzymes break down fibrin-rich clots and help to prevent further clot formation. An exciting development from the research on these enzymes is that one specific recombinant fibrinolytic enzyme derived from fibrolase called alfimeprase is progressing through clinical trials for the treatment of peripheral arterial occlusions. Phosphodiesterase has been found in the venoms of all families of poisonous snakes. It acts as an exonucleotidase, attacking DNA and RNA. Acetylcholinesterase, found in the cobra, catalyzes the hydrolysis of acetylcholine to choline and acetic acid thereby facilitating tetanic paralysis and capture of prey. Phospholipase A_2 is widely distributed in snake venoms, and this enzyme family interacts with other venom components often resulting in synergistic reactions.

The snake venom metalloproteinases (SVMP) are enzymes that disrupt the hemostatic system that blocks the function of integrin receptors, a function that could alleviate a variety of pathological conditions such as inflammation, tumor angiogenesis and metastasis, and thrombosis. SVMPs degrade proteins such as laminin, fibronectin, type IV collagen, and proteoglycans from the endothelial basal membrane; degrade fibrinogen and von Willebrand factor enhancing the hemorrhagic action; and inhibit platelet aggregation and stimulate release of cytokines.

Polypeptides—Snake venom polypeptides are low-molecular-weight proteins that do not have enzymatic activity. More than 80 polypeptides with pharmacologic activity have been isolated from snake venoms. Most of the lethal activity of the poison of the sea snake *Laticauda semifasciata* involves erabutoxins. Erabutoxin-a and α-cobratoxin are curamimetic at the mammalian neuromuscular junction. Disintegrins are a family of short cysteine-rich polypeptides that exhibit affinity for many

ligand receptors. The small basic polypeptide myotoxins are widely distributed in *Crotalus* snake venoms. The specific agent crotamine from *Crotalus durissus terrificus* venom induces skeletal muscle spasms and paralysis by changing the inactivation process of sodium channels leading to depolarization of the neuromuscular junction.

Toxicology—In general, the venoms of rattlesnakes and other New World crotalids produce alterations in the resistances and often in the integrity of blood vessels, changes in blood cells and blood coagulation mechanisms, direct or indirect changes in cardiac and pulmonary dynamics, and—with crotalids such as *C. durrissus terrificus* and *C. scutulatus*—serious alterations in the nervous system and changes in respiration. In humans, the course of the poisoning is determined by the kind and amount of venom injected; the site where it is deposited; the general health, size, and age of the patient; the kind of treatment; and those pharmacodynamic principles noted earlier in this chapter. Death in humans may occur within less than 1 h or after several days, with most deaths occurring between 18 and 32 h. Hypotension or shock is the major therapeutic problem in North American crotalid bites.

Snakebite Treatment—The treatment of bites by venomous snakes is now so highly specialized that almost every envenomation requires specific recommendations. However, three general principles for every bite should be kept in mind: (1) snake venom poisoning is a medical emergency requiring immediate attention and the exercise of considerable judgment; (2) the venom is a complex mixture of substances of which the proteins contribute the major deleterious properties, and the only adequate antidote is the use of specific or polyspecific antivenom; and (3) not every bite by a venomous snake ends in an envenomation. Venom may not be injected. In almost 1000 cases of crotalid bites, 24% did not end in a poisoning. The incidence with the bites of cobras and perhaps other elapids is probably higher (see www.toxinology.com).

ANTIVENOM

Antivenoms have been produced against most medically important snake, spider, scorpion, and marine toxins. Antivenom consists of venom-specific antisera or antibodies concentrated from immune serum to the venom. Antisera contain neutralizing antibodies: one antigen (monospecific) or several antigens (polyspecific). Monovalent antivenoms have a high neutralization capacity, which is desirable against the venom of a specific animal. Neutralization capacity of antivenom is highly variable as there are no enforced international standards. Antivenom may cross-react with venoms from distantly related species and may not react with venom from the intended species. Nevertheless, in general, the antibodies bind to the venom molecules, rendering them ineffective.

All antivenom products may produce hypersensitivity reactions. Type I (immediate) hypersensitivity reactions are caused by antigen cross-linking of endogenous IgE bound to mast cells and basophils. Binding of antigen by a mast cell may cause the release of histamine and other mediators, producing an anaphylactic reaction. Once initiated, anaphylaxis may continue despite discontinuation of antivenom administration. Type III hypersensitivity (serum sickness) may develop several days after antivenom administration. In these cases, antigen–antibody complexes are deposited in different areas of the body, often producing inflammatory responses in the skin, joints, kidneys, and other tissues. Fortunately, these reactions are rarely serious. The risks of anaphylaxis should always be considered when one is deciding whether to administer antivenom.

POTENTIAL CLINICAL APPLICATION OF VENOMS

Toxin specificities for receptors and channels that facilitate the interface and coordination of neuromuscular activity are utilized and manipulated to study, model, diagnose, and sometimes treat acute and degenerative conditions. On closer examination of α-bungarotoxin and candoxin nicotinic acetylcholine receptor specificity, plans are under way to utilize the reversible and irreversible receptor binding in muscular and neuronal tissues, respectively, in Alzheimer patients. In addition to treating neurological diseases, specific α-toxins (longer chained) are also studied for their antiangiogenic capabilities in treating malignant tumor growth in patients suffering from small-cell lung carcinoma. In cases such as this, there is an inherent trade-off between promoting some degree of neurological deficit in light of combating tumor growth. Toxins such as the snake venom thrombin-like enzymes are valuable tools in both research and therapeutic applications. Fibrin(ogen)olytic enzymes that break down fibrin-rich clots preventing further clot formation may be useful as controls in blood clotting research or to treat heart attacks and strokes.

Animal venoms contain components that can reduce pain, can selectively kill specific cancers, may reduce the incidence of stroke via effects on blood coagulability, and function as antibiotics. Other venom components act as enzyme inhibitors. Finally, leeches, earthworms, helminths, snails, centipedes, spiders, and ticks all produce substances with potential clinical applications, such as osteoarthritis, deep vein thrombosis, antimicrobial action, inflammatory bowel disease, analgesia, and hyperlipidemia. Blood from mongoose, hedgehog, and opossum contains proteins that inhibit the hemorrhagins in snake venoms. These proteins may become valuable as agents of resistance to snakebites.

BIBLIOGRAPHY

Auerbach PS (ed.): *Wilderness Medicine*, 6th ed., Philadelphia, PA: Mosby, 2012.

Bingham J-P, Mitsunaga E, Bergeron ZL: Drugs from slugs—past, present and future perspectives of conotoxin research. *Chem Biol Interact* 183:1–18, 2010.

Burrows GE, Tyrl RJ: *Toxic Plants of North America*, 2nd ed., Ames, Iowa: Wiley Blackwell, 2013.

Mackessy SP: *Handbook of Venoms and Toxins of Reptiles*. Boca Raton, FL: CRC Press/Taylor & Francis, 2010.

Mayer AMS, Glaser KB, Cuevas C, et al.: The odyssey of marine pharmaceuticals: a current pipeline perspective. *Trends Pharmacol Sci* 31:255–265, 2010.

QUESTIONS

1. All of the following statements regarding plant toxicity are true EXCEPT:
   a. Genetic variability plays a role in the toxicity of a plant.
   b. Plant toxins are most highly concentrated in the leaves.
   c. Young plants may have a higher toxin concentration than older plants.
   d. The weather can influence the toxicity of plants.
   e. Soil composition can alter a plant's production of toxin.

2. Contact with which of the following plant species would be LEAST likely to cause an allergic dermatitis?
   a. *Urtica.*
   b. *Philodendron.*
   c. *Rhus.*
   d. *Dendranthema.*
   e. *Hevea.*

3. Which of the following statements regarding lectin toxicity is FALSE?
   a. Lectins have an affinity for *N*-acetylglucosamine on mammalian neurons.
   b. Consumption of lectins can cause severe gastrointestinal disturbances.
   c. The fatality rate after ingestion of a fatal dose is very high.
   d. Some toxic lectins inhibit protein synthesis.
   e. A diet high in some lectins has been linked to reduced weight gain.

4. Colchicine, found in lily bulbs:
   a. causes severe dehydration.
   b. is sometimes used as a purgative.
   c. causes a severe contact dermatitis.
   d. inhibits sphingolipid synthesis.
   e. blocks microtubule formation.

5. Activation of a vanilloid receptor is characteristic of which of the following chemicals?
   a. acetylandromedol.
   b. capsaicin.
   c. colchicine.
   d. ergotamine.
   e. linamarin.

6. Which of the following plant species is known to cause cardiac arrhythmias on ingestion?
   a. *Dieffenbachia.*
   b. *Phytolacca americana.*
   c. *Digitalis purpurea.*
   d. *Pteridium aquilinum.*
   e. *Cicuta maculate.*

7. Which of the following plant toxins does NOT affect the neuromuscular junction?
   a. nicotine.
   b. anabasine.
   c. curare.
   d. anatoxin A.
   e. muscimol.

8. Which of the following statements regarding animal toxins is FALSE?
   a. Animal venoms are strictly metabolized by the liver.
   b. The kidneys are responsible for the excretion of metabolized venom.
   c. Venoms can be absorbed by facilitated diffusion.
   d. Most venom fractions distribute unequally throughout the body.
   e. Venom receptor sites exhibit highly variable degrees of sensitivity.

9. Scorpion venoms do NOT:
   a. affect potassium channels.
   b. affect sodium channels.
   c. affect chloride channels.
   d. affect calcium channels.
   e. affect initial depolarization of the action potential.

10. Which of the following statements regarding widow spiders is TRUE?
    a. Widow spiders are exclusively found in tropical regions.
    b. Both male and female widow spiders bite and envenomate humans.
    c. The widow spider toxin decreases calcium concentration in the synaptic terminal.
    d. Alpha-latrotoxin stimulates increased exocytosis from nerve terminals.
    e. A severe alpha-latrotoxin envenomation can result in life-threatening hypotension.

11. Which of the following diseases is not commonly caused by tick envenomation?
    a. Rocky Mountain spotted fever.
    b. Lyme disease.
    c. Q fever.
    d. ehrlichiosis.
    e. cat scratch fever.

12. Which of the following is NOT characteristic Lepidoptera envenomation?
    a. increased prothrombin time.
    b. decreased fibrinogen levels.
    c. decreased partial thromboplastin time.
    d. increased risk of hemorrhaging.
    e. decreased plasminogen levels.

13. Which of the following animals has a venom containing histamine and mast cell–degranulating peptide that is known for causing hypersensitivity reactions?
    a. bees.
    b. ants.
    c. snakes.
    d. spiders.
    e. reduviids.

14. Which of the following enzymes is not typically found in snake venoms?
    a. hyaluronidase.
    b. lactate dehydrogenase.
    c. collagenase.
    d. phosphodiesterase.
    e. histaminase.

15. Which of the following statements regarding snakes is FALSE?
    a. Inorganic anions are often found in snake venoms.
    b. About 20% of snake species are venomous.
    c. Snake venoms often interfere with blood coagulation mechanisms.
    d. Proteolytic enzymes are common constituents of snake venoms.
    e. Snakebite treatment is often specific for each type of envenomation.

Toxic Effects of Calories

Martin J. Ronis, Kartik Shankar, and Thomas M. Badger

- Nutrients can broadly be defined as chemical substances found in food that are necessary for proper growth, development, reproduction, and repair.
- Energy in the body is derived from three main nutrient classes: carbohydrates, protein, and fat, which in turn are made up of sugars, amino acids, and free fatty acids, respectively.
- Hormonal messages generated by the pancreas, adipose tissue, and GI tract orchestrate multiple responses associated with caloric intake and utilization.

- The "set-point" hypothesis proposes that food intake and energy expenditure are coordinately regulated in the central nervous system to maintain a relatively constant level of energy reserve and body weight.
- Dieting is defined as the use of a healthy, balanced diet that meets the daily nutritional needs of the body and that reduces caloric intake with increased moderate exercise.

BIOLOGY OF EATING AND DIGESTION

All biotic organisms derive energy from food to sustain life. This energy "drives" various cellular functions, including digestion, metabolism, pumping blood, and muscle contractions. Nutrients can broadly be defined as chemical substances found in food that are necessary for proper growth and development, reproduction, and repair following injury.

Because most bacteria and higher organisms cannot carry out photosynthesis, they derive their energy by metabolism of preformed organic molecules, such as carbohydrates. In general, bacteria utilize simpler organic molecules and animals and humans require more complex macronutrients (proteins, fats, and carbohydrates) to meet their needs.

Digestion of Foods

The process of digestion is a remarkable orchestration of many complex biochemical and physiologic events. Breakdown of food begins in the mouth via the actions of enzymes in saliva. In the stomach, food is acted upon by gastric juices, which contains high amounts of hydrochloric acid. Numerous enzymes supplied by the pancreas, liver, and gall bladder aid digestion in the small intestine.

The latter parts of the small intestine, the jejunum and ileum, are primary sites of nutrient absorption. The surface area of the intestinal mucosa available for absorption is greatly increased due to a combination of folds called valvulae conniventes (folds of Kerckring) and finger-like projections (villi) that are lined with enterocytes. Digestion of proteins begins in the stomach and continues in the lumen of the small intestine. The jejunum is the site of absorption of amino acids, dipeptides, and tripeptides by amino acid and peptide carriers in the enterocyte brush border. Lipids are hydrolyzed by pancreatic and intestinal lipases. Bile salts, along with phospholipids, facilitate the absorption of lipids. Macronutrient molecules (proteins, sugars, and fatty acids) that end up in the circulation undergo

metabolism in various tissues to be either oxidized to extract energy or stored for future utilization.

Integrated Fuel Metabolism

Energy in the body is derived from three main nutrient classes: carbohydrates, protein, and fat, which in turn are made up of sugars, amino acids, and free fatty acids, respectively. The principal circulating fuels in the body, glucose and free fatty acids, are stored as glycogen and triglycerides, respectively. Triglycerides are stored in specialized cells (adipocytes) within large lipid droplets. Proteins are critical in maintaining structure and function and are catabolized for energy only under extreme conditions.

Maintaining a stable supply of substrate for utilization by the brain is required because the brain has little to no stored energy in the form of glycogen or triglycerides. Unlike the brain, the heart and to some degree the liver and skeletal muscles derive most of their energy needs through the oxidation of fatty acids.

Hormonal messages generated by the endocrine cells of the pancreas, adipose tissue (adipokines), and GI tract (gut neuropeptides) are critical to orchestrating the multiple processes associated with fuel flux and metabolism. Insulin is the principal hormone required to manage nutrient fuels in both fed and fasted states. A rise in glucagon and glucocorticoids (such as cortisol) promote lipolysis and breakdown of glycogen.

Set-Point Theory and Neural Control of Energy Balance

A number of redundant feedback mechanisms that maintain energy homeostasis in living systems regulate the balance between food intake and energy expenditure to maintain fuel reserves at preset levels. Under steady-state conditions, energy is normally utilized to maintain basal metabolic rate and thermogenesis, and to carry out cellular processes, organ-specific functions, and movement (muscle contractions). Excess fuels are converted to triglycerides and stored in adipose tissues. Because adipose tissue is the major depot of preserving energy, signals derived from the periphery communicate with regions in the brain that coordinate energy balance. When total energy consumed equals the total energy required to meet basal metabolic needs, growth, thermogenesis, and physical activity, the individual is in energy balance, and maintaining this balance will result in relatively stable weight and healthy body composition.

One theory called the "set-point" hypothesis proposes that food intake and energy expenditure are coordinately regulated by defined regions in the central nervous system that signal to maintain a relatively constant level of energy reserve and body weight. Implicitly, the model requires the existence of four major components of an energy homeostasis system: (1) afferent signals relaying the levels of energy stores, (2) efferent processes regulating energy storage and expenditure, (3) efferent mechanisms controlling ingestive behavior, and (4) integrative centers in the brain to coordinate these processes. Studies have shown that the hypothalamus plays a central role in the control of energy balance, especially food intake. The hormone leptin, which is secreted in proportion to body fat stores from the adipose tissue, was the first signal to be identified to be a homeostatic regulator of energy balance.

Two populations of neurons involved in appetite control in the brain are sensitive to the action of leptin and other neuropeptides, including orexigenic peptides neuropeptide Y and agouti-related peptide and the anorexigenic peptides proopiomelanocortin and cocaine and amphetamine-regulated transcript. Downstream projections from these neurons interact with the melanocortin receptor neurons and the neurons in the paraventricular nucleus of the hypothalamus. In addition to the hypothalamic control of appetite per se, reward and hedonic processes of "liking" and "wanting" food occur in the ventral striatum of the midbrain in conjunction with the mesolimbic dopamine system. In addition, the corticolimbic system of reward is controlled by areas in the prefrontal cortex, which integrates sensory, emotional, and cognitive information to coordinate behavioral responses. Hence, the homeostatic control of energy balance fits into the larger decision scheme of choice behavior via a complex neural system.

METHODS TO ASSESS ENERGY BALANCE

Assessing Caloric Intake

In animal studies, caloric intake can be quantitatively monitored by measuring the amount of food consumed by animals in metabolic cages. Caloric intake can be derived by multiplying the quantity (g/day) of diets consumed with the caloric density of the diet. A prospective method to collect information about current intake is maintenance of *food records*. These are usually carried out for a specific duration of time (three to seven days, generally including both week and weekend days) during which a written record of all food and beverages

consumed is maintained. Details may include portion sizes, cooking methods, and patterns of eating.

Assessing Caloric Content of Foods

Accurate assessment of the caloric value of foods is essential for effective nutritional management in clinical and public policy arenas. The general calorie factors of 4, 9, and 4 for the major sources of energy—carbohydrate, fat, and protein—have been widely used. The heat released by combustion of a food in a bomb calorimeter is a measure of its gross energy. The truly metabolizable energy can be derived by accounting for energy lost in urine (mainly from nitrogen) and on the body surface. Protein content is mainly determined via estimating nitrogen. Fat content can be assessed by measuring the sum of methanol–chloroform extractable total fatty acids that can be expressed as triglyceride equivalents. Carbohydrate content is generally measured by difference as the remaining energy after accounting for protein, fat, alcohol, and ash.

Assessing Energy Expenditure

The total energy expenditure or metabolic cost for an average adult is primarily composed of three components: (1) basal energy expenditure, (2) thermic effect of food, and (3) energy expenditure associated with physical activity. Basal energy expenditure, also called as resting energy expenditure, is the energy expended when the individual is lying down and at complete rest, generally after sleep in the postabsorptive state. The energy expenditure from physical activity consists of expenditure related to exercise and nonexercise activity thermogenesis.

Components of energy expenditure can be measured using either direct or indirect calorimetry. The basic principle in direct calorimetry is to measure the actual heat produced by the organism in a highly controlled environment as an estimate of energy expenditure. Most commonly used methods to estimate energy expenditure involve indirect calorimetry. By using experimentally derived estimates for energy yields per mole of oxygen, heat production can be calculated based on the quantity of oxygen consumed.

Assessing Body Composition

Body composition assessments permit describing the overall mass of an individual organism in terms of water, fat mass, lean mass, protein, and minerals. In a simple two-compartment model of body composition assessment, total body mass is divided into fat mass (essential and nonessential fat) and fat-free mass (including lean mass and water). Lean mass in this scenario includes protein, carbohydrate, and minerals.

Anthropometric Analysis—Although individuals with greater body weight (mass) per height tend to have greater fat mass, total body weight may also be determined by increased muscle mass. The simplest indirect measure of body fatness is the relative proportion of body weight (in kilograms) to body height squared (meters²), more commonly referred to as body mass index (BMI). BMI, however, is only an estimate: BMI does not always reflect fat mass, and care must be taken when using BMI as an index of body fat.

Hydrodensitometry—Using the density of the whole body and correcting for residual air in the lungs and GI tract, the relative body fat can be estimated using derived equations. This procedure is also known as underwater weighing.

Air Displacement Plesmography—This procedure employs the same principles as underwater weighing described above, except rather than the body displacing water, it displaces air. This is probably the most accurate, precise, and cost-effective measure of total body fat, and is employed widely in clinical research in the United States.

Absorptiometry—In this technique imaging is performed throughout the entire body by a photon beam. This allows imaging of both soft tissues and bone. Percentage of body fat, lean tissue, and bone mineral density can be computed for the whole body or specific sites based on the analysis of images.

Computerized Tomography—The ability to generate three-dimensional cross-sectional images allows regional localization of adipose tissues, muscles, and organs (e.g., liver). Using the image data, percent body fat and lean mass can be calculated.

Nuclear Magnetic Resonance (NMR)—NMR works by interpreting radio-frequency signals of excited nuclei in an external magnetic field. The physical characteristics of the hydrogen atom differ when the hydrogen is located on protein, fat, or water and this can be detected and quantitated to determine body composition.

Electrical Impedance—Bioelectrical impedance analysis and total body electrical conductivity measure total body composition based on measuring electrical impedance (the inverse of conductance) of an electric current passed through the body. Lean mass has more water and greater conductivity than fat mass and predictive equations are employed to derive fat and lean body mass.

Total Body Water—Body fat and lean mass can be calculated by estimating total body water using stable isotopes (either deuterium or O^{18}). Whereas body water occupies 73% of lean mass, fat-free mass can be estimated using appropriate assumptions.

Assessing Physical Activity

Devices such as accelerometers and pedometers can be utilized to empirically estimate activity. An important challenge in utilizing accelerometers is to convert the count data into energy expenditure, which is done using different regression models.

BIOLOGY OF OBESITY

Obesity Risk: Genes and Fetal Environment

Historically, human life was marked by unpredictable access to food. Fitness and survival of an individual were likely to be closely related to the ability to maximally seek, acquire, consume, and store energy (as fat) when food was available, and to select for mechanisms that reduce energy expenditure during times when food is scarce. The advent of agrarian lifestyle and recent industrialization has meant that much of the developed and emerging world now has a drastically altered environment. Food is generally available for most people and our lifestyles require less physical activity and exertion. Hence, our genetic legacy in the context of caloric abundance acts as a powerful engine for weight gain, obesity, and its associated metabolic dysfunction. Natural variation and random mutation in genes controlling hypothalamic energy balance set-points occurred as human beings developed fire and social behaviors and were released from risk of predation. The "drifty gene" hypothesis explains why even in societies where obesity is high, not everyone becomes obese. Obesity is a highly heritable trait and studies comparing monozygotic with dizygotic twins indicate that 40% to 75% of the interindividual difference in trait is accounted for by genetic variability. Several genes whose disruption causes severe monogenic forms of familial obesity have been described. Remarkably, most of these genes impair central control of food intake. However, the genetic basis of non-syndromic (common) obesity has remained elusive.

The incidence of obesity continues to rise, including the prevalence among infants. As for many chronic diseases, it is now widely accepted that increased susceptibility to obesity can be programmed in utero and early postnatal life. Another important influence on risk of obesity in later life is maternal body composition (fat mass) at conception and gestational weight gain.

TOXICITY RELATED TO EXCESS CALORIC INTAKE/OBESITY

Many of the adaptive, physiologic responses to the positive energy balance produced as a result of overeating and inadequate physical activity result in toxicity over the long term. Short-term coordinated changes in metabolic pathways in white adipose tissue in response to overfeeding result in excess energy storage in the form of triglycerides, which leads to increased size of preexisting adipocytes (hypertrophy) and to formation of new adipocytes (hyperplasia). Under conditions of chronic excess ingested energy, the efficiency of energy storage in adipose tissue is decreased and the body stores energy in ectopic sites. Triglycerides begin to accumulate in nonadipose tissues such as liver, skeletal muscle, and the pancreas as lipid droplets resulting in insulin resistance, inflammation, and tissue damage.

In addition, adipose tissue from obese individuals releases chemokines and cytokines, the so-called adipokines, which

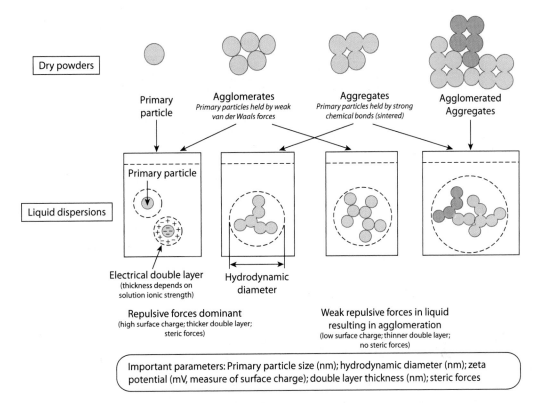

FIGURE 28–3 **Agglomeration and aggregation of nanoparticles in liquids and as dry powders.** (Modified with permission from Jiang JG, Oberdörster E, et al.: Characterization of size, surface charge, and agglomeration state of nanoparticle disperisons for toxicological studies, *J Nanopart Res*, 2009 Jan;11(1): 77–89.)

Surface Chemistry—High surface area and exposed surface atoms or molecules promote increased dissolution and release of ions from metallic or metal oxide NPs relative to bulk particles of the same chemical composition. Metal ions are toxic to bacteria and aquatic organisms by inhibition of enzymes and transport proteins. For example, ZnO NPs are incorporated into sunscreens where they absorb ultraviolet (UV) light; however, in water, Zn^{2+} ions are rapidly released and cause acute toxicity. Surface hydrophilicity of charged NPs increases their ability to be suspended in water, whereas surface hydrophobicity of fullerenes or grapheme repels water and enables these hydrophobic nanomaterials to partition into lipid membranes and enter target cells. In addition, surface defects expose electron active groups that donate an electron to molecular oxygen which generates superoxide anions which are reactive oxygen species (ROS).

CNTs are synthesized in the presence of metal catalysts that can undergo redox cycling and catalyze generation of highly reactive hydroxyl radical groups. Nanomaterials with high surface area can adsorb organic molecules such as polycyclic aromatic hydrocarbons that are potentially carcinogenic and quinones that also participate in generation of free radicals and redox cycling. Cationic NPs that have surface amide groups and cationic dendrimers are especially cytotoxic because they induce membrane damage, especially in lysosomes, that leads to accumulation of water and chloride ions and osmotic rupture.

Unique Quantum and Magnetic Properties—Ferromagnetic NPs less than 10 nm in diameter respond to an external magnetic field. This is exploited for contrast enhancement in diagnostic MRI and for hyperthermia induced by an external magnetic field to kill tumors targeted by magnetic NPs.

Geometry and Dimensions—These are important determinants in cellular uptake, systemic translocation, and potential toxicity. Nanomaterials can enter target cells by passive diffusion, direct physical penetration, or active, receptor-mediated uptake by endocytosis or phagocytosis depending on their size and extent of agglomeration. Small NPs appear to enter cells and organelles by passive diffusion. Single walled CNTs (SWCNTs) have been shown to directly puncture bacterial cells leading to osmotic lysis and death. SWCNTs have also been reported to translocate from the alveoli into the interstitium of the lung where they promote collagen deposition and interstitial fibrosis.

Biopersistence—Biopersistence of ENMs is an important factor in their environmental and biologic toxicity. Biopersistence is related to dissolution, which produces biologically active ionic species as well as has the ability to degrade the particle and clear it from biologic tissue or the environment. The rate of dissolution of metal oxides is increased by natural organic matter in the aqueous environment; therefore, these NPs have low biodurability and it is predicted that they would not bioaccumulate in the environment.

Biopersistence in the lungs and pleural or peritoneal spaces is an important physicochemical characteristic of asbestos and man-made mineral fibers associated with carcinogenicity. Several recent studies have shown that carboxylated SWCNTs do not undergo oxidative degradation in the presence of stimulant fluid that mimics the lysosomal compartment of macrophages. However, oxidatively degraded SWCNTs did not induce lung inflammation or toxicity following pharyngeal aspiration in mice providing proof-of-principle for deliberate design of engineered CNTs that are biodegradable and less likely to induce disease following inhalation or injection for tumor imaging or drug delivery.

THE NANOMATERIAL BIOLOGIC INTERFACE

The high surface area of NPs provides a platform for adsorption of a variety of biologic molecules including proteins, lipids, and nucleic acids. A "protein corona" exists on the NP and governs its initial reaction with target cells. The interaction of nanomaterials with blood plasma proteins has been highly investigated due to its importance in drug delivery, circulation time, organ distribution, and clearance. The consequences of protein adsorption to NPs are not clear; although, depending on the NP surface, proteins may denature resulting in loss of normal structure and function, with altered enzyme activity or unfolding that exposes new antigenic determinants. An important potential pathologic consequence of serum protein adsorption to NPs is binding of fibrinogen leading to formation of blood clots.

NPs that are inhaled or ingested encounter a lipid mucus layer that provides a natural barrier to penetration of particulates and microorganisms. NPs may adhere to mucins causing enlargement of pore size with increased susceptibility to penetration of microorganisms. Smaller, charged NPs may be repelled by the hydrophilic domains and will not be able to penetrate the mucus layer. Aquatic organisms and bacterial biofilms are similarly surrounded.

ENPs also bind nucleic acids and have been proposed as gene delivery devices. Small grapheme oxide nanosheets can also intercalate into double-stranded DNA and induce DNA breaks in the presence of Cu^{2+} ions.

TOXICITY MECHANISMS

The mechanistic pathways associated with toxicity are predictable based on the physicochemical properties of ENMs. Oxidative stress due to direct generation of ROS at the surface of NPs or indirectly by target cells following internalization of NPs is a common mechanism responsible for toxicity of ENMs. The most vulnerable subcellular organelles and physiologic functions that can be perturbed by exposure to ENPs are summarized in Table 28–3.

The cell wall of bacteria and the plasma membrane of eukaryotic cells are the initial barriers to penetration of NPs. Carbon nanomaterials are proposed to act as "nanodarts" creating

TABLE 28–3   In vitro mechanisms of nanoparticle toxicity.

1. Damage to cell wall and plasma membrane
2. Interference with electron transport and aerobic respiration
3. Induction of oxidant stress
4. Activation of cell signaling pathways
5. Perturbed ion homeostasis
6. Release of toxic metal ions from internalized nanoparticles
7. Disruption of lysosomal membrane integrity
8. Incomplete uptake or frustrated phagocytosis
9. Interference with cytoskeletal function
10. DNA and chromosomal damage

holes in the plasma membrane resulting in extracellular release of cytoplasmic contents as assessed by efflux of ribosomal RNA and decreased survival.

A wide variety of NPs have been designed to facilitate delivery of imaging agents, genes, proteins, and drugs into mammalian cells. NPs can also be designed to target specific cell surface receptors triggering internalization. In order to facilitate delivery, NPs can be engineered to escape from endosomes or lysosomes by coating with pH-sensitive polymers, viral caspids, cations, or biodegradable carriers.

NPs that are recognized by surface receptors may activate cell type–specific signaling pathways leading to cell proliferation or death by apoptosis, stress-related signaling, or calcium-mediated signal transduction events. Dysregulated intracellular calcium ion homeostasis may be the consequence of influx across a damaged plasma membrane permeability barrier or release of calcium ion from the major intracellular storage sites. Sustained elevation in intracellular calcium can cause cell death by necrosis.

Macrophages are the initial cells to phagocytize inhaled particulates deposited in the airways or alveoli. If they are longer than the diameter of macrophages, incomplete uptake occurs with prolonged generation of ROS by the respiratory burst mechanism of phagocytes and extracellular release of damaging lysosomal enzymes. In general, incomplete sequestration of NPs that are too large within lysosomes results in physical interference with cytoskeletal function that can cause impaired cell motility.

CAVEATS IN NANOTOXICOLOGIC ASSAYS

Due to their high surface area and hydrophobicity, NPs can adsorb vital dyes, cell culture micronutrients, or released cytokines.

SAFETY CONSIDERATIONS IN NANOMATERIAL DESIGN

In principle, it should be possible to engineer NPs with desirable surface properties for commercial or biomedical applications. Capping or coating of NPs using antioxidants may decrease toxicity. Release of toxic metal ions from quantum dots and iron oxide NPs can be minimized using inorganic shells or biocompatible polymers. In addition, there is some evidence that CNTs are less pathogenic if they are shorter or entangled to hide their fibrous nature.

CASE STUDY: DESIGNING SAFER SUNSCREENS

As previously mentioned, due to its rapid dissolution in water and release of Zn_{2+} ions, ZnO NPs are considered as potential toxicants. TiO_2 NPs are used in sunscreens as well. The potential of ZnO and TiO_2 NPs to induce photo toxicity and penetrate into the dermis has been a major concern for human safety of sunscreens. A series of skin penetration studies using both ex vivo and in vivo models showed that these NPs do not penetrate deeper than the outer most layer, stratum corneum, of intact skin. Thus, it is suggested that the benefits of protection against carcinogenic UV light radiation provided by sunscreens formulated with ZnO or TiO_2 NPs outweigh the minimal risks associated with phototoxicity, DNA damage, and skin penetration.

MAMMALIAN TOXICOLOGY

Introduction

CNTs are a prime example of the two opposing faces of nanomaterials: Many highly desirable properties that are suitable for numerous beneficial applications contrast with reports of serious adverse effects in experimental animals. For example, the excitement of future use of CNTs for delivery of drugs, genes, and biosensors is dampened by reports of inflammatory fibrogenic and even mesothliogenic effects in laboratory rodents.

Concepts of Nanotoxicology

The shape, size, and size distribution are important determinants for the deposition efficiency of inhaled materials throughout the respiratory tract. Uptake into cells is influenced by their surface charge, surface reactivity, the chemistry of surface coatings, and also surface defects to the material as synthesized or introduced during surface functionalization or processing.

Many ENPs are insoluble in the as-produced form and do not undergo simple dissolution but can undergo chemical oxidation in solution, tissue, or the environment to produce soluble species in a process that gradually degrades and eliminates the particle state. Such NPs can act via a "Trojan Horse" mechanism in that they are taken up into cells and subsequently dissolve, thereby creating a very high intracellular, ionic metal concentration that is cytotoxic.

Dosemetrics

Expressing dose–response relationships is most informative utilizing surface area of the NP. Figure 28–4 shows the pulmonary inflammatory dose–response relationship of two sizes of TiO_2 particles induced by intratracheal instillation in rates. A significantly greater influx of inflammatory neutrophils into the lung was induced by 25 nm TiO_2 per unit mass than by 250 nm TiO_2. The result is a very steep dose–response for the nanosized TiO_2 and a flatter dose–response for the larger TiO_2. Likewise there was a clear separation of the dose–response when based on the number as dosemetric; however, when the same data was expressed based on particle surface area, a

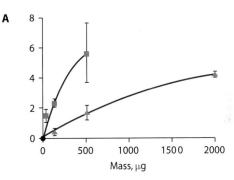

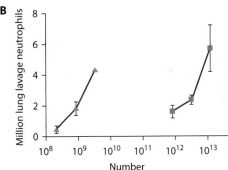

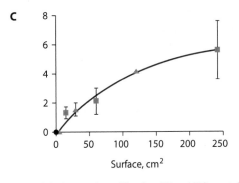

▲ Fine TiO_2 (250 nm)   ■ Ultrafine (25 nm) TiO_2 ● Saline

FIGURE 28–4 Inflammatory cell response (neutrophil number in lung lavage of rats 24 h after intratracheal instillation of two sizes of TiO_2 particles expressed by different dosemetrics. Particle-mass (**A**); -number (**B**); -surface area (**C**). (Reproduced with permission from Oberdörster G, Oberdörster E, Oberdörster J: Concepts of Nanoparticle Dose metric and Response Metric, *Environ Health Perspect*, 2007 Jun;115(6):A290.)

common dose–response relationship emerged. More specifically, although the concept of particle surface area is plausible, the biologically available surface area is of greater value for defining a proper dosemetric.

Volume of NPs has been suggested as another dosemetric. The "particle overload" hypothesis states as follows: When the volume of phagocytized particles in alveolar macrophages exceeds 6% of the normal macrophage volume, their physiologic clearance function becomes impaired; if the volume reaches 60%, clearance no longer functions. This concept has been applied to estimate certain human occupational exposure limits. Dependent upon the situation, either surface area or volume dosemetric may be used. It is also important to remember that chemical properties of NPs are critical determinants of effects resulting from NP–cell interactions (Table 28–2).

Portals of Entry

The respiratory tract, the gastrointestinal (GI) tract, and skin are the main organs of direct exposure of ENM. For medical application, injection will also be an important entry route. Intake via the respiratory tract is the most prevalent exposure route for occupational exposures. Additives of ENM to food and potential contamination of food result in exposure via GI tract. Based on available data, translocation of nanomaterial in vivo across GI-tract epithelial cells seems to be limited; however, DNA damage has been found in bone marrow of cells following very high gavage dosing of rats. Skin exposure via cosmetic and skin-care products occurs, although penetration of healthy skin by NP has not been demonstrated.

Dosing of the Respiratory Tract

Dosing of the respiratory tract of laboratory rodents involve the administration of materials as a bolus in a second or less. However, inhalation is the only physiologic method and should be considered the gold standard for exposure to airborne materials. Major differences between bolus-type and inhalation exposures relate to the dose rate, use of anesthesia, and the distribution of administered material within the respiratory tract.

Bolus delivery occurs within a fraction of a second, whereas inhalation at realistic concentration takes hours to months of exposure in order to deposit the same does in the lung. Treating a dose delivered by bolus to be the same that has accumulated in the lung over a lifelong exposure is not justifiable. Inundating cells abruptly with an extraordinarily high dose overwhelms the cell's defense mechanisms and leaves no time for developing adaptive responses. Consequently, mechanisms of effects induced but unrealistic high doses are different from those induced by relevant dose and dose rates.

Figure 28–5 illustrates a tremendous difference of inducing a pulmonary inflammation by either intratrachially instilling 200 μg of TiO₂ NP versus depositing the same dose by inhalation over a period of four hours for four days. The difference

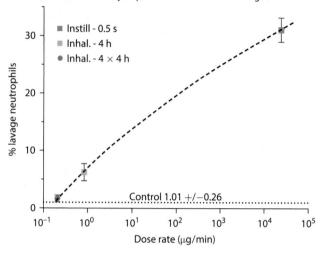

FIGURE 28–5   Dose-rate–response correlation: Deposition of 200 μg nano-TiO₂ in the lungs of rats either by instillation (high dose rate) or by inhalation (low dose rate) induces widely differing pulmonary inflammatory responses as determined by the appearance of inflammatory neutrophils in lung lavage. (Used with permission of G. Oberdörster).

in dose rate is significant with no response at the lowest dose rate of inhalation. This supports that adaptive responses are an important physiologic protective mechanism, which need to be considered when interpreting results of nanomaterial toxicity testing. Despite the limitations of bolus-type delivery, they may be viewed as "proof of principle" with the findings to be confirmed by subsequent inhalation studies. The concept of differential adsorption states that the physicochemical properties of nanoparticles such as size, surface properties, shape, dissolution, and others when in contact with media in the different body compartments, such as respiratory tract lining fluid, gastrointestinal secretions, etc., determine protein and lipid adsorption and thereby influence biodistribution across barriers and in target tissues and cells.

Respiratory Tract Deposition

Inhalation of ENMs results in significant deposition in the three compartments of the respiratory tract: the nasopharyngeal region from the nose/mouth to the larynx, the tracheobronchial region from the larynx to terminal bronchioles, and the alveolar region from the first generation of respiratory bronchioles to the last generation of alveolar ducts. The deposition efficiency depends on particle characteristics, anatomical structure of the airways, and breathing parameters. Particle size, size distribution, density, and shape are the most important because they govern deposition in the respiratory tract by inertial impact, gravitational settling, and displacement by diffusion.

Studies have been performed involving nasal inhalation in rats and humans. Obvious differences between rats and humans are the maximum size of particles that are respirable, that is, will reach the alveolar region. In rats this is about 5 μm aerodynamic size, in humans about 15 μm. Although these sizes are outside the range of single NP, airborne NP occurs for the most part as agglomerates.

It should be noted in a reminder that realistic in vivo doses to cells of the respiratory tract are mostly orders of magnitude lower than doses that are typically applied in vitro to lung epithelial cell cultures. In the alveolar region where the airflow is very low, no deposition hotspots for NPs exist. This nonhomogeneous deposition and formation of hotspots seem to correlate with predilection sites for bronchial carcinoma, which is further enhanced by less effective mucociliary clearance at carnal ridges.

Respiratory Tract Clearance and Disposition of NP: Nanomaterials

Once NPs are deposited in the respiratory tract they will encounter clearance mechanisms. However, there are several differences that separate NP from larger particles. Alveolar macrophages generally are attracted to deposited particles by chemotactic signals generated at the site of deposition. NPs may be too small to generate such signals leading to uptake into the pulmonary interstitium. Translocation into the interstitium and subsequently into blood and lymph circulation distinguishes NPs from microparticles. Figure 28–6 depicts the blood compartment as a plenum from which any tissue or organ can be reached by circulating NP. However, the amount of NP translocating from the lung to the blood circulation and accumulation in secondary organs is very low. Long-term retention studies with radioactive NPs have shown that clearance in extrapulmonary organs following the initial accumulation is very efficient, so after six months, with the exception of liver and spleen, only minor amounts were still present. Despite the low translocation rates, it has to be considered that continuous exposure may result in significant accumulation in some secondary organs.

Nanomaterials and the Brain

Organs with tight endothelial junctions, in particular the CNS, will not likely accumulate blood-borne NPs, unless the tight blood–brain barrier is damaged or NP surface has been specially modified. The most efficient pathway of NP translocation to the CNS appears to be via olfactory sensory neurons from the nasal olfactory mucosa directly to the olfactory bulb. Results of epidemiologic studies of impaired cognitive function and of neurodegenerative brain pathology associated with exposure to traffic-related particles raised the question as to whether ambient UFPs as constituents of urban air pollution may be etiologically involved.

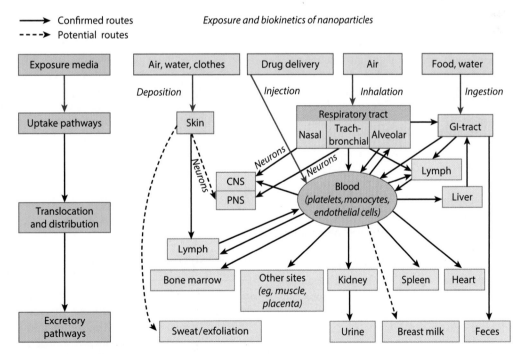

FIGURE 28–6 **Exposure and biokinetics of nanoparticle routes of exposure and biokinetics (uptake, distribution, elimination) of nanomaterials. Translocation rates in general are very low (see text).** (Reproduced with permission from Oberdörster G, Oberdörster E, Oberdörster J: Nanotoxicology: an emerging discipline evolving from studies of ultrafine particles, *Environ Health Perspect*, 2005 Jul;113(7):823–839.)

Elimination of Nanomaterials

Elimination pathways for ENM from the body include mainly feces and urine. Urinary excretion is restricted to nanostructures <5.5 nm in size for metal-based NP. Circulating fibrous structures of ENM, such as large MWCNTs, can collect in the urine of rats following intravenous application. This phenomenon may be explained by a hydrodynamic lining of nanotubes so they will pass through glomerular pores. The fecal excretory clearance pathway consists of several inputs: one is mucociliary clearance of deposited particles from the airways into the GI tract; another is the hepatobiliary clearance of blood-borne ENM via liver and bile into the small intestine. This elimination pathway is also a well-known excretory path for heavy metals in the blood.

Another clearance pathway of deposited ENM in the lung involves translocation via interstitium or lymph to the pleura and subsequent elimination via lymphatic openings on the parietal pleura to mediastinal lymph nodes from where NP may enter the blood circulation via the thoracic ducts. This pathway is of particular importance for fiber-shaped ENM because the size of the parietal stomata prevents efficient clearance of structures >10 μm in length. As a consequence, the interaction of the retained fibers in the pleural cavity with mesothelial cells induce inflammatory and granulomatous responses and in long-term potentially mesothelioma.

CASE STUDY: MWCNTS

Bolus-type Exposures

Bolus-type delivery of CNTs to the respiratory tract of rats and mice revealed induction of dose-dependent significant inflammatory, granulomatous, and fibrogenic responses; they showed also that MWCNTs can reach subpleural and intrapleural sites. In addition, intraperitoneal injection studies clearly show the potential of CNTs, specifically MWCNTs, to induce severe adverse length-dependent effects at mesothelial sites once they reach the pleural cavity.

Inhalation Studies

Relatively few inhalation studies with CNTs in rodents have been reported. The most meaningful and best justified for the risk assessment process would be a subchronic multiconcentration study with sufficient postexposure observation. However, short-term exposure to a relevant concentration is useful for dosimetric purposes when determining the biodistribution from deposition sites in the lung to secondary organs. Parameters varied, but within these variations outcomes ranged from no significant effects to severe pulmonary inflammation/oxidative stress responses.

Critical Appraisal of CNT In Vivo Studies

Given the importance of the physicochemical properties of CNTs for inducing adverse effects, it is of utmost importance

to determine these properties, in particular as they appear in the airborne state at sites of human exposures, at occupational sites, or for the consumer. Adding dispersants for testing purposes will change surface properties; conceptually, inhalation studies in experimental animals for purposes of hazard identification should mimic human exposure conditions with regard to airborne size distribution. Of course, differences in respirability between humans and rodents must be considered and adjustments be made without use of surface altering dispersants.

Appropriately designed multiconcentration, subchronic inhalation studies, including a longer recovery period, are essential for deriving no observed adverse effect levels (NOAELs); results can be used as basis for deriving occupational exposure levels (OELs) by applying rodent/human dosemetric adjustments. Using results from bolus-type studies is difficult and raises questions, although national institute for occupational safety and health has combined results of fibrotic responses from diverse bolus-type and inhalation studies to derive a provisional recommended exposure level of 7 μg/m³. This REL is based on dose–response data from the available studies with bolus-type and short-term inhalation exposures and a subchronic inhalation study.

There has been no conclusive data regarding carcinogenic effects of realistic exposure to CNTs. Thus, exposure should be avoided with appropriate measures (ventilation, filtration, personal protective equipment). There is an obvious and urgent need to perform additional long-term inhalation studies to assess carcinogenic potential.

Biologic Degradation of Carbon Nanomaterials— CNTs have been generally regarded as stable nondegradable materials, which has important implications for long-term health effects following inhalation into the lungs. Recently, however, SWCNT degradation has been observed in acellular assays that stimulate the phagolysosome of macrophages, but only if the tubes have been surface carboxylated, which introduces collateral defects in the side walls. Graphene oxide is also susceptible to oxidative attack by hydrogen peroxide and horseradish peroxidase. These observations may enable design of safer carbon materials that are potentially biodegradable in order to minimize adverse environmental and human health impacts. However, degradation of CNTs in vivo is still to be confirmed.

TOXICITY TESTING

In order to perform risk assessment, exposure and hazard data are required. To identify and characterize a hazard, in vitro and in vivo studies will be useful, and results should be derived via well-designed dose–response relationships. Key considerations include physicochemical characterization of the ENM to be tested, justification of the method(s) of dosing, selection of target cells, tissues, or animal species, and appropriate end points.

has the potential to act as a carrier of certain irritant gases. However, carbon in the ultrafine mode ($< 0.1 \mu m$) has been suggested to be more toxic than the fine mode ($2.5 \mu m$) form, perhaps due to enhanced surface reactivity or tissue penetration. Composition of the ultrafine particle also contributes to its effects and behavior. Ultrafine particles in the environment exist in extremely high numbers but contribute negligibly to mass. Recent commercial introduction of "engineered" nanoparticles brings many of the same concerns as ultrafines by virtue of their similar sizes. Additionally, being "engineered" particles, they may possess design features that "natural" combustion ultrafine (or nano) particles do not.

Chronic Effects and Cancer—The role of air pollution in human lung cancer is difficult to assess because the vast majority of respiratory cancers result from cigarette smoking. VOCs and nitrogen-containing and halogenated organics account for most of the compounds that are derived from combustion sources ranging from tobacco to power plants to incinerators to motor vehicles with potential carcinogenic effects. Human exposure to airborne toxicants is highly complex compositionally as well as in its temporal and spatial heterogeneity.

The lung cancer risk of any individual is some function of the carcinogenic nature of the substance, the amount of material deposited in the lungs, which is itself a function of the concentration in the ambient air, the physical and chemical properties of the inhalant that may determine deposition efficiency, and the cumulative volume of air inhaled. Of course, the innate susceptibility of the individual (including genotype and environmental factors such as diet, etc.) is also likely to be important. The majority of lung cancer risk from ambient air pollution lies within the PM fraction, including the polycyclic organic chemicals, along with the less volatile (semivolatile) nitroaromatics. These persistent organics associate with the PM matrix and thus could have a prolonged residence time at deposition sites within the respiratory tract. Genetic bioassays have revealed the potent mutagenicity, and presumably carcinogenicity, of various chemical fractions of ambient aerosols. Some of these compounds require metabolic transformation to activate their potency while others may be detoxified by their metabolism. Carcinogenic vapors such as benzene are inhaled but target the bone marrow producing leukemia.

The cells lining the respiratory tract turn over relatively quickly, since they interface with the ambient environment with every breath. Conceptually, their DNA would thus be vulnerable to carcinogenic or oxidant-induced replication errors that, when fixed as mutations, could give rise to tumors. Copollutants, such as irritant gases, that initiate inflammation may promote carcinogenic activity by damaging cells and further enhancing their turnover.

Photochemical Air Pollution

Photochemical air pollution (notably O_3) arises secondarily from a series of complex reactions in the troposphere activated by the ultraviolet (UV) spectrum of sunlight. In addition to O_3, it comprises a mixture of nitric oxides (NO_x), aldehydes, peroxyacetyl nitrates (PAN), and a myriad of aromatics and alkenes along with analog reactive radicals. If SO_2 is present, sulfates may also be formed and, collectively, they yield "summer haze." Likewise, the complex chemistry can generate organic PM, nitric acid vapor, and various condensates.

From the point of view of the toxicology of photochemical air pollutant gases, O_3 is by far the toxicant of greatest concern. It is highly reactive and more toxic than NO_x, and because its generation is fueled through cyclic hydrocarbon radicals, it reaches greater concentrations than the hydrocarbon radical intermediates. Although O_3 is of toxicological importance in the troposphere, in the stratosphere it plays a critical protective role. About 10 to 50 km above the earth's surface, UV light directly splits molecular O_2 into atomic $O^\bullet$, which then combines with O_2 to form O_3. The O_3 also dissociates back but much more slowly. The result is an accumulation of O_3 to several ppm within a relatively thin strip of the stratosphere forming an effective "permanent" barrier by absorbing the short-wavelength UV in the chemical process. This barrier had in recent years been threatened by various anthropogenic emissions (Cl_2 gas and certain chlorofluorocarbons) that enhance O_3 degradation (creation of an "O_3 hole"), but recent restrictions on the use of these degrading chemicals seem to have been effective in reversing this process. The benefits are believed to be a reduction of excess UV light infiltration to the earth's surface and reduced skin cancer risk.

This protective issue is quite different in the troposphere, where accumulation of O_3 serves no known purpose and poses a threat to the respiratory tract. Near the earth's surface, NO_2 arising from combustion processes efficiently absorbs longer-wavelength UV light, from which a free O atom is cleaved, initiating the following simplified series of reactions:

$$NO_2 + h\nu \,(\text{UV light}) \rightarrow O^\bullet + NO^\bullet \qquad (29\text{–}1)$$

$$O^\bullet + O_2 \rightarrow O_3 \qquad (29\text{–}2)$$

$$O_3 + NO^\bullet \rightarrow NO_2 \qquad (29\text{–}3)$$

This process is inherently cyclic, with NO_2 regenerated by the reaction of the $NO^\bullet$ and O_3. In the absence of unsaturated hydrocarbons (olefins and substituted aromatics) arising from fuel vaporization or combustion, as well as biogenic terpenes, this series of reactions would approach a steady state with little buildup of O_3. The free electrons of the double bonds of unsaturated hydrocarbons are attacked by free atomic $O^\bullet$, resulting in oxidized compounds and radicals that react further with $NO^\bullet$ to produce more NO_2. Thus, the balance of the reactions sequence shown in Eqs. (29–1) to (29–3) is tipped to the right, leading to buildup of O_3. This reaction is particularly favored when the sun's intensity is greatest at midday, utilizing the NO_2 provided by morning rush-hour traffic. Carbonyl compounds (especially short-chained aldehydes) are also by-products of these reactions. Formaldehyde and acrolein account for about 50% and 5%, respectively, of the total aldehyde content in urban atmospheres. Peroxyacetyl nitrate (CH_3COONO_2), often referred to as PAN, and its homologs also arise in urban air, most likely from the reaction of the peroxyacyl radicals with NO$_2$.

Chronic Exposures to Smog

Epidemiological studies in human populations as well as empirical studies in laboratory animals have attempted to link degenerative lung disease with chronic exposure to photochemical air pollution. Cross-sectional and prospective field studies have suggested an accelerated loss of lung function in people living in areas of high pollution. However, as with many studies of this type, there were problems with confounding factors (meteorology, imprecise exposure assessment, and population variables). Studies have been conducted in children living in modern-day Mexico City, which has high oxidant and PM levels, noted severe epithelial damage and metaplasia as well as permanent remodeling of the nasal epithelium. When children migrated into Mexico City from cleaner, nonurban regions, even more severe damage was observed, suggesting that the tissue remodeling in the permanent residents imparted some degree of incomplete adaptation. Because the children were of middle-class origin, these observations were less likely confounded by socioeconomic variables. In fact, the epithelial cell damage in the nasal cavity of Mexico City children was inversely correlated with glutathione peroxidase, a marker of oxidative stress.

Ozone

General Toxicology—Ozone is the primary oxidant of concern in photochemical smog because of its inherent bioreactivity and its concentration relative to other reactive species. Current mitigation strategies for O$_3$ have been only largely unsuccessful owing to sustained population growth. With suburban sprawl and the downwind transport of air masses from populated areas to more rural environments, the geographic distribution of those exposed has also expanded, as has the temporal profile of individual exposure. In other words, ambient O$_3$ exposures are no longer stereotyped as brief 1 to 2 h peaks. Instead, there is more typically a prolonged period of exposure of 6 h or more at or near the NAAQS level.

Ozone induces a variety of effects in humans and experimental animals at concentrations that occur in many urban areas. These effects include morphologic, functional, immunologic, and biochemical alterations. Because of its low water solubility, a substantial portion of inhaled O$_3$ penetrates deep into the lung, but its reactivity is such that about 17% and 40% are scrubbed by the nasopharynx of resting rats and humans, respectively. Nevertheless, regardless of species, the region of the lung that is predicted to have the greatest O$_3$ deposition (dose per surface area) is the centriacinar region, from the terminal bronchioles to the alveolar ducts, also referred to as the proximal alveolar ductal region. Because O$_3$ penetration increases with increased tidal volume and flow rate, exercise increases the dose to the target area. Thus, it is important to

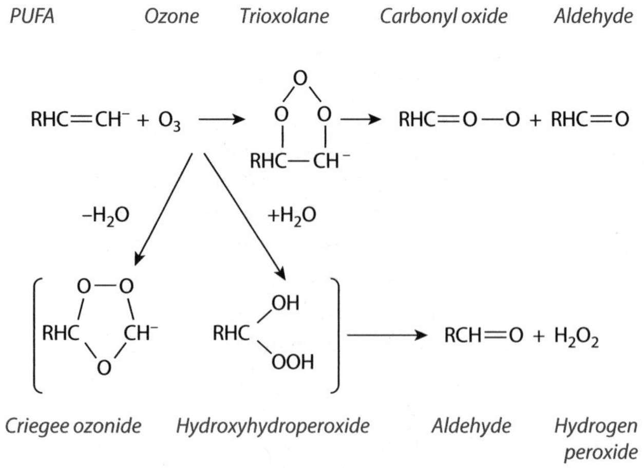

FIGURE 29–6 **Major reaction pathways of O$_3$ with lipids in lung lining fluid and cell membranes.** (Adapted with permission from the *Air Quality Criteria Document for Ozone and Photochemical Oxidants*, U.S. EPA, 1996.)

consider the role of exercise-associated dosimetry in a study of O$_3$ or any inhalant before making cross-study comparisons, especially if that comparison is across species.

As a powerful oxidant, O$_3$ seeks to extract electrons from other molecules. The surface fluid lining the respiratory tract and the cell membranes that underlie the lining fluid contain a significant quantity of polyunsaturated fatty acids (PUFA), either free or as part of the lipoprotein structures of the cell. The double bonds within these fatty acids have a labile, unpaired electron that is easily attacked by O$_3$ to form ozonides that progress through a less stable zwitterion or trioxolane (depending on the presence of water); these ultimately recombine or decompose to lipohydroperoxides, aldehydes, and hydrogen peroxide. These pathways are thought to initiate propagation of lipid radicals and auto-oxidation of cell membranes and macromolecules (Figure 29–6).

Pulmonary Function Effects—Exercising human subjects exposed for 2 to 3 h to 0.12 to 0.4 ppm O$_3$ experience reversible concentration-related decrements in forced exhaled volumes (FVC and forced expiratory volume in one second [FEV$_1$]). It is not clear what mechanisms underlie the altered lung function (in terms of changes in FEV$_1$) produced by O$_3$. There is also evidence that the decrements in lung function are vagally mediated, and that the response can be abrogated by analgesics, such as ibuprofen and opiates, which also reduce pain and inflammation. Thus, pain reflexes involving C-fiber networks may be important in the reduction in forced expiratory volumes along with changes in vagal reflexes that alter airway reactivity and bronchoconstriction.

Airway responsiveness to specific (e.g., allergen) and nonspecific (e.g., cold air, inhaled methacholine) bronchoconstriction is another commonly used test of the pulmonary response to inhaled pollutants such as O$_3$. These types of tests are very important because airway hyperresponsiveness is a central feature of asthma and asthmatics are a sizeable subpopulation

(7% to 9% of the total population in the United States) that may be particularly sensitive to the adverse respiratory effects of inhaled pollutants.

Ozone Interactions with Copollutants—An approach simplifying the complexity of synthetic smog studies, yet addressing the issue of pollutant interactions, involves the exposure of laboratory animals or humans to binary or more complex synthetic mixtures of pollutants that occur together in ambient air. The most frequent combination involves interactions of O_3 and NO_2 or O_3 and PM (e.g., sulfuric acid or diesel particles). Not surprisingly, study design adds a level of complexity in interpretation such that evidence exists supporting either augmentation or antagonism of lung function impairments, lung pathology, and other indices of injury. This apparent conflict in the findings only emphasizes the need to carefully consider the myriad of factors that might affect studies involving multiple determinants and the nature of the exposure that is most relevant to reality.

As the number of interacting variables increases, so does the difficulty in interpretation. Studies of complex atmospheres involving acid-coated carbon combined with O_3 at near-ambient levels also show varied evidence of interaction on lung function and macrophage receptor activity. The statistical separation of the interacting variables and responses from the individual or combined components is difficult. However, it is indeed the complex mixture to which people are exposed that we wish to evaluate. Creative approaches to understanding mixture responses must be addressed in the future.

Nitrogen Dioxide

General Toxicology—Nitrogen dioxide, like O_3, is a deep lung irritant that can produce pulmonary edema if it is inhaled at high concentrations. Potential life-threatening exposure is a real-world problem for farmers, as near-lethal high levels of NO_2 can be liberated from fermenting fresh silage. Being heavier than air, the generated NO_2 and CO_2 displace air and oxygen at the base of silo and diffuse into closed spaces where workers can inadvertently get exposed to very high concentrations perhaps with depleted oxygen. Typically, shortness of breath rapidly ensues with exposures nearing 75 to 100 ppm NO_2, with delayed edema and symptoms of pulmonary damage. Not surprisingly, the symptoms are collectively termed "silo-filler's disease." Nitrogen dioxide is also an important indoor pollutant, especially in homes with unventilated gas stoves or kerosene heaters or in developing countries with the unvented burning of biomass fuels.

The distal lung lesions produced by acute NO_2 are similar among species. Theoretical dosimetry studies indicate that NO_2 is deposited along the length of the respiratory tree, with preferential deposition being in the distal airways. Damage is most apparent in the terminal bronchioles. At high concentrations, the alveolar ducts and alveoli are also affected, with type 1 cells again showing their sensitivity to oxidant challenge.

Pulmonary Function Effects—Exposure of normal human subjects to concentrations of ≤ 4 ppm NO_2 for up to 3 h produces no consistent effects on spirometry. A number of factors appear to be involved (e.g., exercise, inherent sensitivity of the asthmatic subject, exposure method).

Inflammation of the Lung and Host Defense—Unlike O_3, NO_2 does not induce significant neutrophilic inflammation in humans at exposure concentrations encountered in the ambient outdoor environment. There is some evidence for bronchial inflammation after 4 to 6 h at 2.0 ppm, which approximates the highest transient peak indoor levels of this oxidant. Exposures at 2.0 to 5.0 ppm have been shown to affect T lymphocytes, particularly $CD8^+$ cells and natural killer cells that function in host defenses against viruses. Although these concentrations may be high, epidemiological studies variably show effects of NO_2 on respiratory infection rates in children, especially in indoor environments.

Other Oxidants

PAN is thought to be responsible for much of the eye-stinging activity of smog. It is more soluble and reactive than O_3, and hence rapidly decomposes in mucous membranes. The cornea is a sensitive target and is prominent in the burning/stinging discomfort often associated with oxidant smogs.

Aldehydes

Carbonyl compounds, notably short-chained (2-4 C) aldehydes, are common photo-oxidation products of unsaturated hydrocarbons. Two aldehydes are of major interest by virtue of their concentrations and irritancy: formaldehyde (HCHO) and acrolein ($H_2C=CHCHO$). They contribute to the odor as well as eye and sensory effects of smog. Formaldehyde accounts for about 50% of the estimated total aldehydes in polluted air, while acrolein, the more irritating of the two, accounts for about 5% of the total. Acetaldehyde (C_3HCHO) and many other longer-chain aldehydes make up the remainder, but they are not as intrinsically irritating, exist at low concentrations, and have less solubility in airway fluids.

Formaldehyde

Formaldehyde is a primary sensory irritant. Because it is very soluble in water, it is absorbed in mucous membranes in the nose, upper respiratory tract, and eyes. The dose–response curve for formaldehyde is steep: 0.5 to 1 ppm yields a detectable odor, 2 to 3 ppm produces mild irritation, and 4 to 5 ppm is intolerable to most people. Formaldehyde is thought to act via sensory C-fibers that signal locally as well as through the trigeminal nerve to reflexively induce bronchoconstriction through the vagus nerve.

Two aspects of formaldehyde toxicology have brought it from relative obscurity to the forefront of attention in recent years. One is its near ubiquitous presence in indoor atmospheres as an off-gassed product of construction materials such as plywood, furniture, or improperly polymerized urea-formaldehyde foam insulation. In addition, the potential carcinogenicity of formaldehyde is a concern. Formaldehyde is a probable human carcinogen. There is epidemiological evidence that formaldehyde causes nasopharyngeal cancer, strong but not sufficient evidence of leukemia, and limited evidence of sinonasal cancer.

Acrolein

Because acrolein is an unsaturated aldehyde, it is more reactive than formaldehyde. It penetrates a bit deeper into the airways and may not have the same degree of sensory irritancy but it may cause more damage. Concentrations below 1 ppm cause irritation of the eyes and the mucous membranes of the respiratory tract. The mechanism of increased flow resistance appears to be mediated through both a local C-fiber and centrally mediated cholinergic reflexes. Ablation of the C-fiber network and atropine (muscarinic blocker) block this response.

Carbon Monoxide

Carbon monoxide is classed toxicologically as a chemical asphyxiant because its toxic action stems from its formation of carboxyhemoglobin, preventing oxygenation of the blood for systemic transport (see Chapter 11). Motor vehicles still account for two thirds of urban CO emissions. Other sources of CO include both main and sidestream tobacco smoke, and residential and commercial heating systems and mobile auxiliary heating units. No overt clinical human health effects have been demonstrated for COHb levels below 2%, while levels above 40% cause fatal asphyxiation.

Hazardous Air Pollutants

HAPs (so-called air toxics) represent an inclusive classification for air pollutants of anthropogenic origin that are generally of measurable quantity in the air, The HAPs include organic chemicals like acrolein, benzene, minerals like asbestos, polycyclic hydrocarbon such as benzo(*a*)pyrene, various metals and metal compounds like mercury and beryllium compounds, and pesticides such as carbaryl and parathion.

THE MULTIPOLLUTANT REALITY OF AIR POLLUTION

Pollutants in the atmosphere of any community vary considerably in space and time, and are charged by the varied output from a wide range of sources, only to be transformed stoichiometrically by a patterned intensity of sunlight. The reductionist approach examining one pollutant at a time has been successful in diminishing pollutants and improving public health. But there are likely chemical and physiologic interactions between and among pollutants that are of public health consequence that have not been appreciated. Parallel efforts within both the scientific and the regulatory/policy communities need to advance methods for evaluating and managing the effects of air pollution in a multipollutant manner.

CONCLUSIONS

The breadth and complexity of the problem of air pollution—from the development of credible databases to supporting regulatory action and decision making—have been the theme throughout. The classic and still most important air pollutants provide a foundation for understanding and appreciating the nuances of the issues and strategies for air pollution control and protection of public health. The key role of the toxicologist is to develop sensitive methods to assay responses to low pollutant concentrations, apply these methods to relevant exposure scenarios and test species, and develop paradigms to relate empirical toxicological data to real life through an understanding of mechanism. Last, the toxicologist must continually integrate laboratory data with those of epidemiology and clinical study to ensure their maximum utility.

BIBLIOGRAPHY

Foster WM, Costa DL (eds.): *Air Pollutants and the Respiratory Tract*, 2nd ed. Boca Raton, FL: Taylor & Francis, 2005.

Phalen RF, Phalen RN: *An Introduction to Pollution Science: A Public Health Perspective*. Burlington, MA: Jones and Bartlet, 2013.

Vallero DA (ed.): *Fundamental of Air Pollution*, 5th ed. Waltham, MA: Elsevier, 2014.

QUESTION

1. Which of the following compounds is NOT an oxidant-type air pollutant?
   a. NO_2.
   b. SO_2.
   c. O_3.
   d. radical hydrocarbons.
   e. aldehydes.

2. Which of the following pollutants contributes most to nontobacco-smoking lung cancer?
   a. asbestos.
   b. vinyl chloride.
   c. benzene.
   d. products of incomplete combustion.
   e. formaldehyde.

3. Inhalants, such as NO_2 and trichloroethylene, can increase proliferation of opportunistic pathogens in the lungs by:
   a. destroying goblet cells in the respiratory tract.
   b. damaging the alveolar septa.
   c. inactivating cilia in the respiratory tract.
   d. killing alveolar macrophages.
   e. dampening the immune system.

4. Which of the following is NOT a characteristic of SO_2 toxicology?
   a. SO_2 is a major reducing-type air pollutant.
   b. Increased airflow rate increases the amount of SO_2 inhaled.
   c. SO_2 inhalation causes vasoconstriction and increased blood pressure.
   d. SO_2 is predominately absorbed in the conducting airways.
   e. SO_2 inhalation increases mucus secretion in humans.

5. Which of the following would be MOST likely to occur on sulfuric acid exposure?
   a. vasoconstriction.
   b. decreased mucus secretion.
   c. an anti-inflammatory response.
   d. vasodilation.
   e. bronchoconstriction.

6. All of the following statements regarding particulate matter are true EXCEPT:
   a. Metals are most commonly released into the environment during coal and oil combustion.
   b. The interaction of gases and particles in the atmosphere can create a more toxic product than the gas or particle alone.
   c. Solubility does not play a role in the bioavailability of a metal.
   d. The earth's crust is an important source of atmospheric magnesium.
   e. Diesel exhaust contains reducing- and oxidant-type air pollutants.

7. Which of the following statements is NOT true?
   a. Ozone (O_3) combines with a nitric oxide radical to form NO_2.
   b. O_2 combines with an oxygen radical to form ozone.
   c. O_3 can cause damage to the respiratory tract.
   d. Accumulation of O_3 in the stratosphere is important for protection against UV radiation.
   e. Cl_2 gas is known to cause O_2 degradation.

8. Which of the following is NOT a likely symptom of NO_2 exposure?
   a. increased secretion by Clara cells.
   b. pulmonary edema.
   c. shortness of breath.
   d. loss of ciliated cells in bronchioles.
   e. decreased immune response.

9. Which of the following statements regarding aldehyde exposure is FALSE?
   a. The major aldehyde pollutants are formaldehyde and acrolein.
   b. Formaldehyde is found in tobacco smoke, but acrolein is not.
   c. Acrolein causes increased pulmonary flow resistance.
   d. Formaldehyde exposure induces bronchoconstriction.
   e. The water solubility of formaldehyde increases its nasopharyngeal absorption.

10. Carbon monoxide (CO) exerts its toxic effects via its interaction with which of the following?
    a. DNA polymerase.
    b. actin.
    c. kinesin.
    d. hemoglobin.
    e. microtubules.

C H A P T E R

30

Ecotoxicology

Richard T. Di Giulio and Michael C. Newman

INTRODUCTION

Ecotoxicology is the study of contaminants in the biosphere and their effects on constituents of the biosphere. It has an overarching goal of explaining and predicting effect or exposure phenomena at several levels of biologic organization (Figure 30–1). Relevant effects to nonhuman targets range from biomolecular to global. As the need to predict major effects to populations, communities, ecosystems, and other higher level entities has become increasingly apparent, more cause–effect models relevant to these higher levels of biologic organization are added to the conventional set of toxicology models applied by pioneering ecotoxicologists. Contaminant chemical form, phase association, and movement among components of the biosphere are also central issues in ecotoxicology because they determine exposure, bioavailability, and realized dose.

SOME DISTINCT ASPECTS OF EXPOSURE

Ecotoxicology commonly uses sparse information for a few species to predict effects to many species and their interactions. Relevant exposure routes are the conventional ingestion, inhalation, and dermal absorption. But, unique features of exposure pathways must be accommodated for species that ingest a wide range of materials using distinct feeding mechanisms, breathe gaseous or liquid media using different structures, and come into dermal contact with a variety of gaseous, liquid, and solid media.

Prediction of oral exposure can be limited because species feed on different materials; however, conventional principles about oral bioavailability remain relevant. Many techniques applied to determining human oral bioavailability are available to the ecotoxicologist. As an example, some birds are uniquely at high risk of lead poisoning because they ingest and then use lead shot as grit. The birds grind shot in their gizzards under acidic conditions, releasing significant amounts of dissolved lead.

Estimation of chemical speciation is central to predicting bioavailability of water-associated contaminants. Speciation can determine the bioavailability of dissolved metals. Movements of nonionic and ionizable organic compounds across the gut or gills are strongly influenced by lipid solubility and pH partitioning, respectively. Consequently, determination of a compound's lipophilicity or calculation of pH- and pK_a-dependent ionization facilitates some predictive capability for bioavailability.

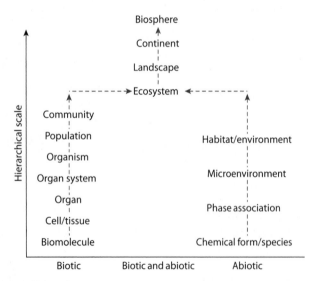

FIGURE 30–1 Ecologic scales relevant to ecotoxicology.
Solely biologic scales relevant to ecotoxicology range from the molecular to the community levels: solely abiotic scales range from the chemical to the entire habitat. Biotic and abiotic components are usually combined at levels above the ecologic community and habitat. The ecologic community and physicochemical habitat combine to form the ecosystem. Ecologic systems can be considered at the landscape scale, that is, the combination of marine, freshwater, and terrestrial systems at a river's mouth. Recently, the continental and biospheric scales have become relevant as in the cases of ozone depletion, acid precipitation, and global warming.

The free ion activity model (FIAM) states that uptake and toxicity of cationic trace metals are best predicted from their free ion activity or concentration, although exceptions exist.

Bioavailability, bioaccumulation, or exposure concentrations for sediment-associated toxicants are also approached by considering chemical speciation and phase partitioning. Metals in sediments are either incorporated into one of the many solid phases or dissolved in the interstitial waters surrounding the sediment particles. Bioavailable metals have been estimated by normalizing sediment metal concentrations to easily extracted iron and manganese concentrations because solid iron and manganese oxides sequester metals in poorly bioavailable solid forms.

Another issue of importance to the ecotoxicologist is the possibility of biomagnification, the increase in contaminant concentration as it moves through a food web. Biomagnification can result in harmful exposures to species situated high in the food web such as birds of prey.

TOXICANT EFFECTS

One approach to this complex topic of ecotoxicologic effects is to organize effects according to biologic levels of organization. One may consider effects, in ascending order, at the subcellular (molecular and biochemical), cellular, organismal, population, community, and ecosystem levels of organization. Ecotoxicology deals with, theoretically at least, all species, and in line with other aspects of natural resource management, the primary concern is one of sustainability. The policies and regulations surrounding chemical effects in natural ecosystems are designed to protect ecologic features such as population dynamics, community structures, and ecosystem functions.

Molecular and Biochemical Effects

This lowest level of organization includes fundamental processes associated with the regulation of gene transcription and translation, biotransformation of xenobiotics, and the deleterious biochemical effects of xenobiotics on cellular constituents including proteins, lipids, and DNA.

Gene Expression and Ecotoxicogenomics

Xenobiotics can affect gene transcription through interactions with transcription factors and/or the promoter regions of genes. In the context of environmental toxicology, perhaps the most studied xenobiotic effects involve ligand-activated transcription factors. These intracellular receptor proteins recognize and bind specific compounds, thus forming a complex that binds to specific promoter regions of genes, thereby activating transcription of mRNAs, and ultimately translation of the associated protein.

Estrogen Receptor—The dominant natural ligand for this nuclear receptor is estradiol (E2). Binding of E2 with estrogen receptor (ER) produces a complex that can then bind to estrogen response elements (ERE) of specific genes that contain one or more EREs, thereby causing gene transcription. Genes regulated in this manner by E2–ER play various important roles in sexual organ development, behavior, fertility, and bone integrity.

A number of chemicals can serve as ligands for ER; in most cases these "xenoestrogens" activate gene transcription acting as receptor agonists. Some of these xenoestrogens include diethylstilbestrol (DES), DDT, methoxychlor, endosulfan, surfactants (nonyl-phenol), some PCBs, bisphenol A, and ethinyl E2, a synthetic estrogen observed in municipal effluents and surface waters. Environmental exposures to these chemicals are sufficient to perturb reproduction or development. Moreover, endocrine disruption by environmental xenoestrogens appears to be stronger for wildlife than for humans, likely due to instances of elevated exposures that are less prone to confounding factors than is typically the case for human exposures. Egg-laying vertebrates provide a biomarker of estrogen exposure—vitellogenin production, which is produced in the liver and transferred to the ovary to become a key component of yolk protein. Increased vitellogenin production in males is useful biomarker of estrogenic chemical exposures.

Aryl Hydrocarbon Receptor—The aryl hydrocarbon receptor (AHR) is a member of the basic helix–loop–helix Per ARNT Sim (bHLH-PAS) family of receptors/transcription factors that is involved in development, as sensors of the internal and external environment in order to maintain homeostasis, and in establishment and maintenance of circadian clocks. Characterized genes that are upregulated by the AHR system code for enzymes involved in the metabolism of lipophilic chemicals, including organic xenobiotics and some endogenous substrates such as steroid hormones. These enzymes include mammalian CYP1A1, 1A2, and 1B1 and their counterparts in other vertebrates, glutathione transferase, glucuronosyltransferase, alcohol dehydrogenase, and quinone oxidoreductase.

Some ubiquitous pollutants that act as AHR ligands and markedly upregulate gene transcription via the AHR–ARNT signaling pathway include the polycyclic aromatic hydrocarbons (PAHs) and the polyhalogenated aromatic hydrocarbons (pHAHs). In general, pHAH-type AHR ligands are more potent AHR ligands and enzyme inducers than PAHs.

Ethoxyresorufin O-deethylase (EROD) activity is often used as a biomarker for AHR-related changes. Elevated activities of hepatic EROD have been associated with exposures to PCBs, dioxins, PAHs, and complex mixtures of these associated with harbor sediments, municipal effluents, paper mill effluents, refinery effluents, and oil spills.

Genomics and Ecotoxicogenomics—Ecotoxicogenomics has great potential for elucidating impacts of chemicals of ecologic concern and ultimately for playing an important role in ecologic risk assessments (ERAs) and regulatory ecotoxicology. Genome sequencing of many species has set the stage for genome-wide analysis of gene expression (transcriptomics), changes in protein production (proteomics), and metabolite profiles (metabolomics). Appropriate bioinformatic analysis can help reveal biologically meaningful patterns of gene expression after exposures to various toxicants. Specific areas to which these emerging fields can contribute include prioritization of chemicals investigated in ERAs, identification of modes of action of pollutants, identification of particularly sensitive species, and effect prediction at higher levels of organization.

Protein Damage—Acetylcholinesterase (AChE) degrades the neurotransmitter acetylcholine, and controls nerve transmission in cholinergic nerve tracts. The widely used organophosphate and carbamate classes of insecticides kill by inhibiting AChE, and this mechanism is operative for "nontarget" organisms including invertebrates, wildlife, and humans. Of particular ecologic concern has been the ingestion of AChE-inhibiting insecticides with food items or granular formulations (mistaken as seed or grit) by birds and aquatic animal exposures from agricultural run-off. Another example is the inhibition of delta-aminolevulinic acid dehydratase after lead exposure. Studies of this enzyme have been exploited as a biomarker for lead exposure in humans and wildlife. In addition to enzyme inhibition, chemicals can damage proteins in other ways, including oxidative damage and the formation of stable adducts similar to those formed with DNA.

Oxidative Stress—Oxidative stress has been defined as the point at which production of ROS exceeds the capacity of antioxidants to prevent damage. Numerous environmental contaminants act as prooxidants and enhance production of ROS. The resulting oxidative damage can account wholly or partially for toxicity. Mechanisms by which chemicals enhance ROS production include redox cycling, interactions with electron transport chains (notably in mitochondria, microsomes, or chloroplasts), and photosensitization. Redox cycling chemicals include diphenols and quinones, nitroaromatics and azo compounds, aromatic hydroxylamines, paraquat, and certain metal chelates, particularly of copper and iron.

Photosensitization is an important mechanism in aquatic systems. Ultraviolet (UV) radiation (specifically UV-B and UV-A) can penetrate surface waters to varying depths, depending on the wavelength of the radiation and the clarity of the water. The UV radiation generates ROS and other free radicals via excitation of photosensitizing chemicals, including common pollutants of aquatic systems.

ROS can drive redox status to a more oxidized state, potentially reducing cell viability. These ROS-mediated impacts and others have been associated with several human diseases including atherosclerosis, arthritis, cancer, and neurodegenerative diseases such as Alzheimer's disease, Parkinson's disease, and amyotrophic lateral sclerosis. With the exception of cancer, the role of ROS in specific diseases in wildlife has received little attention. It is reasonable to assume that oxidative stress accounts in part for the toxicity of diverse pollutants to free-living organisms.

DNA Damage—The importance of DNA as a molecular target was discussed in Chapter 9, and the most important human health issue is associated with cancer. Cancer is an important health outcome associated with chemical exposures in wildlife, particularly for bottom-dwelling fishes. In the context of ecotoxicology, the most widely studied form of damage has been the formation of stable DNA adducts, DNA strand breaks, and oxidized DNA bases. Adduct formation is particularly common with exposure to PAHs. PAHs must be activated to reactive metabolites to form these adducts.

Cellular, Tissue, and Organ Effects

Cells—Most free-living organisms routinely experience energy deficits. For example, food resources are often scarce during the winter for many animals, which adapt by conserving energy (by hibernating or lowering metabolism) or by storing energy beforehand (as is the case for many migratory birds). Thus, the effects of pollutants on mitochondrial energy metabolism can be of particular importance to wildlife.

Lysosomes, which are involved in the degradation of damaged organelles and proteins, sequester many environmental contaminants, including metals, PAHs, and nanoparticles. The accumulation of xenobiotics by lysosomes can elicit membrane damage, which warns of pathologic effects in both invertebrates and vertebrates.

Chemical effects on nuclei have been examined in ecologic contexts. Micronuclei are chromosomal fragments that are not incorporated into the nucleus at cell division, and chemical exposures can markedly increase their frequency. Elevated micronuclei numbers have been observed in erythrocytes in fish and in hemocytes in clams from a PCB-polluted harbor.

Target Organs—An important target organ in ecotoxicology of nonmammalian aquatic vertebrates and many invertebrates is the gill, which is the major site of gas exchange, ionic regulation, acid–base balance, and nitrogenous waste excretion. Gills are immersed in a major exposure medium for these animals (surface water), so metabolically active epithelial cells are in direct contact with this medium. They also receive blood supply directly from the heart. Common structural lesions in gills include cell death (via necrosis and apoptosis), rupture of the epithelium, hyperplasia, and hypotrophy of various cell populations that can lead to lamellar fusion, epithelial swelling, and lifting of the respiratory epithelium from the underlying tissue. Chloride cells have a major role in ionic homeostasis, and they can be compromised after exposure to metals, such as cadmium, copper, lead, silver and zinc. In some cases, this may be due to inhibition of ATPases and/or increased membrane permeability.

Organismal Effects

Mortality—Chemical pollution of the environment does not generally attain levels sufficient to outrightly kill wildlife. The ecotoxicologic concerns are the long-term, chronic impacts of chemicals on organismal variables such as reproduction and development, behavior, and disease susceptibility, and how such impacts parlay into effects at the population and higher

and this process is often tedious and inefficient, with poor recovery of the analyte. Immunoassay may permit avoidance of extractions and facilitate quantification.

7. Miscellaneous—This category covers the large number of compounds that cannot be detected by routine application. Venoms and other toxic mixtures of proteins or uncharacterized constituents fall into this class.

ROLE IN GENERAL TOXICOLOGY

It is universally acknowledged that the chemical under study must be either pure or the nature of any contaminant well-characterized to enable interpretation of the experimental results with validity. Chemicals may degrade when in contact with air, by exposure to ultraviolet or other radiation, by interaction with constituents of the vehicle or dosing solution, and by other means. Developing an analytical procedure by which these changes can be recognized and corrected is essential in achieving consistent and reliable results over the course of a study.

Finally, analytical methods are necessary to determine the bioavailability of a compound that is under study. Some substances with low water solubility are difficult to introduce into an animal, and a variety of vehicles may be investigated. However, a comparison of the blood concentrations for the compound under study provides a simple means of comparing the effectiveness of vehicles.

ROLE IN FORENSIC TOXICOLOGY

The duties of a forensic toxicologist in postmortem investigations include the qualitative and quantitative analysis of drugs or poisons in biologic specimens collected at autopsy and the interpretation of the analytical findings with respect to the physiologic and behavioral effects of the detected chemicals on the deceased at the time of injury and/or death. The cause of death in cases of poisoning cannot be proved beyond contention without toxicologic analysis that confirms the presence of the toxicant in either body fluids or tissues of the deceased.

Additionally, the results of postmortem toxicologic testing provide valuable epidemiologic and statistical data. Forensic toxicologists are often among the first to alert the medical community to new epidemics of substance abuse and the dangers of abusing over-the-counter drugs. Similarly, they often determine the chemical identity and toxicity of novel analogs of psychoactive agents that are subject to abuse, including "designer drugs" such as "china white" (methylfentanyl), "ecstasy" (methylenedioxymethamphetamine), and GHB (gamma-hydroxybutyric acid).

TOXICOLOGIC INVESTIGATION OF A POISON DEATH

The toxicologic investigation of a poison death may be divided into three steps: (1) obtaining the case history and suitable specimens, (2) the toxicologic analyses, and (3) the interpretation of the analytical findings.

Case History and Specimens

Today, thousands of compounds are readily available that are lethal if ingested, injected, or inhaled. Usually, a limited amount of specimen is available on which to perform analyses; therefore it is imperative that before the analyses are initiated, as much information as possible concerning the facts of the case be collected. The age, sex, weight, medical history, and occupation of the decedent as well as any treatment administered before death, the gross autopsy findings, the drugs available to the decedent, and the interval between the onset of symptoms and death should be noted. In a typical year, a postmortem toxicology laboratory will perform analyses for such diverse poisons as over-the-counter medications (e.g., analgesics, antihistamines), prescription drugs (e.g., benzodiazepines, opioids), drugs of abuse (e.g., cocaine, marijuana, methamphetamine), and gases (e.g., inhalants, carbon monoxide).

Specimens of many different body fluids and organs are necessary, as drugs and poisons display varying affinities for body tissues. It is paramount that the handling of all specimens be authenticated and documented. Fluids and tissues should be collected before embalming, as this process will dilute or chemically alter the poisons present, rendering their detection difficult or impossible. Although forensic toxicology laboratories typically receive blood, urine, liver tissue, and/or stomach contents for identification of xenobiotics, they have been increasingly called upon to meet the analytical challenges of many alternative types of samples. Nontraditional matrices, such as bone marrow, hair, vitreous humor, and nails, among others, may be submitted to the laboratory. For example, on occasion, toxicologic analysis is requested for cases of burned, exhumed, putrefied, or skeletal remains. Finally, in severely decomposed bodies, the absence of blood and/or the scarcity of solid tissues suitable for analysis have led to the collection and testing of maggots (fly larvae) feeding on the body.

Toxicologic Analysis

Before the analysis begins, several factors must be considered, including the amount of specimen available, the nature of the poison sought, and the possible biotransformation of the poison. In cases involving oral administration of the poison, the gastrointestinal (GI) contents are analyzed first because large amounts of residual unabsorbed poison may be present. The urine may be analyzed next, as the kidney is the major organ of excretion for most poisons and high concentrations of toxicants and/or their metabolites often are present in urine. After absorption from the GI tract, drugs or poisons are carried to the liver before entering the general systemic circulation; therefore, the first analysis of an internal organ is conducted on the liver.

A thorough knowledge of drug biotransformation is often essential before an analysis is performed. The parent compound and any major pharmacologically active metabolites should be isolated and identified. Many screening tests, such as immunoassays, are specifically designed to detect not the parent drug but its major urinary metabolite.

The analysis may be complicated by the normal chemical changes that occur during the decomposition of a cadaver. The autopsy and toxicologic analysis should be started as soon after death as possible. However, many poisons—such as arsenic, barbiturates, mercury, and strychnine—are extremely stable and may be detectable many years after death.

Forensic toxicology laboratories analyze specimens by using a variety of analytical procedures. Initially, nonspecific tests designed to determine the presence or absence of a class or group of analytes may be performed directly on the specimens. Examples of tests used to rapidly screen urine are the FPN (ferric chloride, perchloric, and nitric acid) color test for phenothiazine drugs and immunoassays for the detection of amphetamines, benzodiazepines, and opiate derivatives, among others. Today, gas chromatography-mass spectrometry (GC-MS) and liquid chromatography-mass spectrometry (LC-MS) are the most widely applied methodology in toxicology and are generally accepted as unequivocal identification for all drugs.

Interpretation of Analytical Results

Once the analysis of the specimens is complete, the toxicologist must interpret his or her findings with regard to the physiologic or behavioral effects of the toxicants on the decedent at the concentrations found. Specific questions may be answered, such as the route of administration, the dose administered, and whether the concentration of the toxicant present was sufficient to cause death or alter the decedent's actions enough to cause his or her death. Assessing the physiologic or behavioral meanings of analytical results is often the most challenging aspect confronted by the forensic toxicologist.

In determining the route of administration, the toxicologist notes the results of the analysis of the various specimens. As a general rule, the highest concentrations of a poison are found at the site of administration. Therefore, the presence of large amounts of drugs and/or poisons in the GI tract and liver indicates oral ingestion, while higher concentrations in the lungs than in other visceral organs can indicate inhalation or intravenous injection.

The physiologic effects of most drugs and poisons are generally correlated with their concentrations in blood or blood fractions such as plasma and serum. The survival time between the administration of a poison and death may be sufficiently long to permit biotransformation and excretion of the agent. Blood values may appear to be nontoxic or consistent with therapeutic administration. Death from hepatic failure after an acetaminophen overdose usually occurs at least three to four days after ingestion. Postmortem acetaminophen concentrations in blood may be consistent with the ingestion of therapeutic doses. Therefore, fatal acetaminophen overdose is determined by case history, central lobular necrosis of the liver, and, if available, analysis of serum specimens collected from the decedent when he or she was admitted to the emergency department.

A new extension of forensic toxicology is the analysis of impurities of illicit drug synthesis in biologic specimens. Many drugs of abuse, particularly methamphetamine, are illicitly manufactured in clandestine laboratories. There are several popular methods of methamphetamine synthesis; when these are applied in clandestine laboratories, side reactions or incomplete conversion of the reactants yield an impure mixture of methamphetamine and synthetic impurities. These impurities can be characteristic of a particular synthetic method and suggest the synthetic method that was used to produce the drug; point to a possible common source of illicit production; and provide a link between manufacturers, dealers, and users.

CRIMINAL POISONING OF THE LIVING

Over the past few decades, forensic toxicologists have become more involved in the analysis of specimens obtained from living victims of criminal poisonings. Generally, this increase in testing is a result of two types of cases: (1) administration of drugs to incapacitate victims of kidnapping, robbery, or sexual assault and (2) poisoning as a form of child abuse.

While alcohol is still often a primary factor in cases of alleged sexual assault, common drugs of abuse or other psychoactive drugs are often involved (Table 32–1). Of particular concern are the many potent inductive agents medically administered prior to general anesthesia. Many of these drugs, such as benzodiazepines and phenothiazines, are available today through illicit sources or legal purchase in foreign

TABLE 32–1 Distribution of drugs of abuse encountered in urine specimens in 1179 cases of alleged sexual assault.*

Rank	Drug/Drug Group	Incidence
1	No drugs found	468
2	Ethanol	451
3	Cannabinoids	218
4	Benzoylecgonine (cocaine metabolite)	97
5	Benzodiazepines	97
6	Amphetamines	51
7	Gamma-hydroxybutyrate (GHB)	48
8	Opiates	25
9	Propoxyphene	17
10	Barbiturates	12

*Thirty-five percent of the drug-positive specimens were positive for more than one drug.
Data from ElSohly MA, Salamone SJ: Prevalence of drugs used in cases of alleged sexual assault. *J Anal Toxicol*, 1999;23(3):141–146.

countries. When administered surreptitiously, they cause sedation and incapacitate the victim while also producing amnesia in the victim as to the events while drugged, without causing severe central nervous system depression. These cases often present a difficult analytical challenge to the toxicologist. Usually, the victim does not bring forth an allegation of assault until 24 h to several days after the attack. Thus, the intoxicating drug may have been largely eliminated or extensively metabolized such that extremely low concentrations of drug or metabolites are present in the victim's blood, urine, and/or hair specimens.

Poisoning as a form of child abuse involves the deliberate administration of toxic or injurious substances to a child, usually by a parent or other caregiver. Common agents used to intentionally poison children have included syrup of ipecac, table salt, laxatives, diuretics, antidepressants, sedative-hypnotics, and narcotics. As in the case of sexual assault, sophisticated MS testing methods may be required to detect such agents as emetine and cephaeline, the emetic alkaloids in syrup of ipecac.

FORENSIC URINE DRUG TESTING

Concerns regarding the potentially adverse consequences of substance abuse for the individual, the workplace, and society have led to widespread urine analysis for controlled or illicit drugs. Currently, such testing is conducted routinely by the military services, regulated transportation and nuclear industries, many federal and state agencies, public utilities, federal and state criminal justice systems, and numerous private businesses and industries. Significant ethical and legal ramifications are associated with such testing. Those having positive test results may not receive employment, be dismissed from a job, be court-martialed, or suffer a damaged reputation.

Forensic urine drug testing (FUDT) differs from other areas of forensic toxicology in which urine is the only specimen analyzed and testing is performed for a limited number of drugs and metabolites. Under the federal certification program, analyses are performed for a limited number of classes or drugs of abuse. Initial testing is performed by immunoassays on rapid, high-throughput chemistry analyzers. A confirmation analysis in FUDT-certified laboratories is performed by GC-MS and LC-MS/MS. FUDT results are reported only as positive or negative for the drugs sought.

Many individuals who are subject to regulated urine testing have devised techniques to mask their drug use either by physiologic means such as the ingestion of diuretics or by attempting to adulterate the specimen directly with bleach, vinegar, or other products that interfere with the initial immunoassay tests. Thus, specimens are routinely tested for adulteration by checking urinary pH, creatinine, and specific gravity and noting any unusual color or smell. Recently a mini-industry has developed to sell various products that are alleged to "beat the drug test" by interfering with the initial

or confirmatory drug test. Thus, FUDT laboratories now routinely test not only for drugs of abuse, but also for a wide variety of chemical adulterants. In most instances, a positive test result for adulteration has as serious a consequence as a positive drug test.

HUMAN PERFORMANCE TESTING

Forensic toxicology activities also include the determination of the presence of ethanol and other drugs and chemicals in blood, breath, or other specimens and the evaluation of their role in modifying human performance and behavior. The most common application of human performance testing is to determine impairment while driving under the influence of ethanol or drugs. Several studies have demonstrated a relatively high occurrence of drugs in impaired or fatally injured drivers. These studies tend to report that the highest drug-use accident rates are associated with the use of such illicit or controlled drugs as cocaine, benzodiazepines, marijuana, and phencyclidine. Before driving under the influence of drugs is as readily accepted by the courts as ethanol testing, legal and scientific problems regarding drug concentrations and driving impairment must be resolved.

COURTROOM TESTIMONY

The forensic toxicologist often is called upon to testify in legal proceedings as an "expert witness." An expert witness may provide two types of testimony: objective testimony and "opinion." Objective testimony by a toxicologist usually involves a description of his or her analytical methods and findings. When a toxicologist testifies as to the interpretation of his or her analytical results or those of others, that toxicologist is offering an "opinion." Whether a toxicologist appears in criminal or civil court, workers' compensation, or parole hearings, the procedure for testifying is the same: direct examination, cross-examination, and redirect examination. Regardless of which side has called for the expert witness, the toxicologist should testify with scientific objectivity. An expert witness is called to provide informed assistance to the jury, not to judge the case.

ROLE IN CLINICAL TOXICOLOGY

Analytical toxicology in a clinical setting plays a role very similar to its role in forensic toxicology. As an aid in the diagnosis and treatment of toxic incidents, as well as in monitoring the effectiveness of treatment regimens, it is useful to clearly identify the nature of the toxic exposure and measure the amount of the toxic substance that has been absorbed. Frequently, this information, together with the clinical state of the patient, permits a clinician to relate the signs and symptoms observed to the anticipated effects of the toxic agent. This may permit a clinical judgment as to whether the treatment must be vigorous and aggressive or whether simple observation and symptomatic treatment of the patient are sufficient.

A cardinal rule in the treatment of poisoning cases is to support vital cardiopulmonary function and to remove any unabsorbed material, limit the absorption of additional poison, and hasten its elimination. Although the instrumentation and the methodology used in a clinical toxicology laboratory are similar to those utilized by a forensic toxicologist, a major difference between these two applications is responsiveness. In emergency toxicology testing, results must be communicated to the clinician within hours to be meaningful for therapy. Primary examples of the usefulness of emergency toxicology testing are the rapid quantitative determination of acetaminophen, salicylate, alcohols, and glycol serum concentrations in instances of suspected overdose.

Ethanol is the most common chemical encountered in emergency toxicology. Although relatively few fatal intoxications occur with ethanol alone, serum values are important in the assessment of behavioral, physiologic, and neurologic function, particularly in trauma cases where the patient is unable to communicate and surgery with the administration of anesthetic or analgesic drugs is indicated. Intoxications from accidental or deliberate ingestion of other alcohols or glycols—such as methanol from windshield deicer or paint thinner, isopropanol from rubbing alcohol, and ethylene glycol from antifreeze—are often encountered in emergency departments. Following ingestion of methanol or ethylene glycol, patients often present with similar neurologic symptoms and severe metabolic acidosis due to the formation of toxic aldehyde and acid metabolites. A rapid quantitative serum determination for these intoxicants will indicate the severity of intoxication and the possible need for dialysis or therapy with an alcohol dehydrogenase inhibitor (fomepizole).

ROLE IN THERAPEUTIC MONITORING

Historically, the administration of drugs for long-term therapy was based largely on experience. A dosage amount was selected and administered at appropriate intervals based on what the clinician had learned was generally tolerated by most patients. If the drug seemed ineffective, the dose was increased; if toxicity developed, the dose was decreased or the frequency of dosing was altered. At times, a different dosage form might be substituted. Establishing an effective dosage regimen was particularly difficult in children and the elderly.

The factors responsible for individual variability in responses to drug therapy include the rate and extent of drug absorption, distribution, and binding in body tissues and fluids, rate of metabolism and excretion, pathologic conditions, and interaction with other drugs. Monitoring of the plasma or serum concentration at regular intervals will detect deviations from the average serum concentration, which, in turn, may suggest that

TABLE 32–2 Drugs commonly indicated for therapeutic monitoring.

Antiarrythmics
Digoxin
Digitoxin
Lidocaine
Procainamide and *N*-acetylprocainamide
Quinidine
Antibiotics
Amikacin
Chloramphenicol
Gentamicin
Tobramycin
Vancomycin
Anticancer
Methotrexate
Anticonvulsants
Carbamazepine
Gabapentin
Lamotrigine
Phenobarbital
Phenytoin
Primidone
Topiramate
Valproic acid
Zonisamide
Antidepressants
Amitriptyline/nortriptyline
Desipramine/imipramine
Doxepin/nordoxepin
Antipsychotics
Clozapine
Pimozide
Bronchodilators
Caffeine
Theophylline
Immunosuppressants
Azathioprine
Cyclosporine
Mycophenolic acid
Sirolimus
Tacrolimus
Mood stabilizing
Lithium

one or more of these variables need to be identified and corrected. Drugs that are commonly monitored during therapy are presented in Table 32–2.

SUMMARY

The analytical techniques employed by forensic toxicologists have continued to expand in complexity and improve in reliability and sensitivity. Many new analytical tools have been applied to toxicologic problems in almost all areas of the field, and the technology continues to open new areas of research. Forensic toxicologists continue to be concerned about conducting unequivocal identification of toxic substances in such a manner that the results can withstand a legal challenge. The issues of substance abuse, designer drugs, increased potency of therapeutic agents, and widespread concern about pollution, and the safety and health of workers present challenges to the analyst's knowledge, skills, and abilities. As these challenges are met, analytical toxicologists will continue to play a substantial role in the expansion of the discipline of toxicology.

BIBLIOGRAPHY

Levine B: *Principles of Forensic Toxicology*, 4th ed. Washington, DC: AACC Press, 2013.

Negruz A, Cooper G: *Clarke's Analytical Forensic Toxicology*. London: Pharmaceutical Press, 2013.

QUESTIONS

1. Which of the following is most commonly used as a drug of sexual assault?
   a. narcotics.
   b. amphetamines.
   c. benzodiazepines.
   d. ethanol.
   e. antidepressants.

2. All of the following statements regarding analytic/forensic toxicology are true EXCEPT:
   a. Analytic toxicology uses analytic chemistry to characterize a chemical's adverse effect on an organism.
   b. Medical examiners and coroners are most important in determining cause of death.
   c. Tissues and body fluids are vital in forensic toxicology.
   d. Forensic toxicology is used for purposes of the law.
   e. Chapuis first characterized a system for classifying toxic agents.

3. Which of the following criteria is NOT routinely used to check for adulteration of drug urine analysis?
   a. urea.
   b. pH.
   c. color.
   d. specific gravity.
   e. creatinine.

4. Which blood alcohol concentration (BAC) is most commonly used as the statutory definition of DUI?
   a. 0.04.
   b. 0.06.
   c. 0.08.
   d. 0.12.
   e. 0.16.

5. Which of the following drugs is NOT properly matched with its most common analytic method?
   a. benzodiazepines—GC/MS.
   b. ibuprofen—TLC/HPLC.
   c. amphetamines—immunoassays.
   d. barbiturates—GC/immunoassays.
   e. ethanol—immunoassays.

6. For which of the following drugs is serum NOT used during toxicology testing?
   a. ethanol.
   b. cocaine.
   c. aspirin.
   d. barbiturates.
   e. ibuprofen.

7. Which of the following is LEAST important in determining variability in response to drug therapy?
   a. drug interactions.
   b. distribution in body tissue.
   c. body mass index.
   d. pathologic conditions.
   e. rate of metabolism.

8. Which of the following statements is FALSE regarding steady state?
   a. Steady-state concentrations are proportional to the dose/dosage interval.
   b. Steady state is attained after approximately four half-lives.
   c. The steady-state concentrations are proportional to F/Cl.
   d. Monitoring of steady-state drug concentration assumes that an effective concentration is present.
   e. Fluctuations in concentration are increased by slow drug absorption.

9. Which of the following is an indirect method of measuring a chemical or its metabolite?
   a. blood test.
   b. hair sample.
   c. urinalysis.
   d. hemoglobin adduct detection.
   e. breath analysis.

10. Which of the following statements regarding analytic/forensic toxicology is TRUE?
    a. Antidepressants are commonly used to incapacitate victims.
    b. It is easy to test for and prove that marijuana is a factor in an automobile accident.
    c. Heroin is the drug most commonly encountered in emergency toxicology.
    d. Toxicologists can play an important role in courtroom testimonies.
    e. Ethanol intoxication often results in death.

Clinical Toxicology

Louis R. Cantilena Jr.

KEY POINTS

- Clinical toxicology encompasses the expertise in the specialties of medical toxicology, applied toxicology, and clinical poison information.
- Important components of the initial clinical encounter with a poisoned patient include stabilization of

the patient, clinical evaluation (history, physical, laboratory, and radiology), prevention of further toxin absorption, enhancement of toxin elimination, administration of antidote, and supportive care with clinical follow-up.

HISTORY OF CLINICAL TOXICOLOGY

The history of poisoning and poisoners goes back to ancient times. Formulas for creating poisonous and noxious vapors have been found in Chinese writings dating back to 1000 BC. Documentation regarding the use of antidotes can be found in Homer's Odyssey and Shastras from 600 BC. Additional history is found in Chapter 1.

INTRODUCTION OF THE POISON CONTROL CENTER

In the United States, poison control centers are staffed by a medical director (medical toxicologist), administrator, specialists in poison information, and educators for poison prevention programs. Personnel provide direct information to

patients with expert recommendations for medical treatment, critical diagnostic and treatment information for health care professionals, education for health care professionals, and poison prevention activities through public education. Poison control centers serve as a potential early-warning system for a potential chemical or biologic terrorist attack.

CLINICAL STRATEGY FOR TREATMENT OF THE POISONED PATIENT

The following general steps represent important components of the initial clinical encounter with a poisoned patient:
1. Stabilization of the patient
2. Clinical evaluation (history, physical, laboratory, and radiology)
3. Prevention of further toxin absorption

TABLE 33–1 Clinical features of toxic syndromes.

	Blood pressure	Pulse	Temperature	Pupils	Lungs	Abdomen	Neurologic
Sympathomimetic	Increase	Increase	Slight increase	Mydriasis	NC	NC	Hyperalert, increased reflexes
Anticholinergic	Slight increase or NC	Increase	Increase	Mydriasis	NC	Decreased bowel sounds	Altered mental status
Cholinergic	Slight decrease or NC	Decrease	NC	Miosis	Increased bronchial sounds	Increased bowel sounds	Altered mental status
Opioid	Decrease	Decrease	Decrease	Miosis	NC or rales (late)	Decreased bowel sounds	Decreased level of consciousness

4. Enhancement of toxin elimination
5. Administration of antidote (if available)
6. Supportive care and clinical follow-up

Clinical Stabilization

The first priority in the treatment of the poisoned patient is stabilization. Initial assessment of airway, respiration, and circulation is crucial. Some toxins or drugs can cause seizures early in the course of presentation. The steps and clinical procedures incorporated to stabilize a critically ill, poisoned patient are numerous and include, if appropriate, support of ventilation, circulation, and oxygenation. In critically ill patients, sometimes treatment interventions must be initiated before a patient is truly stable.

Clinical History in the Poisoned Patient

The primary goal of taking a medical history in poisoned patients is to determine, if possible, the substance ingested or the substance to which the patient has been exposed as well as the extent and time of exposure. In the setting of a suicide attempt, patients may not provide any history or may give incorrect information so as to increase the possibility that they will successfully bring harm to themselves. Information sources commonly employed in this setting include family members, emergency medical technicians who were at the scene, a pharmacist who can sometimes provide a listing of prescriptions recently filled, or an employer who can disclose what chemicals are available in the work environment.

In estimating the level of exposure to the poison, one generally should maximize the possible dose received. That is, one should assume that the entire prescription bottle contents were ingested, that the entire bottle of liquid was consumed, or that the highest possible concentration of airborne contaminant was present in the case of a patient poisoned by inhalation.

With an estimate of dose, the toxicologist can refer to various information sources to determine what the range of expected clinical effects might be from the exposure. The estimation of expected toxicity greatly assists with the triage of poisoned patients. Estimating the timing of the exposure to the poison is frequently the most difficult aspect of the clinical history in the setting of treatment of the poisoned patient.

Taking an accurate history in the poisoned patient can be challenging and in some cases unsuccessful. When the history is unobtainable, the clinical toxicologist is left without a clear picture of the exposure history. In this setting, the treatment proceeds empirically as an "unknown ingestion" poisoning.

Physical Examination

A thorough physical examination is required to assess the patient's condition, determine the patient's mental status, and, if altered, determine possible additional causes such as trauma or central nervous system infection. Whenever possible, the patient's physical examination parameters are categorized into broad classes referred to as *toxic syndromes (toxidromes)*, constellations of clinical signs that, taken together, are likely associated with exposure from certain classes of toxicologic agents. Categorization of the patient's presentation into toxic syndromes allows for the initiation of rational treatment based on the most likely category of toxin responsible, even if the exact nature of the toxin is unknown. Table 33–1 lists clinical features of the major toxic syndromes. Occasionally a characteristic odor detected on the poisoned patient's breath or clothing may point toward exposure or poisoning by a specific agent (Table 33–2).

TABLE 33–2 Characteristic odors associated with poisonings.

Odor	Potential Poison
Bitter almonds	Cyanide
Eggs	Hydrogen sulfide, mercaptans
Garlic	As, organophosphates, DMSO, thallium
Mothballs	Naphthalene, camphor
Vinyl	Ethchlorvynol
Wintergreen	Methylsalicylate

DMSO, dimethyl sulfoxide.

Laboratory Evaluation

Table 33-3 lists drugs or other chemicals that are typically available for immediate measurement in a hospital facility. As one can see, the number of agents for which detection is possible in the rapid-turnaround clinical setting is extremely limited compared with the number of possible agents that can poison patients. This further emphasizes the importance of recognizing clinical syndromes for poisoning and for the clinical toxicologist to initiate general treatment and supportive care for the patient with poisoning from an unknown substance.

For the substances that can be measured on a rapid-turnaround basis in an emergency department setting, the quantitative measurement can often provide both prognostic and therapeutic guidance.

Predictive relationships of drug plasma concentration and clinical outcome and/or suggested concentrations that require therapeutic interventions are available for several agents including salicylates, lithium, digoxin, iron, phenobarbital, and theophylline. Some authors have identified "action levels" or toxic threshold values for the measured plasma concentrations of various drugs or chemicals. Generally, these values represent mean concentrations of the respective substance that have been retrospectively shown to produce a significant harmful effect.

Because of the limited clinical availability of "diagnostic" laboratory tests for poisons, toxicologists utilize specific, routinely obtained clinical laboratory data—especially the anion gap and the osmol gap—to determine what poisons may have been ingested. An abnormal anion or osmol gap suggests a differential diagnosis for significant exposure. Both calculations are used as diagnostic tools when the clinical history suggests poisoning and the patient's condition is consistent with exposure to agents known to cause elevations of these parameters (i.e., metabolic acidosis, altered mental status, etc.).

The anion gap is calculated as the difference between the serum Na ion concentration and the sum of the serum Cl and

TABLE 33-3 List of tests that are commonly measured in a hospital setting on a stat basis.

Acetaminophen	Osmolality
Acetone	Phenobarbital
Carbamazepine	Phenytoin
Carboxyhemoglobin	Procainamide/NAPA
Digoxin	Quinidine
Ethanol	Salicylates
Gentamicin	Theophylline
Iron	Tobramycin
Lithium	Valproic Acid
Methemoglobin	

NAPA, *N*-acetylprocainamide.

TABLE 33-4 Differential diagnosis of metabolic acidosis with elevated anion gap: "AT MUD PILES".

A	Alcohol (ethanol ketoacidosis)
T	Toluene
M	Methanol
U	Uremia
D	Diabetic ketoacidosis
P	Paraldehyde
I	Iron, isoniazid
L	Lactic acid
E	Ethylene glycol
S	Salicylate

HCO_3 ion concentrations. A normal anion gap is <12. When there is laboratory evidence of metabolic acidosis, the finding of an elevated anion gap would suggest systemic toxicity from a relatively limited number of agents (Table 33-4).

The second calculated parameter from clinical chemistry values is the osmol gap. The osmol gap is calculated as the numerical difference between the measured serum osmolality and the serum osmolarity calculated from the clinical chemistry measurements of the serum sodium ion, glucose, and blood urea nitrogen (BUN) concentrations. The normal osmol gap is <10 mOsm. An elevated osmol gap suggests the presence of an osmotically active substance (methanol, ethanol, ethylene glycol, and isopropanol) in the plasma that is not accounted for by the sodium ion, glucose, or BUN concentrations.

Although calculation of both the AG and the osmol gap can provide very useful information from readily available clinical chemistry measurements, these determinations must be interpreted cautiously in certain clinical settings. For example, even though a patient may have ingested a large, significantly toxic amount of methanol, if measured late in the clinical course of the exposure, the osmol gap may not be significantly elevated as most of the osmotically active methanol has left the plasma and has been biotransformed or cleared but is still producing serious clinical effects.

Radiographic Examination

The use of clinical radiographs to visualize drug overdose or poison ingestions is relatively limited due to lack of radiopacity. Generally, plain radiographs can detect a significant amount of ingested oral medication containing ferrous or potassium salts. In addition, certain formulations that have an enteric coating or certain types of sustained release products are radiopaque as well.

The most useful radiographs ordered in a case of overdose or poisoning include the chest and abdominal radiographs and the computed tomography (CT) study of the head. The abdominal radiograph has been used to detect recent lead paint ingestion in children, and ingestion of halogenated hydrocarbons, such as carbon tetrachloride or chloroform, that may be visualized as a radiopaque liquid in the gut lumen. Abdominal plain radiographs have been helpful in the setting where foreign bodies are detected in the gastrointestinal tract, such as would be seen in a "body packer," or one who smuggles illegal substances by swallowing latex or plastic storage vesicles filled with cocaine or some other substance. Occasionally these storage devices rupture and the drug is released into the gastrointestinal tract, with serious and sometimes fatal results.

Plain radiography and other types of diagnostic imaging in clinical toxicology can also be extremely valuable for the diagnosis of toxin-induced pathology. For example, the detection of drug-induced noncardiac pulmonary edema is associated with serious intoxication with salicylates and opioid agonists. Another example of the use of radiologic imaging in clinical toxicology is with CT of the brain. Significant exposure to carbon monoxide (CO) has been associated with CT lesions of the brain consisting of low-density areas in the cerebral white matter and in the basal ganglia, especially the globus pallidus.

Prevention of Further Poison Absorption

During the early phases of poison treatment or intervention for a toxic exposure via the oral, inhalational, or topical route, a significant opportunity exists to prevent further absorption of the poison by minimizing the total amount that reaches the systemic circulation. For toxins presented by the inhalational route, the main intervention used to prevent further absorption involves removing the patient from the environment where the toxin is found and providing adequate ventilation and oxygenation for the patient. For topical exposures, clothing containing the toxin must be removed and the skin washed with water and mild soap taking care not to cause cutaneous abrasions that may enhance dermal absorption.

The four primary methods to prevent continued absorption of an oral poison are induction of emesis with syrup of ipecac, gastric lavage, oral administration of activated charcoal, and whole bowel irrigation. Although potentially indicated for individuals who are hours away from a medical facility, syrup of ipecac use for induction of emesis in the treatment of a potentially toxic ingestion has declined. Risk of cardio- and neurotoxicity and lower effectiveness at removing the toxicant than desired limit its use. Likewise, gastric lavage, which involves placing an orogastric tube into the stomach and aspirating fluid, and then cyclically instilling fluid and aspirating until the effluent is clear, is limited by the risk of aspiration during the lavage procedure and evidence of limited effectiveness.

For many years, orally administered activated charcoal has been routinely incorporated into the initial treatment of a patient poisoned by the oral route. The term *activated* means

that the charcoal has been specially processed to be more efficient at adsorbing toxins.

The usefulness of whole bowel irrigation for a poisoned patient is very limited. Considerable absorption of the toxicant can occur before the procedure "washes" the lumen of the GI tract clear of unabsorbed material. The best evidence for efficacy of this procedure in the setting of poisoning is for removal of ingested packets of illegal drugs swallowed by people smuggling the material and hoping to avoid detection by concealing the agents in their intestines.

Enhancement of Poison Elimination

There are several methods available to enhance the elimination of specific poisons or drugs once they have been absorbed into the systemic circulation. The primary methods employed for this use today include alkalinization of the urine, hemodialysis, hemoperfusion, hemofiltration, plasma exchange or exchange transfusion, and serial oral activated charcoal.

The use of urinary alkalinization results in enhancement of the renal clearance of weak acids. The basic principle is to increase the pH of urinary filtrate to a level sufficient to ionize the weak acid and prevent renal tubule reabsorption of the molecule (ion trapping). Although there are potentially similar advantages to be gained from acidification of the urine in order to enhance the clearance of weak bases, this method is not used because acute renal failure and acid–base and electrolyte disturbances are associated with acidification.

The dialysis technique, either peritoneal dialysis or hemodialysis, relies on passage of the toxic agent through a semipermeable dialysis membrane so that it can subsequently be removed. Hemodialysis incorporates a blood pump to pass blood next to a dialysis membrane, which allows agents permeable to the membrane to pass through and reach equilibrium. Some drugs are bound to plasma proteins and so cannot pass through the dialysis membrane; others are distributed mainly to the tissues and so are not concentrated in the blood, making dialysis impractical. Hemodialysis has been shown to be clinically effective in the treatment of poisoning by the drugs and toxins shown in Table 33–5.

The technique of hemoperfusion is similar to hemodialysis except there is no dialysis membrane or dialysate involved in the procedure. The patient's blood is pumped through a perfusion cartridge, where it is in direct contact with adsorptive material (usually activated charcoal). Protein binding does

TABLE 33–5 Differential diagnosis of elevated osmol gap.

Methanol
Ethanol
Ethylene glycol
Isopropanol

not significantly interfere with removal by hemoperfusion. Because of the more direct contact of the patient's blood with the adsorptive material, the medical risks of this procedure include thrombocytopenia, hypocalcemia, and leukopenia.

The technique of hemofiltration is relatively new in clinical toxicology applications. As in the case of hemodialysis, the patient's blood is delivered through hollow fiber tubes and an ultrafiltrate of plasma is removed by hydrostatic pressure from the blood side of the membrane. The perfusion pressure for the technique is generated either by the patient's blood pressure (for arteriovenous hemofiltration) or by a blood pump (for venovenous hemofiltration). Needed fluid and electrolytes removed in the ultrafiltrate are replaced intravenously with sterile solutions.

The use of either plasma exchange or exchange transfusions has been relatively limited in the field of clinical toxicology. Although the techniques afford the potential advantage of being able to remove high-molecular-weight and/or plasma protein-bound toxins, their clinical utility in poison treatment has been limited. Plasma exchange, or pheresis, involves removal of plasma and replacement with frozen donor plasma, albumin, or both with intravenous fluid. The risks and complications of this technique include allergic-type reactions, infectious complications, and hypotension. Exchange transfusion involves replacement of a patient's blood volume with donor blood. The use of this technique in poison treatment is uncommon and mostly confined to inadvertent drug overdose in a neonate or premature infant.

Serial oral administration of activated charcoal, also referred to as multiple-dose activated charcoal (MDAC), has been shown to increase the systemic clearance of various drug substances. The mechanism for the observed augmentation of nonrenal clearance caused by repeated doses of oral charcoal is thought to be transluminal efflux of the drug from the blood to the charcoal passing through the gastrointestinal tract. The activated charcoal in the gut lumen serves as a "sink" for the toxin. A concentration gradient is maintained and the toxin passes continuously into the gut lumen, where it is adsorbed to charcoal. In addition, MDAC is thought to produce its beneficial effect by interrupting the enteroenteric–enterohepatic circulation of drugs. The technique involves continuing oral administration of activated charcoal beyond the initial dosage every 2 to 4 h. An alternative technique is to give a loading dose of activated charcoal via an orogastric tube or nasogastric tube, followed by a continuous infusion intragastrically. A list of agents for which MDAC has been shown to be an effective means of enhanced body clearance is given in Table 33–6.

Use of Antidotes in Poisoning

A relatively small number of specific antidotes are available for clinical use in the treatment of poisoning. The U.S. Food and Drug Administration (FDA) has placed incentives for sponsors to develop drugs for rare diseases or conditions through the Orphan Drug Act.

TABLE 33–6 Chemicals for which hemodialysis has been shown effective as a treatment modality for poisoning.

Alcohols	Meprobamate
Antibiotics	Metformin
Boric acid	Paraldehyde
Bromide	Phenobarbital
Calcium	Potassium
Chloral hydrate	Salicylates
Fluorides	Strychnine
Iodides	Theophylline
Isoniazid	Thiocynates
Lithium	Valproic acid

The mechanism of action of various antidotes is quite different. For example, a chelating agent or Fab fragments specific to digoxin will work by physically binding the toxin, preventing the toxin from exerting a deleterious effect in vivo, and, in some cases, facilitating body clearance of the toxin. Other antidotes pharmacologically antagonize the effects of the toxin. Atropine, an antimuscarinic, anticholinergic agent, is used to pharmacologically antagonize at the receptor level the effects of organophosphate insecticides that produce lethal cholinergic, muscarinic effects. Certain agents exert their antidote effects by chemically reacting with biologic systems to increase detoxifying capacity for the toxin. For example, sodium nitrite is given to patients poisoned with cyanide to cause formation of methemoglobin, which serves as an alternative binding site for the cyanide ion, thereby making it less toxic to the body.

Supportive Care of the Poisoned Patient

The supportive care phase of poison treatment is very important. Not only are there certain poisonings that have delayed toxicity, but there are also toxins that exhibit multiple phases of toxicity. Close clinical monitoring can detect these later-phase poisoning complications and allow for prompt medical intervention.

Another important component of the supportive care phase of poison treatment is the psychiatric assessment. Generally, a patient who has attempted suicide should be constantly monitored until he or she has been evaluated by the psychiatric consultant and judged to be at low risk for being without constant surveillance. In many cases, it is not possible to perform a psychiatric interview of the patient during the early phases of treatment and evaluation. Once the patient has been stabilized and is able to communicate, a psychiatric evaluation should be obtained.

CASE EXAMPLES OF SPECIFIC POISONINGS

Acetaminophen

A 16-year-old female patient arrives in the ED by ambulance after being found by a parent in what appeared to be an intoxicated state with empty pill bottles scattered about her room. The parent reports the patient was despondent recently after breaking up with her boyfriend. The patient is tearful and reports abdominal pain and admits to drinking alcohol and taking over-the-counter (OTC) pills in an apparent suicide attempt. The estimated time of ingestion is 6 h prior to arrival in the ED. The patient does not use prescription, OTC medications, or dietary supplements and is not known to have a history of regular consumption of alcoholic beverages or use illicit drugs.

On physical examination the blood pressure was 118/80 mm Hg, pulse 88/min and regular, respiratory rate 18/min, and temperature 37.0°C. She was awake and oriented, responded to questions appropriately with slightly slurred speech. Other pertinent findings included normal bowel sounds with mild epigastric tenderness. The neurologic examination was only significant for slightly slurred speech.

The patient was given 1.5 g/kg oral activated charcoal as a slurry in a sorbitol cathartic. Forty minutes later, the laboratory results showed a mildly increased white blood cell count, liver transaminase values elevated to approximately three times the upper limit of normal, and an acetaminophen concentration was 308 μg/mL. Based on the Rumack–Matthew nomogram, which plots acetaminophen plasma concentration versus hours of after ingestion, one can discern whether hepatic toxicity is probable. For example, a plasma acetaminophen concentration of 308 μg/mL at approximately 6 h after ingestion was well within the "probable hepatic toxicity" range, and treatment with *N*-acetylcysteine NAC was initiated.

The patient received the first dose of IV NAC in the ED and was admitted to the medical ward to complete the treatment course of IV NAC. Transient increases of hepatic transaminases were measured over the ensuing two days of the hospitalization. The psychiatry consultation service determined she was not actively suicidal; she was discharged from the hospital two days after admission with scheduled psychiatric and medical follow-up appointments.

The clinical presentation of patients poisoned with acetaminophen is sufficiently confusing in some cases; it is difficult to estimate the time of ingestion. Due to the paucity of clinical symptoms with acute overdose, most clinicians will request an acetaminophen concentration be measured for any patient suspected of having a toxic exposure to any substance. The paucity of signs and symptoms associated with an acetaminophen overdose makes inadvertent missing of a potentially fatal overdose until the window for maximum antidote effectiveness has passed.

Acetaminophen in normal individuals is inactivated by sulfation and glucuronide conjugation, with about 4% biotransformed by CYP2E1 to a toxic metabolite that is normally detoxified by conjugation with glutathione and excreted as the mercapturate. Patients who are concurrently using, or have recently used, agents that induce CYP2E1 may produce more than 4% of the toxic metabolite. When there is evidence (medical history) of concurrent chemicals that induce CYP2E1, the treatment nomogram from acetaminophen should be modified to a lower threshold for treatment with NAC.

Follow-up liver biopsy studies of patients who have recovered three months to a year after hepatotoxicity have demonstrated no long-term sequelae or chronic toxicity. A very small percentage (0.25%) of patients in the national multiclinic study conducted in Denver may progress to hepatic encephalopathy with subsequent death. The clinical nature of the overdose is one of a sharp peak of serum glutamic-oxaloacetic transaminase (SGOT) by day 3, with recovery to less than 100 IU/L by day seven or eight. Patients with SGOT levels as high as 20 000 IU/L have shown complete recovery and no sequelae one week after ingestion.

Laboratory evaluation of a potentially poisoned patient is crucial in terms of both hepatic measures of toxicity and plasma levels of acetaminophen. Accurate estimation of acetaminophen in the plasma should be done on samples drawn at least 4 h after ingestion, when peak plasma levels can be expected.

Once an accurate plasma level has been obtained, it should be plotted on the Rumack–Matthew nomogram to determine if NAC therapy is indicated. This nomogram is based on a series of patients with and without hepatotoxicity and their corresponding measured plasma acetaminophen concentrations.

Ethylene Glycol

A 37-year-old female was brought to the ED after being found unresponsive in her home. At the scene, emergency medical personnel administered oxygen and naloxone and performed a finger stick for glucose (standard procedure for a person with altered mental status and suspected toxic ingestion), which showed a normal value of 95 mg/dL. The patient's spouse reported that she had been depressed and despondent with the recent loss of her job. No empty pill bottles or liquid containers were found with her at home.

Upon arrival to the hospital, she remained comatose. Her vital signs were: blood pressure 105/65 mm Hg, pulse 78/min, respiratory rate elevated at 32/min, and her body temperature was normal. The remainder of the physical examination was significant as her pupils were 3 mm and sluggishly reactive to light; the lung and heart examinations were normal; the abdominal examination revealed diminished but present bowel sounds, and no tenderness, organomegaly, or masses were detected. The rectal examination was normal; the stool was without detectable gross or occult blood. Neuro examination was nonfocal with a diminished gag reflex.

The patient was placed on a cardiac monitor, an IV line was started, clinical laboratory specimens were obtained, and she was placed on oxygen, given naloxone, thiamine, and dextrose (50%) intravenously. Chest and abdominal radiography was without abnormality. A 12-lead ECG was also normal. Faced with the uncertainty of oral ingestion versus topical and inhalation exposure, a decision was made to proceed with gastric decontamination. The patient was endotracheally intubated to protect her airway before an orogastric tube was placed. Gastric lavage was performed and no blood was found. The fluid withdrawn from the stomach was bright yellow in appearance and slightly viscous. When a Wood's lamp illuminated this fluid in a darkened room, fluorescence was observed. This finding suggests the presence of automotive antifreeze that contains ethylene glycol. Activated charcoal (2.0 g/kg) was placed via the orogastric tube into the stomach with a cathartic even though the efficacy for binding ethylene glycol is limited; the use of activated charcoal here was for other, potentially unknown coingestants. Clinical laboratory results returned showing the following:

$$Na = 140\,mEq/L \qquad K = 3.1\,mEq/L$$
$$Cl = 94\,mEq/L \qquad HCO_3 = 8\,mEq/L$$
$$BUN = 12\,mg/dl \qquad Glucose = 100\,mg/dl$$

Arterial blood gas:
$$pH = 7.20;\ pCO_2 = 20\,mm\,Hg;\ pO_2 = 98\,mm\,Hg$$

The complete blood count was normal, the urine analysis was normal, measured serum osmolarity was 330 mOsm/kg, and acetaminophen and salicylate levels were below the limits of detection, and the urine toxicology screen was negative.

The laboratory results were interpreted as follows: a metabolic acidosis with elevated AG (AG = 38) and an elevated osmol gap (40 mOsm). These findings are consistent with either methanol or ethylene glycol poisoning (Tables 33–4 and 33–5). The patient was treated with IV fomepizole (4-methylperazole), sodium bicarbonate was given intravenously for the profound metabolic acidosis, and the patient underwent hemodialysis. After 4 h of hemodialysis, the acid–base and electrolyte abnormalities were corrected but the patient remained comatose. The patient underwent a second 4-h course of hemodialysis 8 h later to again correct her metabolic acidosis with the appearance of minor renal injury (serum creatinine increased to 1.8 mg/dL). She regained normal consciousness within 18 h and her renal function recovered completely within three days. Subsequently, the patient admitted that she intentionally drank more than half a container of antifreeze with the intent of harming herself. She was evaluated by the psychiatry consultation service and transferred to their service for further care.

Ethylene glycol exerts primary toxicity after undergoing biotransformation by alcohol dehydrogenase to glycolic acid and then to glycolic and oxalic acid by the action of aldehyde dehydrogenase. The latter two acid metabolites are thought to be responsible for both the renal and the acid–base toxicity observed during poisoning by ethylene glycol. If untreated or treated too late, ethylene glycol poisoning can result in fatal cerebral edema with seizures as well as irreversible renal damage.

Valproic Acid

A 33-year-old male was brought to the ED after being found unresponsive with two empty prescription pill bottles of extended release valproic acid at his side. He was last seen 8 h prior to being found unresponsive and was then in normal health. The pharmacy confirmed that monthly prescriptions, each containing 30, 250 mg extended release valproic acid tablets, had been dispensed within the preceding three months.

The patient was unresponsive to verbal or tactile stimulation. Vital signs were blood pressure 85/55 mm Hg, pulse 94/min, respiratory rate 20/min, and temperature 33.2°C. Naloxone was administered without effect. A cardiac monitor showed sinus rhythm. The physical examination showed the patient to be without obvious signs of trauma; the skin was cool and without track marks; the pupils were 2 mm and poorly reactive to light; bowel sounds were diminished. The rectal examination was negative for occult blood. The neurologic examination revealed coma without focal motor abnormalities and an absent gag reflex.

Initial laboratories showed mild metabolic acidosis with elevated serum lactate, an increased anion, slightly increased serum ammonia, normal glucose, liver function tests, and renal function tests. The chest and abdominal radiographs were normal. The 12-lead ECG showed a prolonged QT interval without arrhythmia. The patient was endotracheally intubated to protect his airway prior to gastric lavage that yielded some pill fragments only. The patient was placed on a ventilator to support his respiration. Activated charcoal (1.5 g/kg) was administered via the orogastric tube immediately following the lavage procedure. The blood pressure continued to remain low despite IV fluid administration. A STAT valproic acid serum measurement showed the concentration was 572 µg/mL.

Blood pressure responded to low-dose vasopressors (IV dopamine) with continued IV fluid administration. A repeat serum valproic acid concentration was 890 µg/mL at 2 h postadmission. Serial oral activated charcoal (every 4 h) was initiated via the orogastric tube and hemodialysis was started 3 h after admission. IV L-carnitine was given when a repeat serum ammonia concentration was further elevated at 94 mg/dL. Subsequent measured plasma concentrations of valproic acid gradually declined to <100 µg/mL over the next 48 h after one additional hemodialysis session was conducted. The patient regained consciousness 24 h after admission and made a full recovery by the fourth hospital day. The psychiatry consultation service accepted the patient in transfer to their inpatient service after he was medically cleared by the toxicology service.

The increasing plasma concentrations of the toxic substance despite gastric decontamination procedures can occur after ingestion of an extended release formulation, which is pharmaceutically designed to slowly dissolve in the gastrointestinal tract and provide for ongoing sustained release of the active drug product as opposed to immediate release of the agent. Drug substances that demonstrate the "slow release" profile without having been formulated in a sustained release dosage form include salicylates and barbiturates as well as formulations of iron supplements. The presence of a drug bezoar or concretion can be dangerous because the treating team could erroneously stratify a patient based on the initial measured plasma concentration and be unprepared for severe toxicity or a prolonged toxicity time course.

Moderate to severe valproic acid intoxication leads to depletion of L-carnitine, which may cause the observed hyperammonemia. The FDA has recently approved the use of IV L-carnitine for the treatment of valproic acid poisoning in the setting of hepatotoxicity, hyperammonemia, large overdoses of valproate by history, or measured serum concentrations of valproic acid exceeding 450 μg/mL.

CONCLUSION

Clinical toxicology encompasses the expertise in the specialties of medical toxicology, applied toxicology, and clinical poison information specialists. The clinical science has significantly evolved to the present state of the discipline over the past 50 years or more. The incorporation of evidence-based, outcome-driven practice recommendations has significantly improved the critical evaluation of treatment modalities and methods for poison treatment. A careful diagnostic approach to a poisoned patient is essential, as important medical history is often absent or unreliable. Skillful use of antidotes is an important component of the practice of medical toxicology. Continued research will increase the repertoire of effective treatments for poisoning and ultimately improve clinical practice.

BIBLIOGRAPHY

Barile FA: *Clinical Toxicology: Principles and Mechanisms*, 2nd ed. New York: Informa Healthcare, 2010.

Hoffman RS, Howland MA, Lewin NA, et al. (eds.): *Goldfrank's Toxicologic Emergencies*, 10th ed. New York: McGraw-Hill, 2014.

Tintinalli JE, Stapczynski JS, Ma OJ et al. (eds.): *Emergency Medicine: A Comprehensive Study Guide*, 7th ed. New York: McGraw-Hill, 2010.

QUESTIONS

1. What is the primary goal in taking a history in a poisoned patient?
   a. determining drug allergies.
   b. determining susceptibility to drug overdose.
   c. determining likelihood of an attempted suicide.
   d. determining the ingested substance.
   e. determining the motive behind the poisoning.

2. Who is most likely to give incorrect information while taking a history of a poisoned patient?
   a. patient.
   b. EMT.
   c. employer.
   d. pharmacist.
   e. family members.

3. Which of the following sets of clinical features characterizes an anticholinergic toxic syndrome?
   a. increased blood pressure, decreased heart rate, decreased temperature.
   b. decreased blood pressure, increased heart rate, decreased temperature.
   c. increased blood pressure, increased heart rate, increased temperature.
   d. decreased blood pressure, decreased heart rate, decreased temperature.
   e. increased blood pressure, decreased heart rate, increased temperature.

4. Which of the following sets of clinical features characterizes a sympathomimetic toxic syndrome?
   a. miosis, decreased bowel sounds, decreased alertness.
   b. decreased heart rate, increased temperature, mydriasis.
   c. hyperalertness, decreased blood pressure, miosis.
   d. increased temperature, increased heart rate, miosis.
   e. mydriasis, increased blood pressure, hyperalertness.

5. Which of the following drugs CANNOT be tested for in a hospital on a stat basis?
   a. ethanol.
   b. cocaine.
   c. aspirin.
   d. phenytoin.
   e. digoxin.

6. Which is NOT included in the differential diagnosis of an elevated anion gap?
   a. ethanol.
   b. methanol.
   c. diabetes.
   d. ethylene glycol.
   e. diarrhea.

7. An elevated osmol gap might suggest which of the following?
   a. methanol poisoning.
   b. chronic vomiting.
   c. lactic acidosis.
   d. diabetic ketoacidosis.
   e. chronic diarrhea.

8. Which of the following is LEAST likely to prevent further poison absorption?
   a. induction of emesis.
   b. activated charcoal.
   c. gastric lavage.
   d. syrup of ipecac.
   e. parasympathetic agonist.

9. Which of the following would NOT be used to enhance poison elimination?
   a. oral activated charcoal.
   b. hemoperfusion.
   c. acidification of urine.
   d. hemodialysis.
   e. plasma exchange.

10. Which of the following might be used as an antidote for patients with cyanide poisoning?
    a. syrup of ipecac.
    b. atropine.
    c. chelating agents.
    d. sodium nitrite.
    e. quinine.

Answers to Chapter Questions

Chapter 1
1. b.
2. a.
3. a.
4. d.
5. b.

Chapter 2
1. b.
2. c.
3. b.
4. d.
5. e.
6. e.
7. b.
8. c.
9. d.
10. a.

Chapter 3
1. b.
2. e.
3. a.
4. c.
5. d.
6. e.
7. b.
8. a.
9. e.
10. c.
11. b.
12. b.

Chapter 4
1. d.
2. c.
3. c.
4. c.
5. e.
6. c.
7. c.
8. d.
9. c.
10. b.

Chapter 5
1. a.
2. e.
3. d.
4. b.
5. e.
6. c.
7. c.
8. d.
9. b.
10. d.

Chapter 6
1. b.
2. c.
3. c.
4. e.
5. b.
6. d.
7. d.
8. a.
9. e.
10. d.

Chapter 7
1. c.
2. a.
3. d.
4. d.
5. e.
6. c.
7. b.
8. d.
9. b.
10. c.

Chapter 8
1. d.
2. e.
3. e.
4. b.
5. c.
6. a.
7. d.
8. e.
9. c.
10. b.

Chapter 9
1. c.
2. d.
3. b.
4. c.
5. e.
6. b.
7. e.
8. c.
9. c.
10. d.

Chapter 10
1. d.
2. c.
3. a.
4. c.
5. d.
6. b.
7. e.
8. c.
9. e.
10. e.

Chapter 11
1. c.
2. a.
3. d.
4. d.
5. a.
6. c.
7. d.
8. c.
9. e.
10. b.

Chapter 12
1. d.
2. b.
3. c.
4. b.
5. c.
6. d.
7. e.
8. b.
9. d.
10. a.

Chapter 13

1. d.
2. d.
3. b.
4. e.
5. a.
6. c.
7. b.
8. d.
9. e.
10. e.

Chapter 14

1. e.
2. b.
3. c.
4. d.
5. d.
6. a.
7. c.
8. e.
9. d.
10. c.

Chapter 15

1. d.
2. b.
3. d.
4. e.
5. d.
6. b.
7. d.
8. a.
9. c.
10. c.

Chapter 16

1. e.
2. d.
3. c.
4. b.
5. d.
6. b.
7. a.
8. d.
9. c.
10. d.

Chapter 17

1. e.
2. c.
3. b.
4. a.
5. d.
6. a.
7. e.
8. d.
9. e.
10. d.

Chapter 18

1. b.
2. b.
3. d.
4. d.
5. e.
6. c.
7. c.
8. a.
9. d.
10. d.

Chapter 19

1. b.
2. e.
3. a.
4. d.
5. b.
6. c.
7. d.
8. c.
9. c.
10. a.

Chapter 20

1. c.
2. d.
3. b.
4. a.
5. e.
6. b.
7. e.
8. d.
9. b.
10. c.

Chapter 21

1. c.
2. d.
3. b.
4. c.
5. e.
6. b.
7. c.
8. d.
9. a.
10. b.

Chapter 22

1. a.
2. c.
3. b.
4. a.
5. e.
6. d.
7. b.
8. c.
9. d.
10. d.

Chapter 23

1. c.
2. d.
3. d.
4. b.
5. a.
6. e.
7. c.
8. d.
9. a.
10. c.

Chapter 24

1. d.
2. c.
3. c.
4. b.
5. d.
6. b.
7. d.
8. b.
9. a.
10. d.

Chapter 25

1. b.
2. c.
3. a.
4. e.
5. d.
6. c.
7. c.
8. d.
9. a.
10. e.

Chapter 26

1. b.
2. a.
3. c.
4. e.
5. b.
6. c.
7. e.
8. a.
9. d.
10. d.
11. e.
12. c.
13. a.
14. e.
15. a.

Chapter 27

1. a.
2. d.
3. e.
4. b.
5. d.
6. e.
7. a.
8. c.
9. e.
10. d.

Chapter 28

1. e.
2. c.
3. b.
4. e.
5. c.
6. b.
7. e.
8. d.

Chapter 29

1. b.
2. d.
3. e.
4. c.
5. e.
6. c.
7. d.
8. a.
9. b.
10. d.

Chapter 30

1. b.
2. c.
3. a.
4. e.
5. c.
6. c.
7. e.
8. b.
9. e.
10. d.

Chapter 31

1. d.
2. a.
3. b.
4. e.
5. c.
6. d.
7. d.
8. a.
9. e.
10. d.

Chapter 32

1. d.
2. b.
3. a.
4. c.
5. e.
6. b.
7. c.
8. e.
9. d.
10. d.

Chapter 33

1. d.
2. a.
3. c.
4. e.
5. b.
6. e.
7. a.
8. e.
9. c.
10. d.

Chapter 34

1. b.
2. d.
3. c.
4. b.
5. b.
6. a.
7. c.
8. c.
9. e.
10. e.

Index